ACUTE INTERVENTION:

Nursing Process Throughout the Life Span

ACUTE INTERVENTION:

Nursing Process Throughout the Life Span

Edited by
SANDRA C. WARDELL, R.N., M.Ed.

Authored by

CYNTHIA E. DEGAZON, R.N., M.A.
  Assistant Professor, R.N., M.A.
  College of Nursing
  Rutgers—The State University

LINDA K. HARRISON, R.N., M.P.H.
  Assistant Professor
  College of Nursing
  Rutgers—The State University

FANG-LAN WANG KUO, R.N., M.S.
  Assistant Professor
  College of Nursing
  Rutgers—The State University

MARGARET A. MERVA, R.N., M.A.
  Instructor
  College of Nursing
  Rutgers—The State University

ANDREA BRETZ SAVITZ, R.N., M.A.
  Assistant Professor
  College of Nursing
  Rutgers—The State University
  Faculty, The Center for Family Learning
  Certified Family Therapist

SANDRA C. WARDELL, R.N., M.Ed.

Contributors

JEAN R. FISHER, R.N., M.S.N.
  Assistant Professor
  College of Nursing
  Rutgers—The State University

SARAH M. SATTIN, R.N., M.S.
  Instructor
  College of Nursing
  Rutgers—The State University

RUTH RAYSOR WEST, R.N., M.Ed.
  Formerly Assistant Professor
  College of Nursing
  Rutgers—The State University

LYNN SORENSON-LEGGATO, R.N.

 Reston Publishing Company, Inc., Reston, Virginia
A Prentice-Hall Company

Library of Congress Cataloging in Publication Data

Main entry under title:

Acute intervention.

  Includes index.
  Bibliography: p.
  1. Emergency nursing—Case studies.
2. Emergency nursing—Problems, exercises, etc.
I. Wardell, Sandra C. [DNLM: 1. Nursing care.
WY100.3 A189]
RT120.E4A28   610.73′6   79-13582
ISBN 0-8359-0133-5
ISBN 0-8359-0132-7   (pbk)

© 1979 by Reston Publishing Company, Inc.
A Prentice-Hall Company
Reston, Virginia 22090

10 9 8 7 6 5 4 3 2

Printed in the United States of America

This text is dedicated to the College of Nursing faculty members at Rutgers—The State University. Their efforts have made possible the integrated curriculum framework from which this text received its impetus.

Contents

Preface

This text presents case studies of acutely ill clients from a cross section of ethnocultural, religious, and socioeconomic backgrounds. Because the family is recognized as an integral part of the client's care, family histories and genograms are included in many of the case studies.

The case studies depict health services being administered in a variety of settings, including specialized care units in hospitals, outpatient settings, and the client's home. A variety of health care providers work together to meet the needs of the client and his or her family.

Study and discussion questions are provided to assist the learner in applying principles from the biological, physical, behavioral, social, and nursing sciences. Learning activities are suggested to enhance the learner's comprehension of the acute illness situations presented.

This text is intended for the learner who has had academic exposure in the basic nursing specialties, such as medical-surgical, maternal-child, and psychiatric nursing. The case studies may be used in part or in their entirety and are designed for self-study and/or seminar use.

NURSING PROCESS

The authors believe that the nursing process is a systematic approach to analyzing client/family health needs and to facilitating appropriate outcomes. This ongoing process includes the following dynamic activities: assessment, planning, implementation, and evaluation. The authors recommend the use of Dolores E. Little and Doris L. Carnevali's book entitled *Nursing Care Planning,* 2d ed. (Philadelphia: J. B. Lippincott Company, 1976) as a source for understanding the dynamics of the nursing process.

NOTES TO THE LEARNER

The following is a suggested approach to each of the case studies:

1. Read the entire chapter and review the bibliography.
2. Assess the adequacy of your present textbooks for answering the questions.
3. Obtain additional readings from the library to supplement your textbooks where necessary. (The reference books that review current nursing literature and your reference librarian can assist your library search.)
4. Define the terms listed at the beginning of each chapter.
5. Reread each section of the narrative and complete the study questions.
6. Outline your answer for each discussion question and discuss them with your peers, instructors, or appropriate nursing practitioners. (See your instructor for direction.)
7. Complete as many of the suggested activities as possible. (See your instructor for assistance.)
8. File your information cards in alphabetical or chronological order for future retrieval and reference.

INFORMATION CARDS

The Information Cards that follow were designed to assist you in obtaining pertinent data. Enter the information on 5-by-8-inch file cards and keep the cards in alphabetical or chronological order for quick retrieval.

PATHOPHYSIOLOGY CARD (Front)

Condition/Disease:	

Definition:
    Pathologic process organ(s) involved, nature of organ(s) change, physiological functions
    involved, how functions deviate, etc.)	

Etiology:
    causative factor(s)
    incidence
    genetic factors
    predisposing and contributing factors	

Prognosis and Course of Condition/Disease:	
Clinical Manifestations	Bases of Manifestation

Subjective (symptom)
 	
Objective (signs)
    physical examination
    laboratory findings
    other	

PATHOPHYSIOLOGY CARD (Back)

Treatment:
    Dietary
    Pharmacotherapeutics
    Surgical
    Psychosocial
    Other	

Common Complications	Bases for Complication

Preventative Measures:
 	
    Of illness
 	
    Of complications	

GROWTH AND DEVELOPMENT CARD (Front)

Age and sex _____

GROWTH AND DEVELOPMENTAL MILESTONES

I. Physical Development and/or Changes:
    Height (normal range and mean)_____   Pulse_____
    Weight (normal range and mean)_____   Respiration_____
                                           Blood Pressure_____
Development and/or changes by system (musculo-skeletal, neurological,
    gastrointestinal, reproductive, renal, hepatic, integumentary)

GROWTH AND DEVELOPMENT CARD (Back)

II. Motor Skills (abilities, patterns, perceptions, etc.):

III. Cognitive/Analytical Development (intellectual abilities of age group):

IV. Psychosocial/Emotional Development:

V.   Major Interests and Diversions (habits, etc.):

DRUG INFORMATION CARD (Front):

Generic Name: _____   Classification: _____
Trade Name(s): _____
Action: _____

Parameters of Agent	Considerations

Absorption:
 	
Metabolism:
 	
Excretion:
	Precautions:
	    Passage through barriers (placental,
	    lactation, blood-brain, dialysis)
	Drug interactions:
	    Synergistic:
	    Antagonistic:
	Interfering factors:
	    Laboratory tests—causes an abnormal
	    FBS, CPK, urea, or BMR, result)

DRUG INFORMATION CARD (Back)

Agent	Considerations
Indications for use:	Contraindications: Toxic effects:

Administration
    Route: Dosage
                        adult:
                        child:
	Related precautions:
	    Maintaining blood levels
	    Initial and maintenance dose
	    Special procedures (i.e., Z method)
	    Tissue effects (i.e., necrosis)

How supplied:
    dosage and product form
    (tablet, ampule, capsule)
	Precautions:
	    Solubility
	    Can it be crushed?
	    Can it be opened for tube feeding?

Nursing management:
    For each potential side effect
    Necessary patient education
    Other	

ACKNOWLEDGEMENTS

We wish to express our gratitude to the following individuals and/or groups for their encouragement and assistance in completing this endeavor:

- Edward M. Gordon, Ph.D. for assisting the authors in developing clinical approaches to family therapy
- Philip J. Guerin, Jr., M.D. for inspiration and support in the developing of the suicide tool
- Evelyn Hart, R.N., C.N.M., for sharing her knowledge and expertise related to maternity nursing
- Sheila F. Lenihan for sharing her knowledge and expertise related to accidental childhood poisoning
- Lynne Sourenson-Logatto for recommendations to the author after reviewing some of the case studies
- Patricia Rose, R.N., C.N.M., for sharing her knowledge and expertise related to maternity nursing
- Our families and significant others for their patience with the generalized clutter and for their support
- Sarah Karl and other typists who endured our many revisions and spent numerous late hours to help us meet the various manuscript deadlines.

THE AUTHORS

CHAPTER ONE

Premature Newborn in Crisis: Respiratory Distress Syndrome

LINDA K. HARRISON

OVERVIEW

The Westfalls, an American Indian couple, seek the support of their tribe's medicine woman and the modern clinic nearby when Lorene Westfall becomes pregnant. Their infant's premature birth is complicated by respiratory distress syndrome (RDS). Specialized assessment techniques and oxygen therapy equipment are required for the infant. Meanwhile, the family requires assistance in dealing with long periods of separation from their first-born child, particularly since Lorene intends to breast-feed her infant.

CONTENT EMPHASIS

- Prematurity—assessment of gestational age and general health status
- Perinatal nutrition—breast feeding
- Fostering parental bonding with a hospitalized infant
- Facilitating adaptation to extrauterine life
- Identifying common health problems of the premature infant

SETTING

- Maternal / infant clinic
- Labor and delivery rooms
- Observation nursery
- Special care nursery (SCN)

OBJECTIVES

Upon completing this chapter the student will be able to:

1. Contrast the anatomy and physiology of the premature neonate with that of the normal neonate.
2. Design nutritional health care objectives that incorporate the ethnic background of the family and the maturational level of each member.
3. List expected health outcomes for the hospitalized premature neonate in an acute care setting.
4. Create intervention techniques that enhance parental/infant attachment.
5. Designate specific intervention modalities that facilitate the expected health outcomes.
6. Evaluate an ongoing health care plan designed for a premature neonate and its family.

DEFINITION OF TERMS

The following terms are used in this case study and should be defined before proceeding.

Appropriate for gestational age (AGA)
Small for gestational age (SGA)
Large for gestational age (LGA)
Immaturity
Prematurity
Observation nursery
Special care nursery (SCN)
Gestational age (assessment)
Acrocyanosis
Intubation
Intravenous cut-down
Arterial blood gases (ABG's)

Silverman score
Downes score
Radiant warmer
Oxygen hood
Respiratory distress syndrome (RDS)
Subcostal retractions
Intercostal retractions
Circumoral cyanosis
Doptone blood pressure
Apgar score
Nasogastric tube (N/G)
Oxygen concentration (F_1O_2)

FAMILY ASSESSMENT

Johnny and Lorene Westfall are Native Americans of the Laguno Pueblo tribe. They were born on Raintree Reservation near Santa Fe, New Mexico. Life on the reservation, although characterized by poverty, held many good childhood memories of tribal traditions and practices. The Westfalls often recaptured in these memories their conversations with each other. Their marriage announcement was a welcome and joyous occasion for both their families and their tribe. They were married four weeks after high school graduation. The bountiful feast that followed the ceremony was offered to the spirits to ward off evil and to ensure the couple of unlimited happiness. It was an important occasion that would always be remembered by Johnny and Lorene.

The economic situation on the reservation had been worsening for the past few years; consequently there was the incentive for the men to seek jobs away from the tribe. Shortly after their marriage, Johnny accepted a position with the state park commission fifty miles north of the reservation. Although the starting salary was relatively low, the job provided the Westfalls with hospitalization insurance.

It was with some reluctance that Johnny and Lorene moved away from the reservation. They rented a very simple four-room duplex house in the county where Johnny was employed. Although it was in a state of disrepair, the Westfalls felt it was adequate for their needs and within their budget. Lorene especially appreciated the garden space in the backyard where she could raise a few vegetables and herbs. The job suited Johnny as he was always outdoors planting trees and maintaining the park grounds.

PREGNANCY

Lorene's mother was instrumental in convincing her daughter to return to the reservation for a visit to the medicine woman when Lorene had not conceived by the couple's first anniversary. The medicine woman was well known and respected in the tribe. She shared her knowledge of curative practices with her people, but, even more importantly, she understood the power that a person's mind could have on various aspects of their lives. She helped people to recognize and use this inner power in a positive manner.

Lorene finally became pregnant after almost two years of marriage. The pregnancy was a welcome event. Johnny's medical insurance would cover the baby's and Lorene's hospital costs but it would not provide for outpatient costs or the cost of certain complications. Lorene returned to the reservation to seek the advice of the medicine woman on a couple of occasions, during which time the medicine woman encouraged Lorene to see a medical doctor as well. She began attending the nearby maternal and infant clinic in March during her third month of pregnancy.

The main health problem identified by the clinic staff was Lorene's increase in weight. She had gained 11.4 kg (25 lb) during the first seven months of pregnancy. Her hemoglobin level was only 10.0 g%. She attempted to follow the diet the clinic prescribed, but she found it difficult because of her traditional dietary customs and restricted budget. Her diet was low in protein sources—particularly dairy products and red meats. She ate vegetables from her garden, but she found it hard to resist baking and eating breads and sweet cakes. She did, however, take the prenatal vitamins and ferrous gluconate (300 mg tid) as prescribed.

STUDY QUESTIONS

1-1. What philosophical attitudes do the Westfalls exhibit toward health care and their way of life?

1-2. What are some Pueblo values illustrated in this case?

1-3. What are the religious beliefs of the Pueblo culture?

1-4. What are some of the meanings the Pueblo culture attaches to health and illness?

1-5. What are some of the culture's common health problems?

1-6. What kind of health insurance is provided for state employees in your state? What does it cover?

1-7. What is the role of the medicine man/woman as it is portrayed in this case study?

1-8. Describe the typical diet of a southwestern Native American family living on a reservation.

1-9. Complete the following nutrition table for a nineteen-year-old female:

QUANTITY OF FOOD

Food group	19-year-old female	Pregnant 19-year-old Trimester			Rationale for alteration in diet
		1st	2d	3d	
Dairy products (milk, cheese and ice cream)					
Meats					
Eggs					
Vegetables and fruits					
Breads and cereals					
Butter or margarine					
Calories					

1-10. State whether Ms. Westfall is receiving adequate or inadequate amounts of the following nutrients. What nursing measures can be instituted to increase the adequacy of her diet?

Nutrient	(In)adequacy of Ms. Westfall's diet	Nursing measure(s) to increase adequacy
Protein		
Fat		
Carbohydrate		
Vitamins (A, B, C, and D)		
Minerals (calcium and iron)		

1-11. Fill out a drug information card on the following medications: ferrous gluconate, prenatal vitamins.

1-12. What side effects of ferrous gluconate should Ms. Westfall be told about? Why?

1-13. Why is the clinic concerned about Ms. Westfall's weight gain?

1-14. What are the possible causes for the alteration in Ms. Westfall's hemoglobin level?

Laboratory Test	Normal range for adult females	Ms. Westfall's level	Amount of deviation from normal	Possible causes for alteration
Hemoglobin				

DISCUSSION QUESTIONS

D-1. What are some of the ways that an American Pueblo might express his or her emotions or feelings? Why?

D-2. Analyze the possible causes for Ms. Westfall's weight gain and low hemoglobin level. What nursing measures can be instituted to correct these alterations?

LABOR AND DELIVERY

Lorene and Johnny found themselves both bewildered and concerned when Lorene's membranes ruptured suddenly at 5 A.M. on September 11. There were no signs of contractions until nearly 8 A.M. Within an hour Lorene was experiencing moderate contractions every 10 to 15 minutes, and each contraction was lasting 25 to 30 seconds. That's when Johnny called Dr. Benson, the clinic's physician. Dr. Benson advised the Westfalls to proceed to the hospital. It took 25 minutes to drive to the Mountainville Hospital. The couple rode in silence, each sensing the other's concern for the safe birth of their first child.

"I should be happy," Lorene repeated to herself. "The medicine woman says that I must have good thoughts," she continued to remind herself.

Following a relatively uneventful labor lasting eight hours, their son, Jonathan, was born at 1:30 P.M. via a low forceps delivery. Lorene noted the baby's small size and weak cry. His Apgar scores were 7 at one minute and 8 at five minutes. However, the newborn did not appear to be in any acute distress.

Mr. Westfall was waiting just outside the labor and delivery suite. As the nurse wheeled the newborn from the delivery area, she explained to Jonathan's father that the baby needed to be carefully observed and kept warm. Upon her invitation Mr. Westfall accompanied her to the nursery, where he could see Jonathan from the nursery window. Fixing his eyes intently upon his newborn son, he watched as the baby was weighed and placed in an incubator. After filing her report in the observation nursery, the nurse returned to Mr. Westfall's side. She was now ready to answer any questions he had regarding his son's condition. Although she encouraged him to ask questions as she explained how the infant would be carefully watched, he simply acknowledged her comments with an occasional nod and remained focused on his son. After a few rather silent minutes, the nurse asked him if he'd like to visit with his wife in the recovery room.

In the recovery room, Johnny comforted Lorene by gently holding her hand and stroking her face lightly. They spoke to one another only briefly and seemed to be comfortable with their shared silence.

STUDY QUESTIONS

1-15. What conditions of pregnancy are associated with premature delivery?

1-16. What health problems or conditions, which are common to the Native American Indian culture, may have contributed to Lorene's complicated pregnancy and early delivery?

1-17. What is the difference between the following newborn classifications:

   a. premature
   b. immature

    c. SGA

    d. AGA

    e. LGA

1-18. Describe the specific physical and neuromuscular characteristics of an infant who is born at 33 weeks gestational age. What are the implications for care?

1-19. What is the purpose of determining the Apgar score on a newborn?

1-20. What is the significance of Jonathan's Apgar scores?

DISCUSSION QUESTIONS

D-3. What might be the reasons for Mr. and Mrs. Westfall's behavior at this time?

D-4. What do you think their reaction might be to their premature son?

D-5. How could a nurse promote effective communication with each parent individually and as a couple?

NEWBORN ASSESSMENT—OBSERVATION NURSERY

Jonathan's condition began to change as he lay in an observation nursery under the careful monitoring of Ms. Franklin, R.N. Her nursing notes read as follows:

1:40 P.M.	Premature male newborn received by the observation nursery in the transport incubator and placed in a warming unit. Temp.—36.2°C; Apical pulse—140/minute; Respirations—60–70/minute. Generally pale color. Weight—1920 g. (4 lb, 4 oz).
2:15 P.M.	Progressively dusky color with marked acrocyanosis developing. Fair air exchange noted upon auscultation. Temp. 36.4°C R—76/minute; AP—120/minute. Resident notified.
2:30 P.M.	Robert Macey, M.D., examined infant. Suctioned for moderate amount of white mucus. Oxygen therapy 30% via mask started. Color improved slightly. Occasional labored respirations at 50/minute.

In light of the newborn's unstable condition, Ms. Franklin postponed parts of the routine nursing assessment for gestational maturity. She prepared for the possibility of emergency procedures, instead. She made certain that intubation and intravenous cut-down equipment were available and near to the infant's incubator.

For the next hour, Jonathan's condition remained unchanged. His respiratory rate ranged from 50–70/minute and as he demonstrated occasional expiratory grunting. Although a normal sinus rhythm could be identified, the apical pulse rate continued to vary from 110–160/minute. He had become less responsive to touch although his general alertness had not varied.

At 3:30 P.M. the following medical orders were written:

Portable chest and abdominal X-rays stat

Arterial blood gases via umbilical artery after X-ray

Electrolytes and hematocrit stat

Dextrostix stat and then q 4 h

Transfer to a radiant warmer

Maintain 30% humidified O_2 concentration (F_iO_2) per oxygen hood

Intravenous infusion of 10% D/W IV via scalp vein to run at 65 ml/kg/24 hr

Ms. Franklin instituted a schedule of vital signs every 15 minutes until stable and Silverman scores q 1 h (see Appendix B). She carefully positioned Jonathan under the radiant warmer before the X-ray technician arrived. An oxygen mask remained the source of oxygen until the X-rays were obtained. Then the oxygen hood, attached to a plastic hose carrying the humidified oxygen, was assembled and regulated. After the X-rays were completed, a thermostatic skin probe was applied. In addition, she put cardiac-monitor leads on Jonathan, and placed him on an apnea mattress. The necessary blood samples were obtained and an intravenous infusion was started via a # 21 butterfly needle in a large scalp vein.

Within the next hour the following X-ray findings were reported to the unit: "A diffuse reticulogranular pattern causing partial opacification of the lung fields." This confirmed the suspected diagnosis of moderate respiratory distress syndrome (RDS).

The stat laboratory results were as follows:

Hct: 48%   Dextrostix: 45 mg %
p_aO_2: 42 mm Hg   Na: 130 mEq/1
p_aCO_2: 42 mm Hg   K: 4.7 mEq/1
pH: 7.27   C1: 110 mEq/1
BE: −3 units CO_2: 30 mEq/1
                             Ca: 8.4 mEq/1

STUDY QUESTIONS

1-21. What are the special problems of a premature infant? What is the physiologic basis of each? What is the nursing management of each problem?

1-22. Describe the "textbook picture" of newborns with (a) mild, (b) moderate, and (c) severe respiratory distress. Compare Jonathan's clinical manifestations with your findings.

Problem	Physiologic Basis	Nursing Management

1-23. Complete the following laboratory grid:

Test	Normal range for newborns	Jonathan's values	Amount of deviation from normal	Possible cause for alteration
Hematocrit				
Dextrostix				
Sodium				
Potassium				
Chloride				
CO_2 combining power				
Calcium				
p_aO_2				
p_aCO_2				
pH				
BE				

1-24. How do dextrostix values differ from serum glucose values?

1-25. Determine the number of drops per minute Jonathan's IV should run with a microdrip (60 gtt/ml) administration set.

1-26. Determine the nursing care priorities for Jonathan. What is the rationale for each?

Nursing care priority	Rationale
1.	
2.	
3.	
4.	
5.	
6.	

1-27. What are the precautions that must be taken when oxygen therapy is administered to a newborn? What assessment parameters should be watched closely?

1-28. Explain how a radiant warmer controls body temperature. What is the advantage of using a radiant warmer instead of an isolette in this case?

DISCUSSION QUESTIONS

D-6. Was it appropriate for Ms. Franklin to postpone parts of the nursing assessment and make preparations for the possible emergency procedures? Explain your reasoning.

D-7. Discuss the purpose of blood-gas studies and how they are used to monitor patients with respiratory difficulty and/or oxygen therapy.

D-8. Since Johnny's hospitalization insurance did not cover the cost of complications in either the mother or infant, how can social service help the Westfalls deal with the financial burden?

ASSESSMENT—SPECIAL CARE NURSERY

The decision was made to transfer Jonathan to an adjoining special care nursery (SCN) where the equipment and specially trained staff were available should the infant require more intensive respiratory assistance. Ms. Thomas, R.N. was assigned to Jonathan Westfall.

In light of the infant's condition and a P_aO_2 of 42 mm Hg, the ambient O_2 concentration was increased to 50% via the oxygen hood. Ms. Thomas carefully assessed the newborn and documented her observations:

4:00 P.M.   Silverman score: 6. Respirations continue to be labored with moderate subcostal and intercostal retractions and occasional grunting. Resp. rate: 64/minute. Apneic spells × 2 within the last half hour lasting for 15–20 seconds. No change in breath or heart sounds. Skin temperature 36.6–36.9° C under radiant warmer. Color pale with transient circumoral cyanosis. AP: 150, BP (doptone): 40. Gestational age assessment reveals that the infant is approximately 33 weeks gestation. Progressively increased lethargy noted, although reacts readily to tactile stimulation.

Meanwhile, the following medical orders were implemented:

Increased F_iO_2 to 60% via oxygen hood

Change IV solution to add Cutter IV solution # 48 electrolytes in 10% dextrose/water at 65 ml/kg/24 hr

ABG's stat and q 30 minutes following changes in oxygen therapy

Then ABG's q 4 h when stable via heelstick

Umbilical artery catheter equipment at bedside

As soon as she had completed the necessary nursing activities and Jonathan's condition stabilized, Ms. Thomas made arrangements for the newborn to be observed by another nurse. Ms. Thomas then visited with Ms. Westfall, who had since been admitted to the postpartum unit. In the few minutes she had, the nurse offered Jonathan's mother simple explanations of her son's present condition and what was being done for him. She also made arrangement for Ms. Westfall to visit Jonathan.

As Ms. Thomas was preparing to leave, Lorene's eyes filled with tears. "I only wish that I knew what it was that I did wrong. I didn't want to harm my baby." The nurse reassured her, "Mrs. Westfall, you probably had very little to do with why your son was born earlier than expected. But most women in your situation do wonder about it, just the same." Ms. Thomas offered Lorene her hand as she encouraged Lorene to further express her concerns.

Jonathan, with the assistance of his health care team, had stabilized considerably by six hours after birth. He was now receiving 50% O_2 under an oxygen hood. His respiratory effort was less labored, although intercostal retractions were still apparent. The following are the laboratory study results taken at 6 P.M.:

p_aO_2: 5 mm Hg	Na: 132 mEq/1
p_aCO_2: 40 mm Hg	K: 4.7 mEq/1
pH: 7.32	C1: 102 mEq/1
BE: −3 units	CO_2: 28 mEq/1
Glucose: 80 mg %	Ca: 8.8 mEq/1

STUDY QUESTIONS

1-29. What are the limitations on the amount of blood that can be taken from a newborn for laboratory exams?

1-30. Compare the laboratory studies on Jonathan given to this point. Analyze the effects of his treatment regime.

Lab test	4:00 P.M.	6:00 P.M.	Treatment	Effect of treatment
Blood gases Electrolytes				

1-31. What is the rationale behind the change in IV solution orders?

1-32. What is the purpose of the Silverman score and the RDS (Downes) score? How are they done? (See Appendices B and C.)

Test	Purpose	Testing technique
Silverman RDS (Downes)		

1-33. Explain the purpose of each of the following, how they operate, and how they are tested before using them on a client:

Equipment	Purpose	Technique of operation	Testing technique
Oxygen hood Isolette Radiant warmer			

1-34. Complications can occur if there is an equipment malfunction or an accidental human error. How do you assess the client and the equipment to prevent these complications? What nursing actions should be instituted in the event of a complication:

Equipment	Potential malfunction	Infant's response to malfunction (signs and symptoms)	Nursing action	Method and frequency of evaluating infant's response
Oxygen hood with tubing to a humidifier				
Isolette				
Radiant warmer				
IV infusion via scalp vein				

DISCUSSION QUESTION

D-9. How might Ms. Thomas encourage Lorene to express her feelings and give her emotional support?

THE PARENTS' VISIT TO THE SPECIAL CARE NURSERY

Ms. Westfall and her husband requested to see their son after supper. Ms. Baylor, Jonathan's evening nurse, indicated that she would first meet the Westfalls in the lounge at 7:00 P.M. to discuss Jonathan's condition. As Ms. Baylor entered the lounge, Lorene was waiting quietly in a wheelchair and Johnny was staring out the window. Ms. Baylor simply described some of the mechanical devices and wires that were attached to their newborn's tiny body, as well as the differences between their premature infant's needs and those of a full-term infant. They listened intently to the nurse's explanations, but they were unable to understand why their baby was so sick or why he needed all those tubes.

Lorene wondered what she had done to bring evil spirits upon her newborn son. She remembered trying very hard to be happy, as the medicine woman had instructed her, but it was so hard, away from the tribe. Lorene also wondered if the evil spirits had befallen her infant because she had missed the appointment with the medicine woman last week. Since it was obvious that Ms. Baylor was not a Native American, Lorene thought it would be better to wait until she could discuss it further with the medicine woman.

Ms. Baylor walked with the Westfall couple into the nursery, where they just stared at Jonathan. His tiny body was barely visible—his head was covered with a foggy box and seemingly endless tubes were going into him. He lay there so still, hardly moving. He didn't look like any newborn they had ever seen. Lorene got up and walked closer to the incubator where Jonathan lay.

Lorene was visibly overwhelmed; her knees grew weak and her hands gripped each other. She thought, "My baby is going to die . . . even if Johnny could get to the medicine woman in time." Her head began to spin as she fainted. Once revived, Lorene found herself sitting in the wheelchair with Ms. Baylor holding something under her nose. Johnny was holding her hand. Lorene began to cry.

STUDY QUESTION

1-35. What items should be discussed with the parents before they see Jonathan? Outline the items in the order in which they should be presented. What would you explain about each?

Item	Explanation
1.	
2.	
3.	
4.	
5.	
6.	

DISCUSSION QUESTIONS

D-10. Could Ms. Westfall have been better prepared to visit Jonathan? If so, describe.

D-11. Do you think Ms. Baylor was aware of the possibility of Lorene having thoughts that she didn't express (i.e., cultural awareness)?

D-12. How can the nurse elicit positive maternal responses toward an infant in jeopardy? What could Mr. and Mrs. Westfall be encouraged to do that might develop parent-infant attachment under these circumstances?

JONATHAN'S STABILIZATION AND GROWTH PHASE

After three days of oxygen therapy with the oxygen hood, Jonathan's condition steadily improved. The following nursing note was recorded:

September 13

7:30 P.M.   Significant increase in muscular activity noted periodically with only occasional acrocyanosis. Respirations: 45–50/minute without apneic episodes or retractions. Lung sounds clear with improved air exchange noted. AP: 130–140 regular per minute; (skin probe) T: 36.8°C; IV continues to infuse at 65 mg/kg/day. Urinary output of 24 ml for 8 h. Weight: 1720 g. Sputum specimen obtained for culture and sensitivity. Mother visited patient twice today.

The arterial blood gas results were:

		F_iO_2	p_aO_2	p_aCO_2	pH	BE
9/13	12 A.M.	50%	88	30	7.38	+2
	6 A.M.	40	62	33	7.33	0
	Noon	40	64	33	7.32	−1
9/14	6 A.M.	30	62	37	7.30	−4
	Noon	30	62	35	7.31	−3

The following medical orders were written for Jonathan:

Transfer to incubator

Maintain F_iO_2 of 30–40% (depending on infant's condition)

Repeat heelstick blood gases after the first 30 minutes and 60 minutes after placement in the incubator, then q 8 h and prn

Pass N/G tube when condition is stabilized in the incubator

Begin N/G feedings with 10 ml of 5% glucose in H_2O q 2 h × 2, then Enfamil (13 cal/30 ml strength) 10 ml q 2 h × 2

Increase Enfamil 1 ml q feeding up to 20 ml as tolerated

Decrease IV to 120 cc/24 hr.

Both parents came to the SCN that evening to visit Jonathan. The physician discussed the newborn's progress at length with the parents. Since it would be the fifth day after delivery, Ms. Westfall would be discharged in the morning from the postpartum unit. Her feelings were mixed about her discharge because she knew she would not be able to visit her son every day. Because of the distance, Johnny would only be able to take her every two or three days.

Lorene was determined to breast-feed, even though her doctor had advised against breast-feeding. She attempted to manually express the milk from her breasts each time she was in the bathroom.

The day after Lorene's discharge, Johnny drove Lorene to their tribal medicine woman. The medicine woman alleviated some of Lorene's fears about Jonathan's unstable condition by giving her an herbal bag for Jonathan to wear and a pouch of cornmeal to sprinkle around the infant's incubator. The medicine woman also showed Lorene how to manually express her milk into clean bottles when her breasts felt full. Lorene manually expressed her milk three times a day and refrigerated the bottles.

Two days later Lorene and Johnny went to the hospital to see their infant. Lorene greeted the puzzled SCN evening nurse, Ms. Baylor, with the bottles of milk. After a few questions, Ms. Baylor realized that Lorene was determined to breast-feed her baby. The nurse then explained the progress that their seven-day-old infant had made.

Jonathan had been weaned off oxygen supplements, but he was still in the incubator. His IV solutions had been discontinued and he was now tolerating 20 ml of Enfamil (20 cal/30 ml) via the nasogastric tube at each feeding. His weight had increased to 1840 g (4 lbs, 1 oz).

Ms. Baylor explained to Lorene and Johnny that Jonathan's suck was still very weak and that this was the reason for feeding their newborn through the tube to his stomach. However, Lorene's breast milk could be fed to Jonathan through the tube and eventually through a special soft nipple designed for premature babies like Jonathan.

Lorene and Johnny watched intently as Ms. Baylor gave Jonathan his tube feeding. After the feeding, the Westfalls stayed with Jonathan for awhile. Before leaving, Lorene quietly slipped the herbal bag under Jonathan's mattress and then she secretively sprinkled a circle of cornmeal on the floor around Jonathan's incubator.

Not noticing the additions Lorene had made, Ms. Baylor talked with the Westfalls before they left. In response to Ms. Westfall's question, Ms. Baylor explained that it would be ten days to two weeks until Jonathan would be strong enough to breast-feed. The nurse promised to keep them both informed as to Jonathan's feeding progress. Ms. Baylor then demonstrated the use of a breast-pump and gave Lorene sterile bottles to put the milk in. She explained that in a few days Jonathan could be fed with the special premature nipple, and she encouraged the Westfalls to arrange their visits for feeding times so that they could give Jonathan the bottled breast milk. This was received with a smile and great anticipation by the couple. Then Mr. and Ms. Westfall left the unit quietly.

STUDY QUESTIONS

1-36. How is a neonate "weaned" off of supplemental oxygen?

1-37. What special considerations are taken into account when an N/G tube is inserted into a premature infant?

1-38. How does one assess a premature infant's tolerance of N/G tube feedings?

1-39. What is the average daily weight gain of a premature infant during the neonatal period? How does Jonathan's weight gain compare to the average weight gain?

1-40. What are the advantages and disadvantages of giving breast milk to a premature newborn? What special considerations are taken?

1-41. What are the various types of breast pumps and how do they operate?

1-42. Design a teaching plan for instructing Ms. Westfall in the following:

Technique	Objectives	Content	Method of evaluating learning
Manual expression of milk			
Breast pump			
Breast-feeding			

1-43. Compare the nutrients in prepared infant formulas with breast milk.

1-44. When a child is ill within the Pueblo tribe, what rituals are performed?

DISCUSSION QUESTIONS

D-13. What are the policies and relevant procedures for parent visitation to nurseries and SCN's in your area? What philosophy do these policies reflect? What changes should be considered?

D-14. When ritualistic actions are performed in the hospital by the client (for example, placing an herbal bag with the infant) how should the SCN staff react? What precautions can the nurse institute to accommodate the tribe's customs?

DISCHARGE

To the Westfalls, it seemed like an eternity until Jonathan was finally placed in an open crib (at 20 days of age) and until he had attained a weight of 2300 g. Jonathan was discharged at 23 days of age, as an apparently healthy infant. He would be followed carefully at the maternal infant clinic near his home once every two weeks.

STUDY QUESTION

1-45. Why are infants kept hospitalized until they weigh 2300 g or more?

DISCUSSION QUESTIONS

D-15. How should the Westfalls be prepared for Jonathan's discharge? Consider (1) the newborn's physical needs, (2) the parents' confidence in caring for their infant, and (3) their possible need for information about the infant's care once the discharge is completed.

D-16. What are the potential roles of the public health nurse and of the maternal infant clinic? What information would you need to provide the public health nurse and/or the clinic so that they might effectively follow-up on Jonathan Westfall?

CHAPTER DISCUSSION QUESTIONS

1. How might the value systems of Native Americans affect their health care? How might some potential conflicts between traditional health care and biomedical health care be overcome?

2. Analyze the nutritional effects of Southwestern American Indian diet for the following individuals:
    a. a pregnant Indian
    b. a lactating mother
    c. a breast-fed infant
3. How can the staff of an SCN encourage parent-infant bonding during the following time periods:
    a. while the newborn is ill
    b. during stabilization and growth
    c. prior to discharge
4. What is the daily charge for a neonate admitted to an SCN in your area? in a normal newborn nursery?
5. What insurance plans cover the SCN charges in your area?
6. What are some of the cultural practices of the Westfalls? How can the nursing staff demonstrate respect and understanding for their culture?
7. What are the criteria for certifying an SCN in your state?
8. How can the Crippled Children's Act help with the Westfall's financial burden for Jonathan's care?

SUGGESTED ACTIVITIES

1. Role play the interaction between the SCN staff and Ms. Westfall.
2. Visit an SCN during feeding time and visiting hours.
    a. Observe the nurse's role
    b. Observe the parental interaction with SCN staff, with infants
    c. Review the criteria for being admitted to the SCN
    d. Observe the treatment rendered to the newborn patients
3. Manipulate an incubator and an oxygen hood. Give a bath to an infant doll in an incubator.
4. Explore the cost and nutritional content of the various commercially available products used for infant gavage feedings.
5. Participate in the care of a premature infant, including feeding, monitoring, and so forth.

BIBLIOGRAPHY

Babson, S. Gorham et al. *Management of High Risk Pregnancy and Intensive Care of the Neonate.* 3d ed. St. Louis: C. V. Mosby Co., 1975.

Barnard, Martha Underwood. "Supportive Nursing Care for the Mother and Newborn Who Are Separated from Each Other." *American Journal of Maternal Child Nursing* 1 (March/April 1976): 107–110.

Clark, Ann L., and Affonso, Dyanne D. *Childbearing: A Nursing Perspective.* Philadelphia: F. A. Davis Co., 1976, pp. 684–697, 719–750, 777–778, 786–793, 843–852.

Eager, Marcia. "Long Distance Nurturing of the Family Bond." *American Journal of Maternal Child Nursing* 2 (September/October 1977): 293–294.

Farris, Lorene Sanders. "Approaches to Caring for the American Indian Maternity Patient." *American Journal of Maternal Child Nursing* 1 (March/April 1976): 80–87.

————. "The American Indian." In *Cultural Childbearing for Health Professionals.* Edited by Ann L. Clark. Philadelphia: F. A. Davis Co., 1978.

Guyton, Arthur C. *Textbook of Medical Physiology.* 5th ed. Philadelphia: W. B. Saunders Co., 1976, pp. 517–518; 1124–1125; 1131–1132.

Jennie, Joe; Gallerito, Cecelia; and Pino, Josephine. "Cultural Health Traditions." In *Providing Safe Nursing Care for Ethnic People of Color,* edited by Marie F. Branch and Phyllis P. Paxton. New York: Appleton-Century-Crofts, 1976.

Kee, Joyce L., and Gregory, Ann P. "The ABC's and MEq's of Fluid Balance in Children." *Nursing '74* 4 (June 1974): 28–36.

Klaus, Marshall H., and Kennell, John H. "Caring for Parents of a Premature or Sick Infant." In *Maternal-Infant Bonding.* St. Louis: C. V. Mosby Co., 1976.

Kniep-Hardy, Mary, and Burkhardt, Margaret A. "Nursing the Navajo." *American Journal of Nursing* 77 (January 1977): 95–96.

Korones, Sheldon B. *High-Risk Newborn Infants—The Basis for Intensive Nursing Care.* 2d ed. St. Louis: C. V. Mosby Co., 1976.

Little, Dolores, and Carnevali, Doris L. *Nursing Care Planning.* 2d ed. Philadelphia: J. B. Lippincott Co., 1976.

McNall, Leota K., and Galeener, Janet T. "Idiopathic Respiratory Distress Syndrome of the Newborn." In *Current Practices in Obstetric and Gynecologic Nursing,* edited by Marsha Fowler. St. Louis: C. V. Mosby Co., 1976.

Miner, Holly. "Problems and Prognosis for the Small-for-Gestational-Age and the Premature Infant." *The American Journal of Maternal Child Nursing* 3 (July/August 1978): 221–226.

Nalepka, Claire D. "Oxygen Hood for Newborns in Respiratory Distress." *American Journal of Nursing* 75 (December 1975): 2185–2187.

Primeaux, Martha. "Caring for the American Indian Patient." *American Journal of Nursing* 77 (January 1977): 91–94.

Scipien, Gladys M. et al. *Comprehensive Pediatric Nursing.* New York: McGraw-Hill, 1975, pp. 209–211, 311–318; 347–353; 498–513.

Stroot, Violet R.; Lee, Carla A.; and Schaper, C. Ann. *Fluid and Electrolytes: A Practical Approach.* 2d ed. Philadelphia: F. A. Davis Co., 1977.

Thompson, Theodore R. "Respiratory Distress: Identification, Evaluation and Stabilization of the Newborn Infant Prior to Transport: Part 1." *Perinatal Press* 1 (November/December 1977): 3–6.

_____. "Respiratory Distress: Identification, Evaluation and Stabilization of the Newborn Infant Prior to Transport: Part II." *Perinatal Press* 2 (January 1978): 3–7.

CHAPTER TWO

Congenital Defect: Pyloric Stenosis

ANDREA BRETZ SAVITZ

RUTH RAYSOR WEST

OVERVIEW

David Stern is the newborn son of an Orthodox Jewish couple, Frank and Ann Stern. At age 25 days, David begins projectile vomiting of his milk and is rushed to the emergency room of the Englewood Hospital. After being admitted to the pediatric unit, an upper GI series confirms the diagnosis of stenosis of the pyloric valve. After conservative management fails, a pyloromyotomy is performed. The nursing staff not only uses a variety of methods to maintain the infant's nutritional status, but they also must assist a Jewish family to cope with the care of their first-born infant.

CONTENT EMPHASIS

- Genograms
- Nutritional status—assessment and maintenance
- Congenital defect—pyloric stenosis
- Management of an infant following surgery—pyloromyotomy
- Teaching parents—infant care

SETTINGS

- Emergency room
- Pediatric unit
- Pediatric intensive care unit

OBJECTIVES

Upon completing this chapter the student will be able to:

1. Analyze the impact of the Jewish culture on the family of an acutely ill infant.
2. Assess the nutritional and fluid balance of an infant with vomiting.
3. Evaluate the nursing management of an infant with pyloric stenosis and the management of its family.
4. Design specific intervention modalities for an infant who has a pyloromyotomy.
5. Conceptualize the teaching role of the nurse in working with parents of first-born infants and infants with pyloric stenosis.

DEFINITION OF TERMS

The following terms are used in this case study and should be defined before proceeding:

Anthropometry
Brith Milah or Bris
Family constellation
Genealogy
Genogram
Kosher foods

Mohel
Pidyon Ha-Ben
Pyloromyotomy
Rule out (R/O)
Talmud
Upper gastrointestinal series (UGS or UGI)

FAMILY ASSESSMENT

Frank and Ann Stern are an Orthodox Jewish couple who have been married two years. They are financially secure. Presently they live in a nine-room house in Englewood, New Jersey. The home was bought with the idea that it would eventually be filled with Stern children. There are five bedrooms. Their yard is enclosed and private.

Both Frank and Ann are in excellent health. They have maintained good physical fitness primarily through swimming. In fact, the Stern's enthusiasm for exercise was in a way responsible for their meeting. They met three years ago at the YMHA of Bergen County during a family swimming hour.

Frank, age 28, is the middle child of Allen and Florence Stern of Leonia, New Jersey (see genogram and Appendix D). He is close to both of his parents; however, over the years he has had difficulty dealing with his father

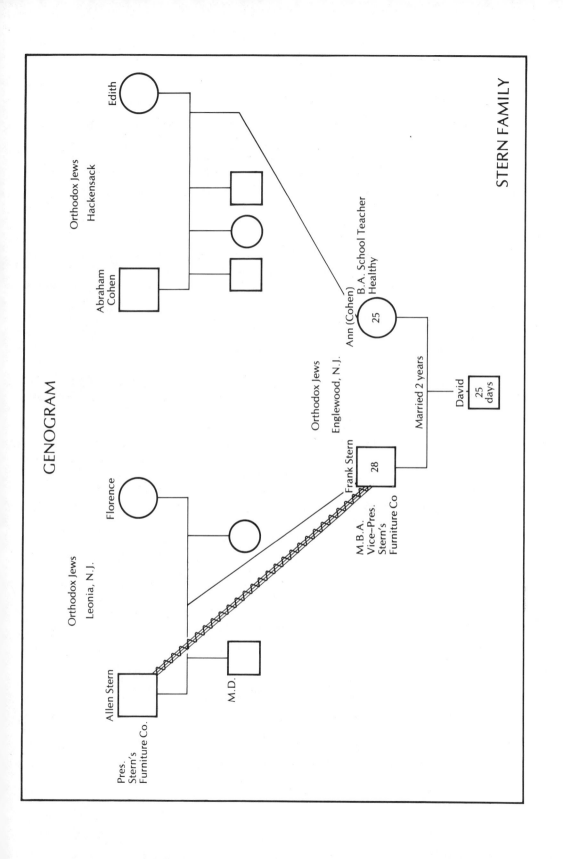

GENOGRAM

Orthodox Jews
Leonia, N.J.

Orthodox Jews
Hackensack

Allen Stern

Pres.
Stern's
Furniture Co.

M.D.

Florence

Frank Stern

28

M.B.A.
Vice–Pres.
Stern's
Furniture Co

Orthodox Jews
Englewood, N.J.

Married 2 years

David

25
days

Ann (Cohen)

25

B.A. School Teacher
Healthy

Abraham
Cohen

Edith

STERN FAMILY

Allen's strong will. Allen had wanted Frank to study one of the traditional professions. Frank's undergraduate cumulative average of 3.3 was not high enough for admission to medical or law school, so he entered graduate school to study business.

When Frank Stern completed his master's in business administration, he joined his father's already well-established furniture company. Frank's desire to please his father, combined with his education and hard work, helped him to increase the company's profits tenfold in five years. Frank is now the Stern Furniture Company's vice-president. His earnings are now in the high income tax bracket.

However, Allen still occasionally comments on how Frank could not make the grade to get into medicine or law. Florence, Frank's mother, is quick to say, "Look Allen, you should be proud of our boy ... see what he has done for the business."

Frank is beginning to be able to kid with his father. In fact Frank has been overheard saying such things to his father as, "A doctor can't sell a couch ... he only buys a couch. Look at the profits, Dad."

Ann (Cohen) Stern, Frank's wife, is an elementary school teacher on a maternity leave of absence. Ann has close ties with her family of origin. She is the youngest child. Edith, Ann's mother, is a major influence on Ann; although the Sterns are the furniture manufacturers, it was Edith Cohen who helped Ann pick her furniture. At least weekly Abraham and Edith Cohen drive over from their home in Hackensack to visit Ann and Frank.

Frank and Ann have a good relationship. They argue infrequently. Ann usually lets Frank take the lead because she has never been comfortable making major decisions alone. Frank, for his part, has said that he is lucky to have found such a wonderful girl as Ann who is anxious to keep a Jewish home.

The senior Sterns and the Cohens were pleased when Ann and Frank announced their intention to marry. The parents knew that their Orthodox Jewish traditions would be continued in such a match. When Frank and Ann's first child, David, was born, a Bris was held in Frank and Ann's home.

STUDY QUESTIONS

2-1. What are the beliefs and religious practices of Orthodox Jews on the following topics?
    a. family size and relationships
    b. marriage
    c. sex of children
    d. health and sanitation

    e. illness
    f. health care providers

2-2. Why are marriages outside of the Jewish religion discouraged by Jews?

2-3. Through whom is the Jewish religion passed down, mother or father? Explain. When does an individual become a Jew?

2-4. How do Orthodox, Conservative, and Reformed Judaism differ? How are they alike?

2-5. What is the Orthodox Jew's view of marriage? sexuality?

2-6. What does keeping the Sabbath mean to a Jew? an Orthodox Jew?

2-7. What are the dietary restrictions of practicing Orthodox Jews?

2-8. What are the principle holidays in the Jewish calendar? What is the meaning of each to a Jew?

2-9. What is the naming system of children born to a practicing Jewish family?

2-10. What is a genogram? What information should be included on a genogram?

2-11. How does a genogram differ from a family tree or genealogy study?

2-12. What are the widely accepted symbols used when drawing a genogram to indicate males, females, marriages, overclose relationships, conflictual relationships and parent-child relationships? (See Appendix D).

2-13. According to Toman, what are the characteristics of the youngest sibling?

2-14. According to Toman, what are the characteristics of the middle sibling?

2-15. What significant traditional heritage does the first-born male child in a Jewish family receive? Explain.

DISCUSSION QUESTIONS

D-1. According to Walter Toman, does Ann fit the character profile of the youngest sibling? Explain.

D-2. Does Frank fit the character profile of the middle sibling according to Toman's research? Explain.

D-3. Are the sibling positions of Frank and Ann compatible for marriage according to the research of Toman? Explain.

D-4. Do you accept that Ann and Edith's relationship was predictable based solely on sibling positions? If you would like other variables considered, what would they be? Explain.

D-5. How can the professional nurse use the genogram to the client's advantage?

D-6. Can the process of taking the genogram be therapeutic for the client? Explain.

D-7. Why would the nurse want to make a special point of frequently checking on a bed-ridden, hospitalized Jew from sundown Friday until sundown Saturday? Explain.

CLIENT ASSESSMENT

After an uneventful pregnancy, David was born in Englewood Hospital, Englewood, New Jersey. David's measurements were recorded on an anthropometric chart (see Appendix E) as follows:

Weight: 3064.5 g

Length: 50 cm

Head circumference: 34.5 cm

Chest circumference: 34.0 cm

Although any healthy infant would have thrilled Ann, Frank and all the grandparents were twice as pleased that a male child had been born.

David and his mother were discharged from the hospital three days after his birth. Just before discharge, David spit up a small amount of his last hospital feeding, which Ann thought was due to the baby being excited.

Edith had come to the hospital to insist that Ann not engage a baby nurse. Edith said, as if to David, "Never mind about your soiled shirt. You'll get a lot of new shirts at your Bris."

David's *Brith Milah* or *Bris* had already been arranged for his eighth day of life by Frank and David's grandparents. During the days preceding the Bris, David started settling into a routine. Edith Cohen had temporarily moved in with Ann to help with David's care. She had said to Ann, "There's no need for a nurse, I'll help you." By the time David was eight days old, Ann was beginning to feel more confident of her parenting ability. After the last guest had left the house following the Bris, Ann told Edith that she felt ready to start parenting on her own. Edith said to Ann, "Your father will be happy to hear the news. Abraham told me yesterday that he doesn't like the life of a 'bachelor.' But am I ever going to miss David."

However, Edith stayed on because David spit up during his next feeding. Ann became upset, saying that "You would think I could at least feed my own child without messing it up." Edith refed David and calmed Ann.

David began to spit up more and more frequently. So Edith was careful to add more formula to compensate for what David had lost, but he was always hungry after each vomiting episode.

The pediatrician, Sol Jacobs, M. D., could find nothing wrong with David. The baby continued to gain weight. Also, Dr. Jacobs hinted that Ann was an "over-anxious" mother, a label Ann did not like.

At home, Ann began to get moody and tired. Ann watched as Edith took over most of David's feedings. Subsequently, Ann confessed to Frank, "I'm beginning to feel like a failure at motherhood. I bubble David, hold him cradled in my arm just so, and still he vomits. David responds better to Mom than to me. I can't understand it... David's hungry, otherwise he wouldn't take formula from Mom after vomiting. Right?"

Frank was baffled, too.

In a few days, David was to have his "ritual of release," called a *Pidyon Ha-Ben.* David was now twenty-five-days-old. Upon feeding, David vomited clear across the floor. Ann almost went into a panic after noting that there were streaks of blood in his vomitus. Ann ran for her coat while shouting to Frank, "Get the car!"

Frank and Edith did not understand Ann's behavior at first. Because it was Friday, Frank was about to say something about it being past sundown. Then Frank saw the blood-speckled vomitus. Frank, Ann, David, and Edith went immediately to Englewood Hospital's emergency room.

STUDY QUESTIONS

2-16. What are the accepted normal ranges of male anthropometric measurements at birth? Are David's measurements normal?

2-17. When is vomiting normal for a neonate? Explain.

2-18. What is considered a normally paced demand feeding routine for most neonates?

2-19. What was the religious significance of David's Bris?

2-20. If a child is born with pyloric stenosis, when do the first symptoms usually appear?

2-21. Complete a pathophysiology information card on pyloric stenosis.

2-22. What is the incidence of pyloric stenosis in the United States?

2-23. Besides blood streaks, what can characteristically be in the vomitus of an infant who has pyloric stenosis?

2-24. What eating behavior would you expect of a normal newborn?

2-25. What motor activity would you expect of the normal neonate?

2-26. What are the developmental tasks of the infant?

2-27. What is the normal daily caloric requirement for a three-week-old neonate?

2-28. What is the normal fluid requirement for a three-week-old neonate?

2-29. What is the weight gain pattern in infancy?

2-30. What is a Mohel? When are his services required?

DISCUSSION QUESTIONS

D-8. What could have accounted for the time lapse between the onset of David's symptoms and the diagnosis?

D-9. As a public health nurse, if you suspected, on history, that a parent was reporting the syndrome of pyloric stenosis, what instruction would you give to protect the infant and to aid the parents in becoming part of the diagnostic team?

Objective	Content	Method of teaching	Evaluation of learning

D-10. Why did the fact that it was past sundown on Friday cause Frank to hesitate before getting the car? Explain.

PREOPERATIVE PERIOD

After arriving in the Englewood Hospital emergency room, the Sterns requested David's pediatrician, Dr. Jacobs. While the Sterns were waiting for Dr. Jacobs, David was admitted to the emergency service by Ms. Laura Murphy, R.N. Ms. Murphy took a brief history on David from his mother. The nurse recorded the following on the emergency room intake sheet:

CHIEF COMPLAINT: Projectile vomiting following completion of last formula feeding approx. 15 min. ago (Red specks in vomitus looked like blood to the infant's mother.)

HISTORY OF PRESENTING PROBLEM: Approximately 2 weeks of vomiting after most formula feeding—followed by immediate refeed. One yellowish-brown stool/day for last 5 days. (Infant had been passing 2 stools/day prior. Infant in no apparent distress.

Ms. Murphy then began her physical assessment of David Stern. The baby was quiet, but had an anxious, alert expression. Ms. Murphy approached David's abdomen first. She recorded the following on David's record:

Abdomen: Olive-sized mass at the rt. costal margin of RUQ
Weight: 3405.0 g

Length: 53 cm

Head circumference: 36.5 cm

Chest circumference: 36.0 cm

Temp.: 37.4°C (rectally)

Pulse: 140

Respirations: 26

The rest of David's physical findings were unremarkable.

When the physical assessment was half over, David began to cry fretfully, and toward the end of the assessment David was screaming. Ann identified his cry as "David's hungry cry." Ann ran her palm over David's brow as she rocked him in her arms. Ann's tense face had a fixed gaze on her son. Edith then demanded that Ms. Murphy attempt to hurry Dr. Jacobs.

In an even, calming voice, Ms. Murphy said, "I'll see what I can do." Moments later, Ms. Murphy reported back to the parents and Edith Cohen that Dr. Jacobs was on his way. He had been held up by an emergency at his office. David continued to cry.

Dr. Jacobs arrived 20 minutes later. He received the report from Ms. Murphy. Then he attempted his own physical exam. However, because David was crying, Dr. Jacobs could not confirm the mass located by Ms. Murphy in David's abdomen. He listed the following tentative diagnosis based on the history obtained by Ms. Murphy:

Pylorospasm

R/O pyloric stenosis

Dr. Jacobs then had David admitted with the following orders:

CBC stat

Electrolytes stat and repeat in 12 hours

PTT stat

Urinalysis stat

NPO

I&O

Daily weight

Upper GI series in A.M.

IV of 5% glucose in 0.45% NaC1 by soluset, 10–15 ml/hr

Vitamin K, 1 mg IM stat

Vitamin D, 400 units IV qd

Vitamin B_1, 1 mg IV qd

Vitamin C, 25 mg qd

Phenobarbital, 6 mg IM q 8 h

On the pediatric unit the Sterns and Edith were met by Ms. Janet Peterson, a nursing student from Rumford University. She noted that the Sterns looked numb, but Edith Cohen was asking questions faster then Miss Peterson could listen. The questions included:

"What's wrong with David?"

"Why does David need intravenous feeding?"

"What do you mean he has to sleep upright in an infant seat?"

"Why do you have his arms tied?"

"When are you going to feed David?"

"What was that blood from when David vomited?"

Ms. Peterson attempted to explain her nursing actions and David's condition as she worked. However, Edith persisted in interrupting. Ann and Frank looked more and more upset by the minute. While Ms. Peterson was finishing making David as comfortable as possible in his infant seat, she said to herself under her breath, "This isn't working very well."

After speaking with her faculty member, Ms. Peterson decided to make time to sit with the family. Shortly after David started to respond to the phenobarbital, Ms. Peterson persuasively invited the family into an empty room to talk.

First, Ms. Peterson assured the Sterns and Edith that David was physically safe. Then she explained that she realized that the family was under a great deal of stress since the discovery of David's illness. Further, Ms. Peterson went on to say that she wanted to help them through this stressful time. Then she emphasized that one way to know how to help people is to first get to know them better. The Sterns and Edith agreed with her logic. Subsequently, Ms. Peterson took a brief genogram of the Sterns and their extended family.

Following the recording of the genogram, Ms. Peterson explained all the details of David's care to the family, while directing her vision toward Ann. Then she gave the family all the time they felt they needed to ask questions. In that way Ms. Peterson was able to control Edith's interruptions while also giving Ann and Frank time to express themselves.

In the meantime, the following laboratory results were received in the pediatric unit:

ELECTROLYTES	
Na: 128 mEq/L	CO_2: 28 mM/L
K: 4.1 mEq/L	Calcium: 6 mEq/L
Cl: 90 mEq/L	Phosphorus: 5 mg/100 ml
	pH: 7.5
	PTT: 75 sec.

URINALYSIS   acetone: neg.
   Sp. gr.: 1.006   protein: 1+
   pH: 6.5
   sugar: neg.

Later that evening, Ann was given a blanket to use while she slept on a chair next to David's crib. Frank, who was noticeably fatigued, took Edith home in a taxi.

The following morning David was given a bottle feeding of barium preceding his X-rays. He was already back in his crib when Frank arrived at 10:00 A.M. Right after asking about his son's welfare, Frank explained that he overslept following a fitful night, and had found the walk to the hospital much longer than he had expected. Ann said, "I'm just glad you are here." Then she leaned into Frank as they both looked helplessly toward their son.

At 6:00 P.M. Dr. Jacobs explained the findings reported from the upper GI series to the Sterns. The report read as follows:

IMPRESSION: There is presence of gastric retention, an elongated, thickened pyloric canal, and delayed pyloric opening time.

Based on the X-ray series, a definite diagnosis of hypertrophied pyloric stenosis was made.

Dr. Jacobs then went on to explain that he had checked David's laboratory studies. David was in excellent health at the present time. However, he could not go back to normal oral feeding until surgery was done to relieve the stenosis. Consent was given for surgery on Monday morning.

The following orders were left on David's chart for the morning of surgery:

Nasogastric tube to intermittent low Gomco suction

Atropine 0.1 mg IM pre-op at 7 A.M.

Continue IV

STUDY QUESTIONS

2-31. Explain the probable cause for the deviations from normal of David's vital signs on admission.

2-32. What happens to the abdominal muscles of an infant when he or she crys? How can this affect David's regurgitation?

2-33. Complete a drug information card on the following medications: vitamin K, vitamin D, vitamin B_1, vitamin C, phenobarbital, atropine.

2-34. Why was David placed on NPO status, I&O, and daily weight?

2-35. What specific areas of the neonate's body can receive intramuscular injections safely? Why?

2-36. What is the rationale for each of the medical orders:

Orders	Rationale
Upon admission Pre-op	

2-37. The technician is about to draw venous blood for David's electrolytes. How would you restrain the infant? What would be the preferable site for venipuncture? Explain.

2-38. Complete the following laboratory grid on David:

Test	Normal range for newborns	David's values	Amount of deviation from normal	Possible cause of alteration

2-39. What anatomical structures are visualized during an upper gastrointestinal series?

2-40. What observations should the nurse make of an infant following an upper gastrointestinal (GI) series?

2-41. How would you position an infant following an upper GI series? Explain why.

2-42. How would you calculate the degree of David's dehydration by using his weight?

2-43. What is the purpose of the insertion of an in-dwelling N/G tube before surgery? What should the nurse monitor once the N/G tube is in place?

2-44. What might be a contributing factor to David's irregular, slow respiratory rate? Consider the lab values.

2-45. What are the working principles underlying the functioning of a nasogastric tube attached to intermittent low Gomco suction?

DISCUSSION QUESTIONS

D-11. Why do you believe Ms. Murphy, R.N., made the judgment to physically assess David's abdomen first, rather than approaching him in a more classical, systematic manner?

D-12. What do you believe accounted for the rather minor dip in David's weight curve as demonstrated by plotting his birth weight and his twenty-five-day-old weight on the infant boy anthropometric chart? How did David's clinical picture deviate from the classical syndrome seen in infants having pyloric stenosis that is not diagnosed immediately after birth?

D-13. What other treatment approach could Dr. Jacobs have tried for David? Explain.

D-14. Based on Ann's ability to label the meaning of David's cry, make a judgment on how the maternal-infant bonding is progressing. Explain.

D-15. Why do you believe Ms. Peterson decided to direct most of her communication to Ann?

PROGRESS

On the morning of surgery, David was taken to the operating room as he slept. His nasogastric tube was in place; his intravenous therapy went uninterrupted. A general anesthetic was given and a pyloromyotomy was performed on David. He tolerated the procedure well.

When admitted to the pediatric intensive care unit, David's postoperative vital signs were as follows:

BP: 80/60

Pulse: 142

Respirations: 30

His IV of 5% glucose in 0.45 NaC1 was infusing well. His nasogastric tube was in place. As prior to surgery, he was wearing elbow restraints. By noon his vital signs had stabilized as follows:

BP: 70/50

Pulse: 130

Respirations: 34

David was returned to the pediatric unit shortly thereafter.

As she started working the evening shift, Ms. Peterson was looking forward to the assignment of David Stern. She had liked the challenge of working with David and his family preoperatively and now she wanted to help the Sterns through the postoperative period.

David was doing well. He was sleeping intermittently in his crib. Ann and Frank were seated in the room. For the first time they had enough emotional energy to ask Ms. Peterson about David's future care.

Aside from frequent checks on David throughout the evening, Ms. Peterson spent her time teaching the Sterns about infant care. Among the subjects reviewed were the following:

Introduction of foods: 1–6 months

Immunization and screening: 1–6 months

Developmental milestones: 1–6 months

Ms. Peterson was careful to reinforce the correct information Ann already knew about infants. Each time she complimented her, Ann's face brightened up with a broad smile.

When Edith Cohen visited after dinner she was surprised to see her daughter Ann's relaxed expression. Edith said, "I didn't expect you to be so relaxed darling, but I'm glad to see it."

On David's first day post-op, his bowel sounds returned. Dr. Jacobs was informed. The physician then indicated that the N/G tube could be removed. David was started on oral feedings of 0.5 oz of 5% glucose water via eye dropper. Aside from a couple of incidences of spitting up, David tolerated the feedings completely. Consequently, the quantity of feedings were increased. By the second post-op day, David was placed on dilute evaporated milk (13 cals/oz) formula by bottle, and his IV was discontinued. On post-op day 3 David was placed back on his original 20 calories per ounce formula, and the Pidyon Ha-Ben was held at his crib side.

The Sterns told their parents that they thanked God for his continued loan of David. David was discharged post-op day 7.

STUDY QUESTIONS

2-46. Complete a drug information card on ether, halothane, and cyclopropane.

2-47. What does the return of bowel sounds after abdominal surgery signify? Explain.

2-48. What is the best position for David when he is eating?

2-49. What observation must the nurse make for the client in restraints? How often?

2-50. Create a nursing care plan for David's post-operative period.

Objective	Rationale	Nursing action	Rationale	Method and frequency of evaluating effectiveness

CHAPTER DISCUSSION QUESTIONS

1. What are the differences between pylorospasm and pyloric stenosis? Why was David's diagnosis late in being recognized?
2. Why do you believe Ms. Peterson took every opportunity available to compliment Ann's parenting judgment and ability?
3. Why was no one alarmed when David vomited a bit in the postsurgical period?
4. Create a teaching plan for the Sterns on infant feeding, immunizations, and development.

Objective	Content	Method of teaching	Evaluation of learning

SUGGESTED ACTIVITIES

1. Take three genograms on members of different families, then compare and contrast them.
2. Interview separately three or four strangers of the same sex. Control for age and sex. Ask each how he or she would handle the same problem. Then, using Toman's research as a guide, predict the participant's sibling position, and check your work.
3. Interview young parents who have had a neonate who underwent surgery. (If you decide to use the genogram method, be sure to ask the parents to whom in the family they went for emotional support.)

BIBLIOGRAPHY

Bergersen, Betty. *Pharmacology in Nursing.* 13th ed. St. Louis: C. V. Mosby Co., 1976.

Blake, Florence G.: Wright, Howell F.; and Waechter, Eugenia. *Nursing Care of Children.* 8th ed. Philadelphia: J. B. Lippincott Co., 1970, pp. 66–76; 216–219.

Brunner, Lillian, and Suddarth, Doris. *Lippincott Manual of Nursing Practice.* 2d ed. Philadelphia: J. B. Lippincott Co., 1978.

Campbell, Claire. *Nursing Diagnosis and Intervention.* New York: John Wiley & Sons, 1978.

Dodge, J. A. "Infantile Hypertrophic Pyloric Stenosis." *Nursing Times* 73 (May 26, 1977): 780ff.

Feinbloom, Richard. *Child Health Encyclopedia.* Boston: Delacorte Press, 1975.

Freeman, N. V. "Pyloric Stenosis." *Nursing Times* 72 (October 7, 1976): 1553–1555.

Garb, Solomon. *Laboratory Tests in Common Use.* 6th ed. New York: Springer Publishing Co., Inc., 1976.

Guerin, Philip J., Jr. *Family Therapy.* New York: Gardner Press, Inc., 1976.

Guyton, Arthur C. *Textbook of Medical Physiology.* 5th ed. Philadelphia: W. B. Saunders Co., 1976.

Kee, Joyce L., and Gregory, Ann P. "The ABC's and MEq's of Fluid Balance in Children." *Nursing '74* 4 (June 1974): 28–36.

Little, Dolores, and Carnevali, Doris. *Nursing Care Planning.* 2d ed. Philadelphia: J. B. Lippincott Co., 1976.

Millgram, Abraham. *Jewish Worship.* Philadelphia: Jewish Publication Society of America, 1971.

Paxton, Phyllis; Ramirez, Martina C.; and Walloch, Esther C. "Nursing Assessment and Intervention." In *Providing Safe Nursing Care for Ethnic People of Color,* edited by Marie Branch and Phyllis Paxton. New York: Appleton-Century-Crofts, 1976.

Pendagast, Eileen G., and Sherman, Charles O. "A Guide to the Genogram Family Systems Training." *The Family* 5 (1977): 3–14.

Petrillo, Madeline, and Sanger, Sirgay. *Emotional Care of Hospitalized Children.* Philadelphia: J. B. Lippincott Co., 1972.

Pumphrey, John. "Recognizing Your Patients' Spiritual Needs." *Nursing '77* 7 (December 1977): 64–70.

Robinson, Corinne, and Lawler, Marilyn R. *Normal and Therapeutic Nutrition.* 15th ed. New York: Macmillan, 1977.

Rothfeder, Barbara, and Tiedeman, Mary. "Feeding the Low-Birth-Weight Neonate." *Nursing '77* 7 (October 1977): 58–59.

Savitri, Kamath. "Nutritional Assessment." In *Health Assessment,* edited by Lois Malasanos et al. St. Louis: C. V. Mosby Co., 1978.

Scipien, Gladys M. et al. *Comprehensive Pediatric Nursing.* New York: McGraw-Hill, 1975.

Smart, Mollie S., and Smart, Russell C. *Children.* 3d ed. New York: Macmillan, 1977.

Spitz, Phyllis, and Sweetwood, Hannelore. "Kids in Crisis: Part I, Bedside Assessment." *Nursing '78* 78 (March 1978): 70–79.

_____. "Kids in Crisis: Part II, Common Emergencies." *Nursing '78* 8 (April 1978): 27–30.

Stroot, Violet R.; Lee, Carla A.; and Schaper, C. Ann. *Fluid and Electrolytes: A Practical Approach.* 2d ed. Philadelphia: F. A. Davis Co., 1977.

Thompson, Jacqueline. "Human Growth and Development: A Basis for Nursing Assessment." In *Nursing Care of the Child with Long Term Illness.* 2d ed. Edited by Shirley Steele. New York: Appleton-Century-Crofts, 1977.

_____. "Current Nutritional Considerations: Manipulation of the Internal Environment and the Role of the Nurse." In *Nursing Care of the Child with Long Term Illness.* 2d ed. Edited by Shirley Steele. New York: Appleton-Century-Crofts, 1977.

Toman, Walter. *Family Constellation: Its Effects on Personality and Social Behavior.* New York: Springer Publishing Company, 1969.

Vaughan, Victor, and McKay, James. *Nelson Textbook of Pediatrics.* 10th ed. Philadelphia: W. B. Saunders Co., 1976.

Ziemer, Mary, and Carroll, Jane S. "Infant Gavage Reconsidered," *American Journal of Nursing* 78 (September 1978): 1543–1544.

CHAPTER THREE

Childhood Poisoning: Accidental Aspirin Ingestion

LINDA K. HARRISON

OVERVIEW

Jason Simpson, a two-year-old toddler, is the oldest of two children. The Simpsons have just moved to a U.S. Army base located in South Carolina, over 500 miles from their family and friends. When Jason's nine-month-old brother has a fever, Jane Simpson unwittingly leaves the baby aspirin on a dresser in the master bedroom. During nap-time Jason discovers the bottle and ingests the "candy." He receives his emergency care at the base hospital and then he is hospitalized for observation and further treatment. The guilt-ridden Jane Simpson has only one support system during this situational crisis.

CONTENT EMPHASIS

- Accidental poisoning—assessment and treatment
- Fostering the building of support systems in situational crises
- Prevention of accidental poisoning

SETTINGS

- Poison control center (ER)
- Pediatric unit
- Home

OBJECTIVES

Upon completing this chapter the student will be able to:

1. Comprehend the incidence, classification, and control of poisoning in various childhood populations.
2. Analyze support systems available to the parents of a nuclear family during periods of stress or crisis.
3. Differentiate the severity of aspirin poisoning based upon symptoms.
4. Analyze the nursing implications and responsibilities in caring for a client following the ingestion of a poison.
5. Design a health education program aimed at the prevention and control of poisoning.
6. Identify the effect of hospitalization on toddlers.

DEFINITION OF TERMS

The following terms are used in this chapter and should be defined before proceeding:

Acetonuria	Salicylate poisoning
Gastric lavage	Serum salicylate level
Nuclear family	Support system
Poisoning	Toddler

ASSESSMENT

Paul and Jane Simpson, ages 24 and 22 years respectively, are the parents of Jason (23 months) and David (9 months). Paul is a private, first class, in the U.S. Army. One month ago he was transferred to a base in South Carolina. The relocation placed the Simpsons over 500 miles away from their hometown, where their familes and close friends still reside. It was difficult to be so far away from their parents and friends, but they were fortunate to have a neighbor who often dropped in to say hello.

A week ago, Paul had been sent out on a survival training maneuver. It was the first time that Jane had managed both her sons without some assistance from either her husband or one of the children's grandparents. Paul would be away from the base for another week. By late evening, David was cranky. He had nasal congestion and his temperature was 38.6°C (101.6°F). That night seemed like an eternity to Jane, as she spent most of the time awake with David. Jane used the orange-flavored children's aspirin from the locked cupboard in the kitchen where she kept all the medicines. She gave David 75 mg of aspirin every 4–5 hours. Jane placed the aspirin bottle on the dresser next to the thermometer in her bedroom so that they'd be more readily available to her through the night. Since David's crying was arousing Jason, Jane wheeled David's crib into her bedroom for the rest of the night. By having him in the same room she could keep an eye on him. It was 3:30 A.M. before Jane was able to get to sleep.

Jason was awake at 6:30 A.M. He had managed to crawl out of his crib—a recent, prized accomplishment. He found his mother and brother sleeping in his parents' bedroom and wasted no time waking them and demanding his usual morning bowl of cereal.

It was a chaotic morning in the Simpson house, and it was compounded by David's crankiness and need for frequent attention. Jason was testing every limit that Jane set for him. In an attempt to gain Jason's cooperation, his mother promised that he could nap on his parents' bed if he would finish his lunch. Jane couldn't wait to get both children in bed for their afternoon naps, since she was beginning to feel the effects of lack of sound sleep herself. It had always been at times like these that she could count on some help from Paul or her mother, but this time she had to manage alone.

Having finally settled the children down for naps, Jane was able to finish a few household chores and take a short nap herself. Occasionally, she heard Jason talking to his toy monkey, which always accompanied him to bed, but she was relieved that he was content to stay on his parents' bed. She knew that he would eventually fall asleep if left alone.

When Jason awoke nearly two hours later, he occupied himself with toys in the living room while Jane continued to iron. It wasn't long before she noticed that Jason was walking somewhat unsteadily and holding his hand near his stomach. Jason admitted to his mother that his "tummy hurts" when she questioned him. He was sweaty to her touch and seemed unusually quiet. Jane thought to herself, "I wonder if he's getting David's cold." She offered him a glass of juice, which he refused. Jane decided to check Jason's temperature. When she went to her bedroom dresser for the thermometer, she was immediately aware of the missing aspirin bottle.

Jane's heart sank as her eyes searched the room. The bottle was sitting on her bed where Jason had napped—nearly empty. She could feel herself on the verge of a panic as she tried to question Jason about the missing aspirin. Jason acted meekly and continued to complain about the pain in his stomach. Remembering the map of the base she had received on arrival, she frantically looked through the desk and found it.

As quickly as she could, Jane gathered David, Jason, and the nearly empty aspirin bottle into the family car and drove to the hospital on the other side of the base.

Upon arriving at the emergency room, she was met by Kathy Walker, R.N. "I think Jason swallowed the aspirin," Jane blurted out while pointing to the bottle. The tears welled in her frightened eyes. Ms. Walker carried Jason and the bottle to an examining room while Jane followed with David in her arms.

Kathy tried to calm Ms. Simpson by reassuring her that she had done the right thing to get help quickly. Ms. Walker performed a brief nursing assessment, recognizing that there was no time to lose. Through careful questioning of the client's mother, Ms. Walker learned that the 13-kg, 23-month-old client had ingested up to twenty 75-mg flavored aspirin tablets 2–3 hours ago. Kathy also ascertained that Jason had eaten tomato soup, a piece of bread, 60 g of bologna, and 90–120 ml of milk about 1–2 hours before the aspirin ingestion.

Dr. Roberts, a pediatrician, came into the room within a few minutes, having just finished with another client. Following his brief examination of Jason and after consulting with Ms. Walker, the following orders were written:

Gastric lavage with clear water. Send first specimen to lab for analysis

Blood specimen for serum salicylate level

Serum calcium and venous pH

Serum electrolytes

Intake and output q 1 h

NPO

Check urine pH with phenistix q 1 h

Vitamin K, 5 mg IM now

Jane sobbed as Dr. Roberts tried to explain how they would treat Jason's condition. Since Ms. Walker was busy with Jason, another ER nurse, Ms. Hartman, R.N., stayed with Jane Simpson in a nearby waiting room. Ms. Hartman offered Ms. Simpson a chair and some tissues in an attempt to comfort her. "What a stupid mother I've been. This should never have happened to my child. I'll never forgive myself for this," Jane declared with frustration. Jason's cry could occasionally be heard by his mother as the blood specimens were obtained and the gastric lavage was being prepared. After Ms. Simpson seemed to calm down, Ms. Hartman responded, "Many mothers feel the very same way you do when things like this happen. You have nothing to blame yourself for. Children get into things when their parents least expect it. But you did the right thing to bring your child here as soon as you realized that he needed help." Ms. Hartman explained what procedures were being done and why they were needed. Then she offered to watch David for a while at the desk, if Jane wanted to stay with Jason during the lavage.

It was about thirty minutes later when the lab results were available.

Serum salicylate: 42 mg %

Blood pH (venous): 7.3

Na: 130 mEq/L

K: 3.9 mEq/L

C1: 100 mEq/L

CO_2: 20 mM/L

Ca: 5.3 mEq/L

Jason was exhibiting an increased depth of respiration, diaphoresis, acetonuria, and he continued to complain of abdominal pain. He apparently had not vomited since the ingestion. His vital signs were: T: 37.78°C rectal, P: 108/min, R: 30 (deep)/min. The decision was made that Jason should be admitted to the pediatric unit for further observation. An intravenous infusion of 5% dextrose in 0.33% isotonic saline with minidrop was started in Jason's right arm. It was calibrated to infuse at 60 ml/hr. Elbow restraints were applied. Dr. Roberts explained his decision to hospitalize Jason to Ms. Simpson. He also indicated that the prognosis was good if Jason received adequate care at this time.

STUDY QUESTIONS

3-1.   Complete a growth and development card for a two-year-old male and for a nine-month-old male.

3-2.   Identify the four classifications of poisoning and a few examples of each type. Which is most common in children? adults?

3-3.   Poisoning by ingestion is identified as a common form of poisoning, especially in children. Such poisoning is categorized as corrosive or noncorrosive, depending upon the substance ingested. Differentiate the probable causes, clinical manifestations, and first aid measures for the two categories of poisoning by ingestion:

Item	Corrosive ingestion	Noncorrosive ingestion
Causes Clinical manifestations First-aid measures		

3-4.   What signs and symptoms are particularly indicative of aspirin or salicylate poisoning?

3-5.   What first-aid measures might Ms. Simpson have taken prior to taking Jason to the hospital?

3-6.   Describe the pathophysiology associated with salicylate poisoning. What are the major effects on each of the body's organ systems?

3-7.   Complete the following laboratory grid:

Test	Normal range for toddlers	Jason's level	Amount of deviation from normal	Possible causes of alteration

3-8.   Is Jason in mild, moderate, or severe salicylate poisoning? Describe the rationale for your answer.

3-9.   Describe the specific types of electrolyte imbalances that may occur during different stages of salicyclate poisoning.

3-10. Why is an intravenous solution such as 5% dextrose in 0.33% normal saline used? What is the purpose of intravenous infusion after ingestion of toxic substances?

3-11. In some instances, sodium bicarbonate is given intravenously to clients who suffer from salicylate poisoning. What is its indication?

3-12. When is a gastric lavage contraindicated for ingestion poisoning?

3-13. What equipment and solutions should be prepared for a lavage? a lavage for salicylate poisoning? What precautions should be taken to prevent complications and what items should be documented?

Equipment	Precautions (before, during, and after)	Rationale for precaution	Nurses notes

3-14. Describe the procedure for passing a lavage tube on a child. What is the proper way to perform a lavage?

3-15. Why is an early specimen of the gastric lavage saved? How should it be transferred to the lab?

3-16. What are some of the means by which a toddler can be restrained to prevent the IV from being dislodged? What is the rationale and nursing action for each?

Type restraint	Rationale	Nursing actions

3-17. What are some of the nursing techniques that can be instituted to prevent infection at the infusion site?

3-18. What potential support systems are available to Jane Simpson?

DISCUSSION QUESTIONS

D-1. As a professional nurse in the emergency unit, how would you handle an incoming phone call from a distressed parent who suspects that their child has ingested a toxic substance?

D-2. What would be the essential components of the nursing assessment of a toddler who has ingested aspirin?

D-3. Ms. Hartman, R.N., is sitting with Ms. Simpson and David in the emergency room unit. How should she respond to Ms. Simpson's emotional upset and her comment ("What a stupid mother I've been . . . ")? Describe a therapeutic interaction that is directed by the nurse.

D-4.   What are Jason's nursing-care problems, needs, and priorities? What is the rationale for each?

Problems	Priorities	Rationale

PEDIATRIC UNIT

Ms. Simpson and David were able to accompany Jason to the pediatric unit. It was now 7:30 P.M. and David was becoming very fussy. A pediatric nurse's aide stayed with David in the unit's family lounge while Ms. Simpson answered the nurse's last-minute questions and Jason was settled in his room. It was obvious even to his mother that Jason was exhausted. Promising Jason that she would come back in the morning, Jane left his room. It was difficult for her to leave Jason as he cried out, "Mommy."

Recognizing that Ms. Simpson could not stay overnight with her son, the nurse, Ms. Black, gave her the unit phone number and reassured her that she would be notified right away if there was any change. Ms. Black informed Ms. Simpson that Jason would be checked frequently during the night.

The following medical orders, written by Dr. Roberts, arrived with Jason Simpson:

NPO

Maintain IV of 5% D/0.33 NS at 60 ml/hr

Temperature, apical pulse and respirations q 4 h

Intake and output q 4 h until A.M.; call M.D. if output is less than 100 ml/4 hrs.

Check urine pH—call M.D. if less than 5.0 or more than 8.0

Clear liquids in A.M. as tolerated

Serum salicylate, Serum pH, Electrolytes at 6:00 A.M. tomorrow

Ms. Black finished her nursing assessment and recorded her findings. Based on her assessment, a nursing care plan was developed for the client. An open-ended pediatric urine collector was applied so that Jason's urine could be monitored more accurately. Jason slept most of the night. The assessment sheet was used during Jason's hospitalization.

ASSESSMENT SHEET

Time	Vital signs			Intake		Output	Comments
	T	P	R	PO	IV	Urine	
7:30 P.M.	37.3°C	144 thready	36 shallow				IV of 5% D/0.33 NS running c̄ 325 ml left c/o abdominal pain, pallor, diaphoresis, lethargic
11:00 P.M.		128	32 Deeper	—	200	175 pH: 7.8	sleeping, moist to touch, 500 ml of 5% D/0.33 NS added at 1:15 A.M.
3:00 A.M.		112	24	—	250	125 pH: 6.5	skin warm and dry
7:00 A.M.	37.1°C	108	26	—	230	170 pH: 6.0	awake and playing quietly; refused liquids. 500 ml of 5% D/0.33 NS added at 9:30 A.M.
11:00 A.M.		102	24	200	240	diaper × 2; pH: 6.2	

Ms. Simpson arrived on the unit at 10:00 the next morning, anxious to spend time with her son. Jane's neighbor had agreed to take David for a few hours. Ms. Lawson, R.N., was changing Jason's hospital gown and diaper. Ms. Simpson seemed anxious as she commented, "Jason has been toilet trained for almost a month. I just can't imagine why he would wet in his bed!"

Jason was none too subtle in expressing his feelings towards his mother. He lay in his bed and turned his head away from his mother and faced the nurse. Ms. Lawson stated that Jason had slept well throughout the night and that many of his symptoms were gone. Jason had refused his clear liquids earlier in the morning, but Ms. Lawson was hoping that Jason's mother might be able to get him to drink. The nurse asked Jason, "Would you like to sit on Mommy's lap to drink your apple juice?" His arms had been restrained during the night because of the IV and he seemed pleased when one of the arm boards was removed by the nurse. Hesitantly, he allowed his mother closer to him. By noon, he had successfully consumed over 300 cc of various juices with considerable maternal encouragement.

Jason's morning blood work results arrived on the unit at 12:30 P.M.

Serum salicylate: 31 mg %
Serum pH: 7.38

Na: 140 mEq/L

K: 3.9 mEq/L

C1: 100 mEq/L

CO_2: 24 mM/L

Ms. Simpson left the unit after Jason fell asleep for his afternoon nap. She left word with the nursing staff that she would try to return in the early evening—assuming that she could find a baby-sitter to look after David.

Dr. Roberts examined Jason at 1 P.M. The following orders were left:

D/C IV when present bottle infuses

Full fluid diet as tolerated—reg. diet in A.M.

May be discharged in A.M.

When Ms. Simpson returned at 7 P.M., she found Jason contentedly playing with Ms. Black. It was still difficult for her to understand Jason's coolness toward his own mother. Since Jason's IV was almost empty, Ms. Black asked Jane if she would like to stay with Jason while the IV needle was removed or wait in the family lounge. Ms. Simpson decided to stay, declaring, "I'll help in any way I can." While Ms. Simpson restrained Jason in her lap, the nurse was able to quickly discontinue the IV. After a few minutes of crying, Jason's attention had turned to the band-aid, which he proudly displayed.

The next morning, Ms. Simpson came to the unit prepared for Jason's discharge. Prior to the discharge, Ms. Lawson met with Ms. Simpson in the unit conference room. Together, they discussed Jason's ingestion, how it might be prevented in the future, and what additional measures she could take at home in the event that one of her children ingested poisons again. Ms. Simpson was helped to gain some understanding of her expressed feelings of guilt, as well as why the incident occurred. Ms. Lawson also explained that a public health nurse would be visiting her in the near future to see how Jason was doing and to answer any of her questions. (A referral is made by the ER nurse in cases of poisoning.) Shortly afterwards, Jason was discharged from the hospital—a fortunately healthy toddler.

STUDY QUESTIONS

3-19. What factors should be monitored frequently on Jason throughout the night?

3-20. What is the rationale for each of Jason's medical orders? What is the nursing action for each?

Order	Rationale	Nursing action

3-21. Determine the number of drops per minute Jason's IV should run with a microdrip (60 gtt/ml) administration set.

3-22. Compare the laboratory studies for Jason. Analyze the effect of his treatment regime.

Test	Treatment	Effect of treatment

DISCUSSION QUESTIONS

D-5.   What information (history) would Ms. Black need when admitting Jason to the pediatric unit? What physical assessments should she obtain? Why?

D-6.   Compare Jason's fluid intake and output through the night. What conclusions can you make?

D-7.   What are Jason's nursing diagnoses? What are the nursing objectives? What is the rationale of each? How can they be evaluated?

Nursing diagnosis	Nursing objectives	Rationale	Method and frequency of evaluating

D-8. Is it appropriate for the pediatric nurse to allow Ms. Simpson to be present and involved in the discontinuance of the IV infusion? Discuss your reasoning.

CHAPTER STUDY QUESTIONS

1. Under what circumstances of ingestion poisoning should vomiting *not* be induced? Give the rationale.
2. What are the indications for and action of activated charcoal? What instructions would you give a lay person who needed to administer it?
3. Describe the indications for syrup of ipecac. What instructions would you give a lay person who needed to administer it? Why do you suppose that it was not given to Jason in the ER unit?
4. What is the goal of treatment with clients who have ingested noncorrosive toxic substances? Corrosive toxic substances?
5. What is the expected effect of hospitalization on a toddler?
6. What is the rationale for keeping Jason NPO, then proceeding to clear fluids and finally a diet as tolerated. What are the nutritional needs of a toddler? Eating habits? Favorite foods?

CHAPTER DISCUSSION QUESTIONS

1. Identify the effect this hospitalization appears to have had on Jason.
2. Are there other ways that the nursing staff and Ms. Simpson might have facilitated Jason's adjustment to the hospitalization? Describe these.
3. Identify the stresses Ms. Simpson is experiencing. How is she coping with these stresses?
4. How can the professional nurse assist Ms. Simpson with
   a. stress
   b. guilt feelings
   c. Jason's hospitalization
   d. lack of support systems
5. Develop a poison accident prevention program for an audience consisting of parents of young children. What would be your objectives, content, and method of evaluating learning?

POISON PREVENTION

Objectives	Content	Method of evaluating learning

6. What are the reasons a toddler, such as Jason, might ingest aspirin?

SUGGESTED ACTIVITIES

1. Visit a poison control center in your area. How does it function? What does it do for aspirin ingestion?
2. Role play the interaction between a poison control center and a parent(s) while discussing the prevention, recognition, and treatment of poisoning.
3. Visit a local community hospital. What actions do they institute when an aspirin ingestion is brought to the ER? Other forms of poison injection?

BIBLIOGRAPHY

Arena, Jay M. "The Treatment of Poisoning." *Clinical Symposia*, C.I.B.A. 30 (1978).

Bergersen, Betty. *Pharmacology in Nursing*. 13th ed. St. Louis: C. V. Mosby Co., 1976.

Brunner, Lillian Scholtis, and Suddarth, Doris Smith. *The Lippincott Manual of Nursing Practice*. 2d ed. Philadelphia: J. B. Lippincott Co., 1978.

Dreisbach, Robert H. *Handbook of Poisoning*. 6th ed. Los Altos: Lange Medical Publishers, 1969, pp. 217–221.

Garb, Solomon. *Laboratory Tests in Common Use*. 6th ed. New York: Springer Publishing Co., Inc., 1976.

Horoshak, Irene. "What to Do in a Poison Emergency." *RN* 40 (July 1977): 44–50.

Little, Dolores E., and Carnevali, Doris L. *Nursing Care Planning*. 2d ed. Philadelphia: J. B. Lippincott Co., 1976.

Lybanger, Patricia. "Accidental Poisoning in Children—An Ongoing Problem." *Issues in Comprehensive Pediatric Nursing* 1 (May 1977): 30–39.

Malasanos, Lois et al. *Health Assessment.* St. Louis: C. V. Mosby Co., 1978.

Mennear, John H. "The Poisoning Emergency." *American Journal of Nursing* 77 (May 1977): 842–844.

Pascoe, Delmer J., and Grossman, Moses, eds. *Quick Reference to Pediatric Emergencies.* Philadelphia: J. B. Lippincott Co., 1973, pp. 299–302, 307, 315–317.

Petrillo, Madeline, and Sanger, Sirgay. *Emotional Care of Hospitalized Children.* Philadelphia: J. B. Lippincott Co., 1972, pp. 19–33.

Scipien, Gladys M. et al. *Comprehensive Pediatric Nursing.* New York: McGraw-Hill, 1975, pp. 124–38, 238–244, 364–375, 935.

Stroot, Violet R.; Lee, Carla A.; and Schaper, C. Ann. *Fluid and Electrolytes: A Practical Approach.* 2d ed. Philadelphia: F. A. Davis Co., 1977.

Vaughan, Victor, and McKay, James R. *Nelson Textbook of Pediatrics.* 10th ed. Philadelphia: W. B. Saunders Co., 1976, pp. 246, 265–266, 1277, 1660–1664, 1717.

CHAPTER FOUR

Intensive Respiratory Imbalance: Croup

LINDA K. HARRISON

RUTH RAYSOR WEST

OVERVIEW

Tanya Wilson is a three-year-old toddler who lives with her widowed father, Safā Wilson, in a poorly heated apartment. Safā has been unemployed for more than two months. Safā, a recent convert to the Muslim faith, resists financial assistance. When a public health nurse visits the Wilsons, Tanya has a severe upper respiratory infection. Safā is encouraged to take Tanya to the neighborhood hospital. Tanya is diagnosed as having acute laryngotracheobronchitis (LTB) and is admitted to the pediatric unit. An emergency tracheostomy is performed and she receives intensive respiratory care. Play therapy is used by the nursing staff to facilitate Tanya's psychosocial adjustment to her temporary tracheostomy and hospitalization.

CONTENT EMPHASIS

- Stress in a single-parent family
- Airway obstruction—tracheostomy
- Intensive respiratory care
- Play therapy

SETTINGS

- Public health nurse—home visit
- Emergency room
- Pediatric unit

OBJECTIVES

Upon completing this chapter, the student will be able to:

1. Identify a crisis response in a single-parent family.
2. Identify the socioreligious values influencing health priorities for American Muslims.
3. Differentiate the pathophysiology of an upper airway obstruction from a lower airway obstruction.
4. Designate specific intervention modalities to support expected health outcomes for a toddler in acute respiratory distress.
5. Evaluate expected health outcomes for a toddler in acute respiratory distress.
6. Analyze the use of play therapy in helping children to adjust to illness and hospitalization.

DEFINITION OF TERMS

The following terms are used in this care study and should be defined before proceeding:

Acute laryngotracheobronchitis (LTB)
Aid to dependent children (ADC)
Child health clinic
Cool mist tent
Croup
Cyanosis
Diphtheria
Dyspnea
Intercostal retractions
Light reflex
Medicaid
Midclavicular line (MCL)

Muslim
Normal sinus rhythm (NSR)
Point of maximal impulse (PMI)
Rule out (R/O)
Supplemental security income (SSI)
Stridor
Substernal retractions
Suctioning
Suprasternal retractions
Tracheostomy
Tracheotomy

ASSESSMENT

Ms. Smith, R.N., is a public health nurse with the City Health Department. A phone call to the agency was referred directly to her one morning. The caller identified herself as Sister Ann, a fellow Muslim and next door neighbor of Safā Wilson and his daughter, Tanya. She stated that she was quite concerned about the three-year-old girl, Tanya, who seemed to be sick a lot lately. Briefly, Sister Ann related the family's situation and requested that someone visit the Wilson home.

Ms. Smith was able to rearrange her schedule that afternoon to accommodate a home visit to the Wilsons. She gathered the following data during her visit:

November 10th:

Safā Wilson, age 23, and his three-year-old daughter Tanya reside in an intermittently heated, one-bedroom apartment on the fourth floor of a low-income housing unit in Newark. The apartment is sparsely furnished, clean and uncluttered.

Mr. Wilson relocated from South Carolina six months ago when he was laid off from his factory job. His wife, Patricia, had died shortly after Tanya's delivery.

Safā was able to obtain a construction job during the summer months, but then he was laid off. He has been unemployed for the last two and one-half months. His financial situation is characterized by no regular income and refusal to accept welfare since his decision to practice the Muslim faith. His rent payments are delinquent by two months.

CURRENT PROBLEM: Safā Wilson admits that Tanya has been ill for the past week with a bad cold; her coughing worsened two days ago and her appetite has been poor since then.

PHYSICAL ASSESSMENT: Appears lethargic and of small size for stated age. Breathing is labored. Has frequent harsh cough.

T = 39° C rectally,   P = 114,   R = 36
Weight: 13.6 kg (30 lbs) estimated by the nurse
Skin: ashen appearance with cyanotic nailbeds.
HEENT: moderate quantity of soft cerumen in ears, good light reflex; tonsils appear enlarged; nonglossy oral mucosa and dry lips; moderate, milkish-colored nasal mucous drainage; frequent bark-like cough noted.
Chest: suprasternal and substernal retractions noted upon inspiration. Breath sounds are diminished in lower lobes of both lungs.
Heart: NSR; PMI at 4th intercostal space, 1 cm left of MCL; 114/min.
Abdomen: soft, no masses or tenderness noted.

Having completed this portion of her assessment, Ms. Smith was quite aware of the urgency of Tanya's health situation. Briefly, she explained to Mr. Wilson that Tanya needed medical care for her condition right away. Safā seemed hesitant to take the nurse's advice, yet he was greatly concerned for his daughter. It took strong encouragement and additional explanation before Safā consented to have Tanya seen in the Oraton Hospital emergency room.

Ms. Smith phoned the hospital to alert them of Tanya Wilson's condition and her pending arrival.

STUDY QUESTIONS

4-1. What are the religious beliefs of Muslims?

4-2. Which of these beliefs and/or religious practices are followed by Mr. Wilson?

4-3. Complete the following nutrition grid on a three-year-old.

Food group	Three-year-old	Three-year-old Muslim	Religious rationale for alternation in diet
Dairy products (milk, cheese and ice cream)			
Meats			
Eggs			
Vegetables and fruits			
Breads and cereals			
Butter or margarine			
Calories			

4-4. Complete a growth and development information card on a three-year-old female.

4-5. How is cyanosis assessed in the black client?

4-6. Compare the pathophysiology of upper and lower airway obstruction.

4-7. How do you assess the client who is diagnosed with an upper respiratory obstruction, for example, croup?

4-8. What are the signs associated with mild, moderate, and severe substernal/intercostal retractions?

4-9. Identify the nursing problems in caring for a client with upper respiratory obstruction. What are the nursing goals for each?

Problem	Nursing goals	Method and frequency of evaluating

DISCUSSION QUESTIONS

D-1. Identify the assistance programs that may be available to aid Mr. Wilson and Tanya.

D-2. What home remedies might have been attempted to ease Tanya's respirations?

D-3. What further assistance might the public health nurse offer Mr. Wilson?

D-4. What possible implications could Mr. Wilson's religious beliefs have on his refusal of welfare assistance? How might his religious community be mobilized to assist his family?

ACUTE CARE

The pediatric resident diagnosed Tanya's condition as acute laryngotracheobronchitis and R/O diphtheria. She was then admitted to the pediatric unit at 12 noon with the following orders:

Aspirin 150 mg rectally or orally for temp > 38.3° C q 4 h prn

Intake and output

Clear fluids as tolerated

Maintain 30% humidified O_2 concentration in cool mist tent

Chloral hydrate suppository 150 mg at 6 P.M. if indicated

Keep emergency tracheotomy set at bedside

Electrolytes, CBC, blood gases stat

Urinalysis

Throat culture stat

Mr. Wilson appeared anxious during the afternoon and evening, pacing up and down the corridors and making frequent trips to the telephone. At 4 P.M., Ms. Johnson, R.N., arrived on duty and noted Tanya resting in the mist tent.

The little girl was breathing with mild substernal retractions, had no cyanosis, and her vital signs were T: 38°C, P: 90, R: 28. Ms. Johnson explained the need for the use of the mist tent to Mr. Wilson. She tried to reassure him that everything possible was being done for Tanya to help her. Mr. Wilson's anxiety was extremely high. Ms. Johnson had difficulty assessing how much he was able to understand. His verbalizations were filled with self-recriminations and doubts. "This is my fault," Mr. Wilson told Ms. Johnson. "If only I had gotten help. I should have left her home in South Carolina with my mother. I can't buy her proper clothes. The apartment is cold. She's just too young to take it. Is my baby going to make it?" Ms. Johnson assured him that Tanya's condition was stable and she would be checking on his daughter frequently—especially during the night.

Later, when Safā's anxiety was lowered, he related the following thoughts to Ms. Johnson, "I don't want handouts from the city. I'm a man, I gotta make my own way!" She related to him that she understood how he felt, and referred him to the social worker to discuss approaches to his financial problems.

Ms. Johnson observed Tanya every 15–20 minutes and explained to Mr. Wilson that she was looking for any signs that showed Tanya was having more trouble breathing or was growing uncomfortable. Mr. Wilson settled down to watch Tanya; he refused to leave even to get something to eat.

At seven o'clock, Sister Ann arrived, having brought a sandwich for Mr. Wilson. Tanya, recognizing her, reached out to her as though asking to be held. Ms. Johnson indicated to Ann that Tanya needed to remain in the tent. Sister Ann was cooperative as she briefly bowed her head in prayer to Allah. After gratefully accepting the sandwich from Sister Ann, Mr. Wilson left the unit explaining that he wanted to go to the mosque and pray to Allah to make Tanya well. When he returned, Sister Ann left the unit promising to return in the morning.

Diphtheria was ruled out after the buccal smear was examined. The following are the results of Tanya's laboratory studies obtained upon admission:

BLOOD GASES (ARTERIAL)
P_aO_2: 70 mm Hg
P_aCO_2: 65 mm Hg
pH: 7.25

ELECTROLYTES
Na: 138 mEq/L
K: 3.5 mEq/L
Cl: 90 mEq/L
CO_2: 27 mM/L
Ca: 8.8 mEq/L

CBC
Hgb: 9 g
Hct: 38%
RBC: 4.4×10^6 mm^3
WBC: 12,000 mm^3

URINALYSIS
Color: dark amber
Sp. gr.: 1.034
pH: 7.25
Glucose: negative
Acetone: negative
Protein: 1+
RBC: negative
WBC: negative

STUDY QUESTIONS

4-10. What is the pathophysiology underlying Tanya's respiratory difficulty?

4-11. Compare the signs and symptoms of LTB with diphtheria.

4-12. Besides diphtheria, what are some other possible diagnoses?

4-13. What organisms are frequently implicated as the cause of LTB?

4-14. Complete the following laboratory grid:

Test	Normal range for 3-year-old	Tanya's values	Amount of deviation from normal	Possible cause for deviation
Hgb				
Hct				
WBC				
RBC				
Na				
Cl				
CO_2				
CA				
p_aO				
p_aCO_2				
pH				

4-15. What is the rationale for each of the medical orders?

Medical order	Rationale

4-16. Complete a drug information card on the following medications: chloral hydrate, and aspirin.

4-17. Why were antibiotics not ordered for Tanya?

4-18. If Tanya's temperature continues to rise, what should the nurse be alert for?

4-19. Why is it important to encourage Tanya to drink large amounts of fluids?

4-20. If Tanya developed unequal chest retractions, what would this suggest? Explain.

4-21. Why was it imperative that Tanya be constantly observed? Explain.

4-22. Based upon the nursing problem list in Question 4-9, what are the nursing interventions for Tanya? What is the rationale for each?

Nursing interventions	Rationale

DISCUSSION QUESTIONS

D-5. What can the nurse do to decrease Tanya's apprehension? To further decrease Mr. Wilson's anxiety?

D-6. Why was Mr. Wilson encouraged to room-in with Tanya?

EMERGENCY TRACHEOSTOMY

At 10 P.M. Mr. Wilson observed that Tanya had become restless and was sitting up in her mist tent. When Ms. Johnson answered Mr. Wilson's call for help, she found Tanya gasping for breath with both substernal and suprasternal retractions. Vital signs were T: 39°C, P: 144, R: 38. Her color appeared ashen gray. Ms. Johnson called Dr. Rothchild stat. The decision was soon made to take Tanya to the OR for an emergency tracheostomy. When Mr. Wilson was informed of this he became extremely agitated, blaming himself again for causing Tanya's condition. It was some time before Ms. Johnson was able to calm him so that Dr. Rothchild could obtain the necessary written permission for the procedure.

Tanya returned from the operating room at 11:30 P.M. with a tracheostomy tube in place. Her breathing was calmer and no cyanosis was noted. Her orders were as follows:

Vital signs q ½ h until stable, then q 1 h × 2, then q 4 h

250 cc 5% D/0.33 NaC1 to run at 35 ml/hr

Check coughing and swallowing reflex q 1 h

Place in croupette with 50% humidified O_2 concentration

Full fluids in A.M. as tolerated

Suction prn

Mr. Wilson sat quietly at Tanya's bedside fingering his worry beads. Ms. Johnson had already explained the reason for the tracheostomy to him, but she took the opportunity to do so again during her rounds.

At 11:45 P.M., Ms. Price, R.N., attempted to suction Tanya's tracheostomy, whereupon Tanya kicked and turned her head away. Mr. Wilson screamed, "Be good or the nurse can't help you; now stop it, Tanya!" Ms. Price talked quietly to Tanya, allowing her to play with the suction tubing. Eventually she was able to suction Tanya's tracheostomy with minimal resistance. Later that evening, while Mr. Wilson walked in the hallway outside Tanya's room, Ms. Price discussed his concern regarding Tanya's behavior and her initial reaction to suctioning.

STUDY QUESTIONS

4-23. Why did Tanya become restless and gasp for breath?

4-24. What caused her substernal and suprasternal retractions?

4-25. What are other symptoms of laryngeal obstruction?

4-26. What is the purpose of performing a tracheostomy on a client such as Tanya? What equipment would be assembled should an emergency tracheostomy be indicated at the client's bedside?

4-27. What is the difference between a cuffed and noncuffed tracheostomy tube? What precautions should be instituted if a cuffed tracheostomy tube were used? Why?

4-28. What is a child's physiological and psychological response to a tracheostomy and what are the nursing actions required for each? What are the ongoing nursing objectives and the related interventions in caring for a child with tracheostomy?

TRACHEOSTOMY

Phase of care	Child's response (psychological and physiological)	Scientific rationale for child's response	Nursing objectives and actions	Method and frequency of evaluating nursing actions
Pre-procedure				
While tracheostomy is being performed				
Daily care				
Care following removal of tracheostomy tube				

4-29. What are the indications for suctioning? What risks are associated?

4-30. Describe the procedure for suctioning.

4-31. In what position is Tanya apt to be most comfortable?

DISCUSSION QUESTIONS

D-7.   What should Mr. Wilson be told about the tracheostomy? What might be done to help him better understand and cope with his daughter's condition?

D-8.   What items should be discussed with Mr. Wilson before seeing Tanya after surgery? Outline the items in the order in which they should be presented. What would you explain about each?

Item	Explanation

D-9.   Discuss possible ways of helping Tanya cope with the tracheostomy and frequent suctioning. How might play therapy techniques be used to help Tanya?

D-10. What should be assessed about Tanya's tracheostomy site? Why?

RECOVERY

Tanya passed the night without further incident. The following morning, Ms. Sensenback, R.N., noted improvement in Tanya's vital signs (T: 38° C, P: 100, R: 30). Tanya followed Ms. Sensenback with her eyes as the nurse recorded Tanya's vital signs and held her hands briefly while suctioning the tracheostomy. She then tested Tanya's gag and swallow reflex. Since they were both present she fed Tanya a dish of green Kosher jello.

By midmorning Mr. Wilson had decided to go down to the hospital cafeteria. He told Tanya, "I'll be right back, you be good now."

Tanya's condition continued to improve over the next few days. Her respirations decreased to 26 per minute and her cough and stridor disappeared. Her temperature on the fifth day was 37.7°C rectally, and she was tolerating a soft diet and drinking adequate quantities of fluids. It was decided to partially occlude her tracheostomy every other hour as tolerated. By the sixth day

Tanya was tolerating continuous closure of the tube. Mr. Wilson had begun to relax. He trusted the nurses enough to leave the ward for longer periods of time. He had even gone to apply for the Job Corps, following up on a referral made by Ms. R. James, M.S.W., of the hospital Social Service department.

On the seventh day Tanya was permitted to spend some time in the playroom with the other children. Ms. P. Smith, a nursing student from Patterson University, accompanied Tanya during her first trip to the playroom.

When Tanya arrived in the playroom, her eyes lit up as she looked around at all the toys. The room was well-equipped. It had been supplied through donations from civic organizations. Ms. Smith held Tanya's hand and they were drawn toward the hospital corner where Ms. Smith had earlier set up a miniature croup tent and placed suction catheters nearby. Tanya chose one of the female dolls and one of the catheters. She placed the doll and catheter inside the croup tent and began frantically poking the doll in the front of its neck, as tears rolled down her cheeks.

Having noted Tanya's behavior with the doll, Ms. Smith squatted down beside her. After a pause, she asked Tanya what she was doing. Tanya replied, "Alice hurts, she is crying. She is calling Daddy." Ms. Smith asked, "Were you hurt like Alice?" Tanya nodded her head affirmatively. Ms. Smith asked, "How can Daddy make it better?" Whereupon Tanya took the doll and hugged it to her chest. Ms. Smith responded by hugging both Alice and Tanya.

STUDY QUESTIONS

4-32. Why was Tanya's gag reflex and swallow reflex tested before encouraging her to eat? How are these reflexes tested?

4-33. Why was green Kosher jello fed to Tanya as her first feeding?

4-34. What is the importance of play as a component of care to children in hospitals? Explain.

4-35. What play activities would be appropriate for Tanya? Explain.

DISCUSSION QUESTIONS

D-11. How is a client weaned off a tracheostomy tube? What precautions should be taken?

D-12. What are the nursing objectives during Tanya's recovery phase? What are the nursing actions and rationale for each? How would you evaluate the effectiveness of care?

Objective	Nursing action	Rationale	Method and frequency of evaluating effectiveness

D-13. What nursing interventions could be implemented to help Safā and Tanya cope with hospitalization and separation anxieties?

DISCHARGE

Tanya's tracheostomy tube was removed on the eighth day and she continued to improve. She was discharged fourteen days after her admission. The pediatric nursing staff sent a summary of Tanya's hospitalization to Ms. Smith, the public health nurse. A request was made for nursing follow-up visits to assess Tanya's recovery and Mr. Wilson's adjustment as a single parent. Ms. James, the social worker, had been notified prior to the discharge and had visited Tanya in the hospital. She also visited Sister Ann and learned that Mr. Wilson's heating problem had been solved. Ms. James had been able to convince and assist Mr. Wilson to apply for financial assistance. In addition, the Job Corps had accepted his application and he expected to begin training as an electrician apprentice the following week.

CHAPTER DISCUSSION QUESTIONS

1. What is the main psychosocial task of the average three-year-old? Explain. What are the potential effects of hospitalization on this task for Tanya?

2. What are the potential residual effects of LTB on Tanya? Explain.

3. What are the motor and sensory capabilities of an average three-year-old? Which ones might be most affected by hospitalization?

4. What forms of humidification could Mr. Wilson provide for Tanya at home? How would you teach Mr. Wilson home methods of humidification in case Tanya has another episode of respiratory difficulty?

5. What are the problems encountered by a single parent? How can the public health nurse assist a single parent?

6. Tanya's stay in the hospital has provided some opportunities for anticipatory guidance. What areas could be discussed with Mr. Wilson? What anticipatory

guidance might better be offered by the public health nurse following Tanya's discharge?

7. As the hospital nurse completing the hospital summary to be sent to the public health nurse, what would you include in your report?

8. As the public health nurse making the home visit to Safā and Tanya Wilson, design your care plan. How many visits might be necessary to carry out the complete plan? How would you determine the frequency of home visits needed? When would you terminate public health nursing services to this family?

9. What services and support mechanisms are available to the members of the Muslim Community?

SUGGESTED ACTIVITIES

1. Manipulate a mist tent and a tracheostomy tube. Observe the functioning of both on a pediatric unit.

2. Develop a teaching plan for the Wilsons incorporating their strengths and weaknesses.

3. Interview a Muslim family to determine the effect of their religion on their health.

4. Interview the parents of a child who developed croup. What were their fears? How did they feel about the hospitalization and subsequent separation from their child?

5. Visit your local financial assistance agency (welfare). Identify the kinds of programs available. Observe the interaction between the agency's employees and the potential clients. What questions are asked and what are the clients' nonverbal responses?

6. Implement the nursing process while caring for a young child with respiratory distress.

BIBLIOGRAPHY

Ablstrom, Sydney E. *A Religious History of the American People.* New Haven: Yale University Press, 1972.

Benson, Evelyn, and McDevitt, Joan. *Community Health and Nursing Practice.* Englewood Cliffs, N.J.: Prentice-Hall, 1975.

Bergersen, Betty. *Pharmacology in Nursing.* 13th ed. St. Louis: C. V. Mosby Co., 1976.

Chadwick, Barbara J.; Pflederer, Diane; and Ray, Mary Alice. "Maintaining the Hospitalized Child's Home Ties." *American Journal of Nursing* 78 (August 1978): 1360–1362.

Coles, H. M. T. "Croup." *Nursing Times* 73 (October 20, 1977): 1634–1635.

Feinbloom, Richard. *Child Health Encyclopedia.* Boston: Delacorte Press, 1975.

Garb, Solomon. *Laboratory Tests in Common Use.* 6th ed. New York: Springer Publishing Co., Inc., 1976.

Geis, D., and Lambertz, C. "Acute Respiratory Infections in Young Children." *American Journal of Nursing* 68 (February 1968).

Horowitz, June A., and Perdue, Bobbie J. "Single-Parent Families." *Nursing Clinics of North America* 12 (September 1977): 503–511.

Isler, Charlotte. "This Technique May Make Tracheostomy Unnecessary." *RN Magazine* 40 (January 1977): 32–33.

Johnston, Dorothy. "Diphtheria." In *Essentials of Communicable Disease.* St. Louis: C. V. Mosby Co., 1969.

Juenker, Donna. "Child's Perception of His Illness." In *Nursing Care of the Child with Long Term Illness.* 2d ed. Edited by Shirley Steele. New York: Appleton-Century-Crofts, 1977.

_____. "Play as a Tool for the Nurse." In *Nursing Care of the Child with Long Term Illness.* 2d ed. Edited by Shirley Steele. New York: Appleton-Century-Crofts, 1977.

Kee, Joyce and Gregory, Ann P. "The ABC's and MEQ's of Fluid Balance in Children." *Nursing '74* 4 (June 1974): 28–36.

Lincoln, Eric. *The Black Muslims in America.* 2d ed. Boston: Beacon Press, 1973.

Little, Dolores E., and Carnevali, Doris L. *Nursing Care Planning.* 2d ed. Philadelphia: J. B. Lippincott Co., 1976.

Luciano, Kathy, and Shumsky, Claire J. "Pediatric Procedures." *Nursing '75* 5 (January 1975), 45–52.

Malasanos, Lois et al. "Assessment of the Pediatric Client." In *Health Assessment.* St. Louis: C. V. Mosby Co., 1978.

_____. "Developmental Assessment." In *Health Assessment.* St. Louis: C. V. Mosby Co., 1978.

McRae, Maureen. "An Approach to the Single Parent Dilemma." *American Journal of Maternal Child Nursing* 2 (May/June 1977), 164–167.

Paxton, Phyllis; Ramirez, Martina C.; and Walloch, Esther C. "Nursing Assessment and Intervention." In *Providing Safe Nursing Care for Ethnic People of Color,* edited by Marie F. Branch and Phyllis P. Paxton. New York: Appleton-Century-Crofts, 1976.

Pendagast, Eileen G., and Sherman, Charles O. "A Guide to the Genogram Family Systems Training." *The Family* 5 (1978): 3–14.

Petrillo, Madeline, and Sanger, Sirgay. *Emotional Care of Hospitalized Children.* Philadelphia: J. B. Lippincott Co., 1972.

Price, Joseph, and Braden, Carrie. "The Reality in Home Visits." *American Journal of Nursing* 78 (September 1978): 1536–1538.

Pumphrey, John B. "Recognizing Your Patients' Spiritual Needs." *Nursing '77* 7 (December 1977): 64–70.

Reeves, Kathryn R. "Acute Epiglottitis: Pediatric Emergency." *American Journal of Nursing* 71 (August 1971): 1539–1541.

Roach, Lora B. "Assessment: Color Changes in Dark Skin." *Nursing '77* 7 (January 1977): 48–51.

Robinson, Corinne, and Lawler, Marilyn R. *Normal and Therapeutic Nutrition.* 15th ed. New York: Macmillan, 1977.

Scipien, Gladys M. et al. *Comprehensive Pediatric Nursing.* New York: McGraw-Hill, 1975, pp. 184–283; 498–506; 515–521; 525–528; 534–535.

Shufer, Shirley. "Teaching Via the Play-Discussion Group." *American Journal of Nursing* 77 (December 1977): 1960–1962.

Smart, Mollie, and Smart, Russell C. *Children.* 3d ed. New York: Macmillan, 1977.

Smith, Elaine C., "Are You Really Communicating." *American Journal of Nursing* 77 (December 1977): 1966–1968.

Smith, Linda Fischer. "An Experiment With Play Therapy." *American Journal of Nursing* 77 (December 1977): 1963–1965.

Spitz, Phyllis, and Sweetwood, Hannelore. "Kids in Crisis—Part I." *Nursing '78* 8 (March 1978): 70–79.

———. "Kids in Crisis—Part II." *Nursing '78* 8 (April 1978): 27–30.

Stroot, Violet R.; Lee, Carla A.; and Schaper, C. Ann. *Fluid and Electrolytes: A Practical Approach.* 2d ed. Philadelphia: F. A. Davis Co., 1977.

Vaughan, Victor, and McKay, James. *Nelson Textbook of Pediatrics.* 10th ed. Philadelphia: W. B. Saunders Co., 1976.

CHAPTER FIVE

Emergency Room Triage: Aftermath of a Fire (Burns)

CYNTHIA DEGAZON

OVERVIEW

A fire in an urban apartment building results in four victims who experience either smoke inhalation, burns, and/or a fracture. The community hospital emergency room staff successfully manages the "mini-disaster" with the assistance of other community and hospital personnel. Emphasis is placed on the six-year-old victim, Carol Jenkins, who sustains extensive burns. After emergency room treatment to stabilize her condition, Carol is transferred to a regional burn center.

CONTENT EMPHASIS

- Triage techniques
- Professional support systems
- Administrative/legal ramifications of emergency care
- Stabilization and transfer of a burn victim

SETTINGS

- Burning apartment building
- Hospital emergency room/trauma center

OBJECTIVES

Upon completing this chapter the student will be able to:

1. Describe the triage management of disaster victims.
2. Evaluate the extent and severity of burns.
3. Create an initial nursing care plan for burn victims based upon scientific rationale.
4. Analyze methods of mobilizing professional support systems for the emergency room during a mini-disaster.

DEFINITION OF TERMS

The following terms are used in this case study and should be defined before proceeding:

Cardiac monitor
Disaster plan
Emergency medical technician
   (EMT)
Endotracheal tube
First-degree burns
Full thickness burn
Indwelling Foley catheter
Levine tube
Low Gomco suction

Occlusive dressings
Papillary edema
Rales
Regional burn center
Rescue squad
Respiratory distress
Rhonchi
Second-degree burns
Third-degree burns

COMMUNITY ASSESSMENT

Cedars is a 520-bed hospital located in a formerly suburban setting in the town of Providence. This community was once a town of great affluence and wealth, but in the last decade it has changed to one of impoverishment. Many of the old wooden mansions have been converted into two- and three-family dwellings. The subsequent maintenance and upkeep of these structures have been greatly neglected. The population is comprised of 40% black, 30% hispanic, and 30% white.

Cedars was once a small community hospital. It has had to expand its service facilities and physical plant constantly. It is the only hospital for a community of approximately 80,000 people. The emergency room (ER) statistics report an average of 3,500 visits per month. Approximately 45 percent of these visits are classified as nonemergency.

D-1. What ER patient diagnoses would you classify as "nonemergency?" What would you classify as "emergency?"

D-2. How might a community be informed of the purpose of an ER? Are there acceptable methods of discouraging misuse of ER services? Explain.

D-3. What factors influence how a community uses its ER services?

AN EMERGENCY ROOM'S RESPONSE TO A MINI-DISASTER

It was 9 A.M. on a Saturday morning, Sheila Len, R.N., charge nurse, was standing at the nurses' station in the emergency room talking with her co-worker, Karen Burke, R.N. Karen was commenting on how slow things were in the ER. Cedars Hospital had seen one patient in its emergency room since 7 A.M., when these nurses had started their tour of duty. Sheila declared that it was always hectic with acutely ill patients when she was the weekend charge nurse. Karen suggested to Sheila that they take their coffee break now while the emergency room was still experiencing a lull. Sheila agreed to accompany her to the coffee shop. At that moment, the yellow phone, which was connected to the local precinct, rang. Sheila answered it. The police dispatcher informed her that a three-alarm fire had broken out in a multiple-family dwelling and that the victims were going to be brought to the Cedars Hospital. Sheila suggested sending the hospital's emergency team to the scene, but was told that the rescue squads were already there and would be arriving at the hospital in a few minutes. The number of victims was unknown.

Plans for coffee breaks were cancelled. Sheila promptly called an emergency staff conference (five registered nurses, two attending physicians, one LPN, and one clerk). They were told of the fire and that victims would begin to arrive momentarily. The staff was directed by Sheila to operate under disaster plan protocol. Assignments were made to reflect the anticipated situation and additional appropriate supplies were obtained.

Within five minutes after the initial dispatcher call, an emergency medical technician from the Providence Rescue Squad radioed that he was en route to the Cedars hospital with two victims. He gave the following information to the charge nurse while Jim Hanson, M.D., the ER staff physician, listened.

... black female, name unknown, about six-years-old, in respiratory distress, with burns of varying severity over arms, legs, chest, and hands. She was pulled from the collapsing building by firemen. Her pulse is 120, weak and thready. Respirations are 44 and shallow. She's receiving O_2 by mask.

The second victim is identified as Tom Adams, thirty-two-year-old black male, also in respiratory distress. He has first- and second-degree burns on his face. His vi are BP: 160/90, P: 124, thready, R: 28. He is also receiving O_2 by mask. He is complaining of severe pain in his hands, legs, and feet. He jumped from a second story window. Anticipated arrival time is five minutes.

A second rescue squad was also reported en route to the hospital with two victims. The driver of that emergency vehicle related the following information about his injured passengers:

Hilda Brown, twenty-five-year-old Caucasian female . . . complains of severe pain with inspiration. Vital signs are BP: 140/85, P: 92, R: 30; no other visible signs of injury.

Melissa Simpson, twenty-six-year-old Caucasian female. Admission vital signs are BP: 124/80, P: 80, R: 22 . . . also complaining of chest pain upon inspiration . . . Arrival time is anticipated at ten minutes from now . . .

An additional pediatrician, an anesthesiologist, and a respiratory therapist were requested for the ER from other parts of the hospital to assist with the victims.

As the first victims arrived at the emergency room entrance, Sheila identified the burned child and instructed that she be taken to Room A, which had been prepared to receive her. The child was covered with blankets with only her face exposed. She was later identified as Carole Jenkins. Her voice could be heard throughout most of the ER hallway as she moaned and called out, "Mommy, Mommy." Dr. Hanson was assisted by the pediatrician and by Karen Burke, R.N., in the evaluation and treatment of the patient.

Sheila made a brief assessment of Tom Adams, the other victim brought in by the same vehicle; she noted a mild respiratory distress, deep abrasions on both hands, and a possible fracture of the right leg. He was taken to Room C, the orthopedic room. Attending physician, Michael Mahon, M.D., evaluated this victim and ordered a Phisohex soak with cool water and X-rays of the right leg and foot, spine, and chest. While waiting for the results, Sheila soaked Tom's abrasions and cleansed the burned areas. Tom was later transferred to the Orthopedic Unit.

When Sheila asked the EMT from the squad vehicle if he could offer any helpful information, he informed her that the fire had probably started in Carole's mother's apartment while the mother was out of the building. It was believed that Carole was making breakfast and may have been attempting to light the stove when it caught on fire. A neighbor heard an explosion and saw the smoke and called the fire department; but the flames had spread quickly through the old wooden structure.

Five minutes later, the other two victims arrived. It was noted that Hilda Brown was drowsy and listless as she complained of being dizzy, having a headache and pain with inspiration. She was placed in Bed 2 in Room D, the six-bed unit. Hilda was placed on a cardiac monitor, and had blood drawn for electrolytes and enzymes stat. An EKG and chest X-ray were performed. The decision was later made to transfer Hilda to the cardiac unit because her monitor showed premature ventricular contractions.

Melissa Simpson was placed in Bed 3, next to Hilda Brown. Sheila Allen, R.N., briefly assessed that this victim was not in any acute distress nor did she have any visible signs of injury. When questioned, Melissa denied having any physical complaints except for an occasional discomfort with deep respirations. Her respirations were generally unlabored at 24 breaths per minute. Melissa told the nurse that she was Hilda's roommate at the apartment. One nurse, Anne White, R.N., was assigned to Room D—Beds 2 and 3. Melissa was discharged after the result of her chest X-ray was obtained.

As Sheila scanned the emergency room situation, she noted that Karen Burke, R.N., in Room A appeared extremely busy. To provide her with some assistance, Sheila assigned Patricia Murphy, L.P.N., to work with Karen.

Six additional walk-in patients were also being treated in the emergency room including one for a deep laceration in the hand who was in Room B, and an eighteen-month-old child who had a reportedly high fever with vomiting was in Room D, Bed 6. Each of these patients required a registered nurse.

Because of the volume of medical orders being written and the overwhelming paperwork that was resulting, Sheila phoned the nursing office and requested that an additional trained clerk be sent to the ER. She was informed that a clerk could not be sent immediately; but that they would do their best to send someone as soon as possible. In the meantime, Sheila helped out the regular ER clerk by prioritizing the orders to be completed "stat" and those which could wait for a short while. This action expedited patient care.

STUDY QUESTIONS

5-1. What is a disaster plan (protocol)? Who is involved in formating it? What should be included?

5-2. What is an emergency medical technician? What is their educational preparation? What are they prepared to do?

5-3. Triage requires prompt, accurate clinical judgment. What are the four classifications of treatment? Give examples of each. Who is qualified to do triage?

5-4. Identify the principles of emergency management that are applicable to any injured or disaster victim.

5-5. Develop an emergency room nursing protocol for each of the following: burns, respiratory distress related to smoke inhalation, chest pain, fracture.

5-6. What are the legal implications of implementing verbal orders? What is the appropriate way to document verbal orders?

5-7. What are the responsibilities of an ER charge nurse? What factors must be evaluated when nursing staff assignments are made?

5-8. What additional supplies should be obtained when preparing for victims of a fire? Which department supplies these items?

Items	Department

DISCUSSION QUESTIONS

D-4. What are the pressures related to the role of the charge nurse? How well do you think that Sheila Len, R.N., carries out that role in this case study?

D-5. Discuss the emotional impact upon hospital personnel who work with emergency-room patients on a regular basis. What are some of the coping mechanisms used by the personnel, especially during a time of crisis (disaster)?

D-6. What other health professionals might be called upon to assist in an ER during a disaster?

D-7. Would you make any changes in Sheila's staff assignment for the disaster? Explain. Ideally, what personnel should be available for this situation?

D-8. Discuss the emergency room management and the impact of the disaster as perceived by Sheila Len.

ASSESSMENT AND TREATMENT OF BURNS

All personnel in Room A were attired in masks, caps, gowns, and gloves. Shortly after the victim, Carole, was transported to the room, the anesthesiologist and pediatrician arrived. In the meantime, Carole's clothing was removed and an assessment continued in a systematic manner, recognizing and treating priorities.

Karen assessed Carole's burns to be: third-degree over the chest and the hands; second-degree over the arms, some areas of the face, including the ears, and first-degree over other areas of the face and arms. Despite the 50% humidified oxygen being given her by mask, Carole's respirations were 40 per minute and labored. Her lips were becoming increasingly cyanotic. "Let's get an ET tube in right away," the anesthesiologist declared. While he proceeded with this, the pediatrician performed an intravenous cut-down procedure in the saphenous vein. Karen assessed the vital signs and prepared the IV solution and medications for administration. Pat Murphy, L.P.N., assisted the physician with positioning the patient and easing Carole's anxiety. Within a twenty-minute period an endotracheal (ET) tube was in place, the IV was initiated, and an in-dwelling Foley catheter was inserted. Humidified oxygen (40%) was continued. A verbal order for "5 mg Morphine sulfate IV" was given. The medication was administered IV by the anesthesiologist. Karen Burke, R.N., carefully monitored for any changes in the patient's conditon.

All data was recorded on a "Burn Summary Sheet." The following medical orders were given verbally and later signed by the pediatrician.

ET tube stat c̄ 40% humidified O_2

IV cutdown in saphenous vein. Hang 1,000 ml Lactated Ringers. Administer 4 ml/kg/24 hr with ½ total in first 8 hr, ¼ in second 8 hr, and ¼ in third 8 hr (client's approximate weight: 22 kg).

In-dwelling Foley catheter

VS q 15 mins, temp q 1 h

Morphine sulfate 5 mg slow IV push stat

Blood specimens for type and cross-match, hemoglobin, hematocrit, electrolytes, prothrombin time, blood gases, and BUN stat

Urinalysis

NPO

Strict I & O, check urine output q 1 h

Urine sp. gr. q 1 h

Levine tube to low Gomco suction.

Tetanus toxoid 0.5 cc IM now

Comprehensive assessment of Carole's burns was then made by the physicians.

Dr. Hanson asked Sheila to make arrangements with the regional burn center for a patient transfer. During this activity, Sheila heard a female voice approaching the ER nurse's station. "I'm Carole Jenkin's mother. Where's my baby? Oh, please let me see her," the woman stated loudly.

Melissa Simpson recognized Ms. Jenkin's voice in the hallway. Without a moment's hesitation, she bolted out of bed and ran into the hallway yelling, "If you would stay home and take care of that kid of yours this wouldn't have happened. We could have been killed you know!" Anne White, R.N., came out from behind Bed 2's curtains. She was gentle but firm with Melissa as she led the patient back to her bed. Ms. Jenkins was quite upset by this incident. Sheila escorted her to a nearby conference room and she explained, "Yes, your daughter is here. The staff is doing everything possible to make her comfortable. If you'll wait here, I'll have one of the doctors who's caring for Carole speak with you. He can tell you more specifically about Carole's condition." Within a few minutes, Dr. Hanson was able to come to the conference room. Ms. Jenkins kept insisting that she wanted to see her daughter. Sheila tried to prepare her before allowing her to enter her daughter's room. Dr. Hanson and Ms. Jenkins donned gowns, gloves, caps, and masks before entering Room A. Carole's eyes immediately focused upon her mother as she entered the room. As she stared at Carole's body, Ms. Jenkins blurted out, "Oh my poor baby. . . . It's all my fault. How could I have let this happen to you?" Recognizing that Ms. Jenkins was visibly shaken, Karen stayed by her side. After a few minutes, Carole's mother was encouraged to wait outside the room. A hospital social worker soon arrived who would stay with Ms. Jenkins.

The following lab results were phoned to the nursing station within the hour:

Hemoglobin: 11.8 g/100ml
Hematocrit: 45 mg%
Prothrombin time:
—control, 13 seconds
—patient, 15 seconds
BUN: 18 mg/100 ml
Total protein: 6.9 g/100 ml

p_aO_2: 80 mmHg
p_aCO_2: 32 mmHg
pH: 7.31
BE: −2.0

Na: 126 mEq/L
K: 6 mEq/L
Cl: 92 mEq/L
CO_2: 34 mM/L

Urinalysis:
pH: 6.0
Sp. gr.: 1.012
Protein: 2+
Glucose: neg.

Sheila relayed these results to Room A immediately. She also informed the team that the regional burn center would be able to accept Carole for admission by 12 noon. The decision was made to transport Carole to the local airport by ambulance where she would be picked up by the burn center's helicopter. An R.N. from the ER would accompany Carole during the transport.

Meanwhile, Carole was being closely monitored. The burn areas were cleansed with Phisohex and covered with silver nitrate (0.5%) occlusive dressings as advised by the burn center staff. Carole's respiratory status improved as her condition stabilized. She was made as comfortable as possible. Her transfer from the ER was completed at 11 A.M. Carole's mother was driven to the burn center by a close family friend. The center was located fifty miles away.

STUDY QUESTIONS

5-9. How should Emergency Room A be prepared in order to properly manage a burned client?

5-10. Why are all persons who enter Room A instructed to wear gown, mask, gloves, and cap? Explain.

5-11. Complete a growth and development information card on a six-year-old female.

5-12. What equipment should be readily available when an endotracheal tube (ET tube) is going to be inserted into a victim? What is the function of an ET tube?

5-13. What equipment should be readily available when an intravenous cut-down is performed? Why is a cut-down performed for certain intravenous infusions? Why was the saphenous vein used?

5-14. When morphine sulfate is given intravenously what precautions must be taken? What antidote should be immediately available? Why is it the pain reliever of choice in victims who have been seriously burned?

5-15. Identify the purpose for each of the medical orders for the patient.

5-16. Complete drug information cards on the following: morphine sulfate, tetanus toxoid, silver nitrate.

5-17. What are the dangers of administering narcotics, such as morphine, to a burned client? Explain.

5-18. What are the advantages and disadvantages of silver nitrate application in the management of burns?

5-19. When and why are occlusive dressings used on burns?

5-20. How is the "rule of nines" used to assess the percent of burned body surface on an adult client? an infant?

5-21. What are the characteristics of each of the four degrees of burns? What are their clinical implications for nursing activities?

Degree of burn	Characteristics	Pathophysiologic effect on client	Therapy	Nursing objectives and actions	Method and frequency of evaluating effectiveness
First					
Second					
Third					
Fourth					

5-22. Compute the percentage of burns received by Carole.

5-23. Compute the amount of intravenous fluid that Carole should receive in the first eight hours; second eight hours; third eight hours.

5-24. What factors determine whether blood, blood products, or plasma are prescribed for a burn patient?

5-25. What are the nursing care objectives and actions for Carole's initial care? How is the effectiveness of treatment evaluated?

Objective	Rationale	Nursing action	Rationale	Method and frequency of evaluating effectiveness

5-26. Complete the following laboratory test grid.

Lab test	Normal value range	Client's value	Significance and reason for alteration in burn patient
Hemoglobin			
Hematocrit			
Prothrombin time			
Blood urea nitrogen			
Total protein			
Na			
K			
Cl			
CO_2			
p_aCO_2			
p_aO_2			
Base excess			
Urine			
pH			
specific gravity			
protein			
glucose			

DISCUSSION QUESTIONS

D-9. How might the nurse decrease Carole's anxiety when she is admitted to the ER?

D-10. What determines a burn victim's prognosis, the quantity of body surface burned, the degree of burns or both? Explain.

D-11. Analyze Ms. Jenkins's reaction to her daughter being burned. What methods of communication are most likely to be useful when dealing with situations similar to this?

D-12. How might Ms. Jenkins have been better prepared for her visit to her burned daughter? What topics should be discussed with Ms. Jenkins before she sees Carole? Outline the items in the order in which they should be presented. What would you explain about each?

Topic	Explanation

D-13. In preparation for the transfer of a burn patient to a regional burn center, what information should be sent with the client?

SUGGESTED ACTIVITIES

1. Care for a stable burn patient.
2. Tour a hospital burn unit. Find out their protocol for client admission. Talk to one of the nursing staff about their interactions with patients and their families. If possible, interview a patient who is recovering from burns.
3. Review a hospital disaster plan. What are the roles of the various staff members during a disaster?
4. Participate in a hospital disaster drill.
5. Explore what services are available to disaster victims in your community.
6. Interview an ER charge nurse about her responsibilities, roles, and functions during a mini-disaster.

BIBLIOGRAPHY

Alexander, Mary M., and Brown, Marie Scott. "Physical Examination." *Nursing '75* 5 (January 1975): 44–48.

Artz, C. P., and Monerief, J. A. *The Treatment of Burns.* Philadelphia: W. B. Saunders Co., 1969.

American College of Emergency Room Physicians. "Patient Transfer Guidelines—A Position Paper." *Journal of the American College of Emergency Room Physicians* (October, 1977): 467.

Bowden, Marjorie L., and Feller, Irving. "Family Reaction to a Severe Burn." *American Journal of Nursing* 73 (February 1973): 317–319.

Brunner, Lillian Sholtis, and Suddarth, Doris S. *Textbook of Medical–Surgical Nursing.* 3d. ed. Philadelphia: J. B. Lippincott Co., 1975.

Campbell, Claire. *Nursing Diagnosis and Intervention in Nursing Practice.* New York: John Wiley and Sons, 1978, pp. 817–821.

Cosgriff, James H., Jr., and Anderson, Diann Laden. *The Practice of Emergency Nursing*. Philadelphia: J. B. Lippincott Co., 1975, pp. 37–45, 52–60, 61–70, 244–254.

Esley, Larry, and Reskin, Wayne. "Algorithm-Directed Triage in an Emergency Department." *Journal of the American College of Emergency Room Physicians* (November 1976): 869–876.

Garb, Solomon. *Laboratory Tests in Common Use*. 6th ed. New York: Springer Publishing Co., Inc., 1976.

Jones, Claudella A., and Feller, Irving. "Burns: What to Do During the First Crucial Hours," *Nursing '77* 7 (March 1977): 22–31.

Little, Dolores E., and Carnevali, Doris L. *Nursing Care Planning*. Philadelphia: J. B. Lippincott Co., 1976.

Luciano, Kathy, and Shumsky, Claire J. "Pediatric Procedures," *Nursing '75* 5 (January 1975): 45–52.

Malasanos, Lois et al. *Health Assessment*. St. Louis: C. V. Mosby Co., 1978.

Mancini, Marguerite. "Liability in the Emergency Room." *American Journal of Nursing* 78 (June 1978): 1083–1084.

McLeod, Kathryn A. "Learning to Take the Trauma of Triage." *RN* 75 (July 1975): 23–37.

McManus, William S., and Dain, Joseph C. "Can the Well-trained E.M.T.–Paramedic Maintain Skills and Knowledge." *Journal of the American College of Emergency Room Physicians* (December 1976): 984–986.

Mills, John et al., "Effectiveness of Nurse Triage in the Emergency Department of An Urban County Hospital." *Journal of the American College of Emergency Room Physicians* (November 1976): 877–882.

Peterson, Grace G. "Evaluating the Assignments Head Nurses Make." *American Journal of Nursing* 73 (April 1973): 641–644.

Rogenes, Paula R., and Moylan, Joseph A. "Restoring Fluid Balance in the Patient with Severe Burns." *American Journal of Nursing* 76 (December 1976): 1952–1957.

Scipien, Gladys M. et al. *Comprehensive Pediatric Nursing*. New York: McGraw-Hill, 1975, pp. 842–857.

Spitz, Phyllis, and Sweetwood, Hannelore. "Kids in Crisis: Part I, Bedside Assessment." *Nursing '78* 8 (March 1978): 70–79.

———. "Kids in Crisis: Part II, Emergencies." *Nursing '78* 8 (April 1978): 27–30.

Stroot, Violet R.; Lee, Carla A.; and Schaper, C. Ann. *Fluid and Electrolytes: A Practical Approach*. 2d ed. Philadelphia: F. A. Davis Co., 1977.

Wagner, Mary M. "Emergency Care of the Burned Patient." *American Journal of Nursing* 77 (November 1977): 1788–1791.

Warlick, Sharon. "Sam: The Patient Nobody Wanted to Visit." *Nursing '78* 8 (July 1978): 56–58.

Whorton, M. Donald. "Carbon Monoxide Intoxication: A Review of Fourteen Patients." *Journal of the American College of Emergency Room Physicians* (July 1976): 505–509.

CHAPTER SIX

Fluid and Electrolyte Imbalance: Acute Glomerulonephritis

MARGARET MERVA

OVERVIEW

Peter Kang is the seven-year-old adopted son of John and Sue-Sin Kang. Peter develops acute glomerulonephritis following a streptococcal infection. The school nurse practitioner realizes that Peter is more than just tired when he is sent to her office for sleeping in class. The child is taken to the emergency room by his mother and is later admitted to the pediatric unit, where the diagnosis of acute glomerulonephritis is confirmed based upon the laboratory findings.

CONTENT EMPHASIS

- Adoption
- Fluid and electrolyte—balance/imbalance
- Sequelae of streptococcal pharyngitis
- Assessment and treatment of acute glomerulonephritis

SETTINGS

- School nurse's office
- Emergency room
- Pediatric unit

OBJECTIVES

Upon completing this chapter the student will be able to:

1. Describe the psychosocial characteristics of the adoptive family.
2. Recognize the disruption of fluid and electrolyte balance in acute renal failure.
3. Construct expected health outcomes for children with a fluid and electrolyte imbalance and their families.
4. Understand the epidemiological aspects of streptococcal infections.
5. Select nursing interventions specific to the care of the school-age child with acute glomerulonephritis.

DEFINITION OF TERMS

The following terms are used in this chapter and should be defined before proceeding:

Adoption   Immune complex disease
Anorexia   Infertile family
Antistreptolysin (ASO) titer   Lethargic
Anuric   Micturition
Erythrocyte sedimentation rate   Oliguric
  (ESR)   Peri-orbital edema
Group A beta hemolytic   Pharyngitis
  streptococcus, type 12   Proteinuria
Hematuria   Scarlatiniform rash
Hyperkalemia   School nurse practitioner

FAMILY ASSESSMENT

John and Sue-Sin Kang live in an upper-middle-class suburb of Chicago. Both of their parents live in the surrounding area and visit with the Kangs at least once a month. The Kangs are of Korean extraction and are practicing Methodists. Both families of origin were born in South Korea, but John and Sue-Sin were born in Chicago. John is the oldest of five children while Sue-Sin is the third of four children.

The initial meeting between John Kang and Sue-Sin was arranged by their parents. John was a junior lawyer at the time and Sue was a sophmore in college. They were married soon after Sue graduated from college.

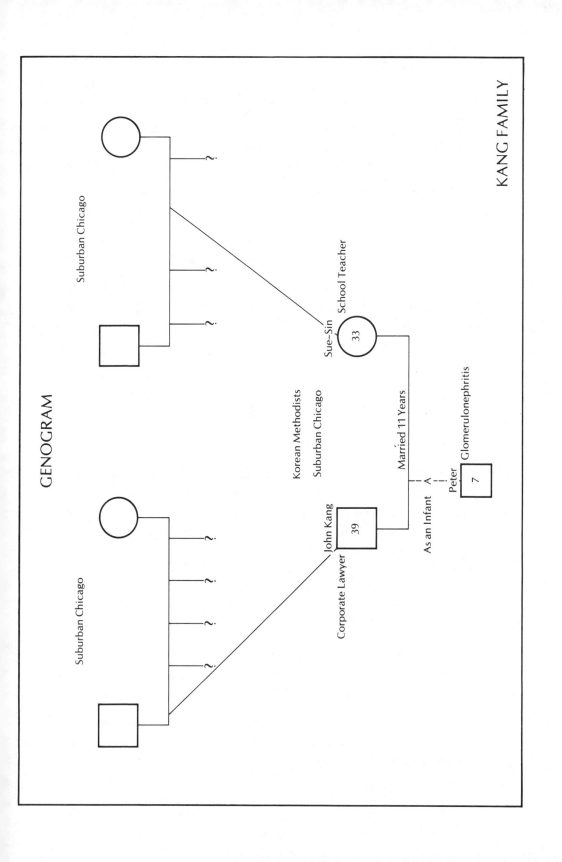

GENOGRAM

KANG FAMILY

Suburban Chicago

Suburban Chicago

Korean Methodists
Suburban Chicago

John Kang
Corporate Lawyer
39

Sue–Sin
School Teacher
33

Married 11 Years

As an Infant

Peter
Glomerulonephritis
7

Shortly after they were married, John was promoted to an executive position in the corporation's legal staff. Meanwhile, Sue obtained a job as an elementary school teacher. In two years the Kangs were able to purchase a four-bedroom home in an upper-middle class suburb of Chicago.

After three years of marriage, Sue was still not pregnant at the age of 25. They were getting pressure and advice from both the Kang and the Sin families. Finally, they applied to the Catholic adoption agency in Chicago for a "healthy Korean male infant." It was only 10 months before an infant was available.

The year of "foster parenting" began, and Sue quit her job to take care of Peter. Finally, the court decision was made and adoption papers were issued. At last Peter was theirs.

The Kangs were warm and loving parents. Sue, and occasionally John, would read stories to Peter at night. They frequently took Peter to museums and various parks on the weekend.

When Peter entered first grade, Sue resumed her previous job as a school teacher. However, the only vacancy at that time was in a school twenty miles away. Both Sue and John's parents were displeased with Sue's working; however, John supported Sue's reemployment.

STUDY QUESTIONS

6-1. What are the beliefs of practicing Methodists on the following topics: family, marriage, alcohol and tobacco, health and illness?

6-2. What are the beliefs of Koreans on the following topics: family, marriage, children, health and illness, infertility, and adoption?

6-3. What are some methods for adopting a child? Explain each.

6-4. What occurs during the three basic phases of adoption from a nonsectarian social service agency? Explain each.
   a. Application phase
   b. Supervision phase (foster parenting)
   c. Adoption phase

DISCUSSION QUESTIONS

D-1. Where can a couple be directed to apply for adoption in your area?

D-2. What restrictions, if any, are placed on the adoptive parents by a social agency? a Catholic agency?

D-3. Why did the Kangs insist on a "healthy Korean male infant?"

D-4. Why were Sue and John's parents displeased with Sue's reemployment? Explain.

D-5. What is the availability of Oriental children for adoption at this time in your area? white children? black children? multiracial?

D-6. Can an agency "guarantee" the health of an infant? What can happen if the infant is found to have a congenital defect during the supervision phase of adoption? Who pays for the medical bills?

D-7. What stressful situations are occurring in the Kang family at this time?

D-8. Should Peter know he is an adopted child? Explain your answer.

CLIENT ASSESSMENT

Peter attends the second grade at the local public school. One day Peter's teacher, Ms. Eaton, noticed that the young lad was having a difficult time staying awake. Since this was unusual behavior for Peter, Ms. Eaton sent Peter to the school nurse.

When Ms. Jones, R.N., read Peter's chart, she noted that Peter had been absent from school for a week with the diagnosis of acute pharyngitis (group A beta hemolytic strep, type 12). The nurse had a note in the file from Peter's pediatrician that confirmed this diagnosis. Ms. Jones realized that Peter could develop complications from this type of acute sore throat. She noted the following significant data while doing the assessment:

General description: age 7 years; height 125 cm, weight 25 kg, brown eyes, black hair

Vital signs: T: 37.4°C. P: 88 and regular. R: 25. BP: 138/80.

Musculoskeletal: Bilateral lumbar flank pain

Neurological: Generally lethargic, related, "I'm sleepy, I want my Mommy; my head hurts."

Skin: Warm and dry, lips dry and cracked, color pale

Abdomen: Enlarged right kidney on palpation

Ophthalmic: bilateral peri-orbital edema

Extremities: tight fitting shoes; nonpitting edema in lower extremities

The nurse comforted Peter and moved him to a bed in the infirmary and covered him with a blanket. She explained the need to remain still and quiet while she called his mother and his pediatrician. Dr. Eng, M.D., indicated that he would see Peter at the community hospital's emergency room. Ms. Kang said that she would pick Peter up in 30 minutes and drive him to the hospital. Sue immediately notified her principal, who relieved her from class.

EMERGENCY ROOM

Since Dr. Eng was still busy on the pediatric unit, Ms. Davis, R.N., took a nursing history and assessed the following data:

CHIEF COMPLAINT: anorexia, fatigue, and headache

HISTORY OF ILLNESS: Streptococcal throat infection 3 weeks ago, treated with oral erythromycin for 10 days. Last visit to M.D.—1 week ago. Mother denies child had any contact with any known communicable disease within or outside of the home. During the period of illness Peter had swollen cervical nodes, a low-grade fever, a scarlatiniform rash, and a poor appetite.

OTHER: Mother denies knowledge of child ingesting poisons, medications, or other toxic substances.

ALLERGIES:
   Drugs—Penicillin
   Food—Lactose intolerance; Mother uses *Lactobacillus* supplement in milk. Child tolerates frozen yogurt, but cannot eat ice cream or frozen milk.

GASTROINTESTINAL: Usually good appetite, enjoys chicken, roast beef, rice, and macaroni. Eats three meals, plus snacks in afternoon and at bedtime. (Salt added in cooking and at the table.)

FLUID INTAKE: 6–7 glasses per day; only 1 or 2 glasses in last 24 hours.

ELIMINATION: Stool q 1–2 days in A.M. following breakfast. Diarrhea and cramping pains occur with ingestion of pure milk products. Child does not complain of burning on micturition. Mother has not observed quality or quantity of child's urine within the past 10 days.

NEUROLOGICAL: lethargic; orientated to time, place, and person.

INTEGUMENT: No rashes prior to the rash accompanying the strep throat. Denies any lesions. Bruises heal normally.

COMMUNICABLE DISEASES AND IMMUNIZATIONS: Had chickenpox, immunized for mumps/measles/rubella; oral polio vaccine and DPT toxoid given x3 and boosters x1. Last tine test prior to school admission—negative.

FAMILY MEMBERS AT HOME:
Father John, age 38 years   health: good   lawyer
Mother Sue, age 32 years   health: good   teacher
Son Peter,   age 7 years   health: generally good
                            second grade in school

Natural Parents   no health history available

CHILD'S DAILY HABITS: Needs minor assistance in dressing.
Sleeps 8–9 hr per night; occasionally wakes to go to the bathroom ×1 per night; no daytime napping. Activities—soccer, wrestling, painting, molds clay. Likes to watch "Sesame Street" and cartoons.

PSYCHOSOCIAL HISTORY: Talks occasionally about parents; exhibits affection toward parents. States that he wishes he had a brother or sister. Child has no playmates at home. Enjoys school. No close friends in school.

HEALTH INSURANCE: Blue Cross/Blue Shield with Major Medical coverage

STUDY QUESTIONS

6-5. Complete a growth and development card on a seven-year-old male.

6-6. Compare Peter to the "average" seven-year-old male.

6-7. What would children Peter's age understand regarding their bodily organs and functions?

6-8. Is complete isolation of children with streptococcocal infections necessary? Explain.

6-9. What is the technique for obtaining a pharyngeal culture and sensitivity? What precautions should be followed to prevent an inaccurate report due to contamination?

6-10. How soon after beginning treatment with antibiotics for a strep infection can the child safely return to school?

6-11. Complete a drug information card on erythromycin.

6-12. Why was Peter given erythromycin for his strep throat instead of a sulfonamide?

6-13. Why was erythromycin prescribed for a ten-day interval? Explain.

6-14. What are the potential complications following a strep throat?

DISCUSSION QUESTIONS

D-9. What additional family history would be useful in assessing and planning your care for this client/family?

D-10. Since Peter developed pharyngitis, should all members of the Kang family see their physician for a throat culture? Explain.

D-11. What measures should the pediatric nurse caring for Peter carry out immediately in order to ensure safety and the prevention of complications?

D-12. What might the nurse suggest to meet Ms. Kang's needs at this time?

D-13. Create a nursing care plan for Peter's initial period of hospitalization; consider the following:

Subjective data	Objective data	Nursing diagnosis	Intervention	Rationale

PEDIATRICS

Peter was admitted to the pediatric unit at 2:30 P.M. by Judy Grass, R.N. The following laboratory tests soon arrived on the unit:

URINALYSIS:
gr.: sp. 1.012
pH: 5.0
WBC: 7
RBC: numerous
Hyaline casts: numerous
Protein: 2+
Glucose: negative

ELECTROYTES:
Na: 150 mEq/L
K: 6.5 mEq/L
C1: 96 mEq/L
CO_2: 14 mEq/L

CBC:
Hbg: 10g%
Hct: 45%
RBC: 4.0×10^6 mm^3
WBC: 13,500 mm^3
Sed. rate: 44 mm/hr

OTHER:
Blood pH (venous): 7.33
BUN: 120 mg/100 ml
Creatinine: 20 mg/100 ml
Serum albumin: 2.9 g/100 ml
C reactive protein: +2
Serum albumin: 2.9 g/100 ml
ASO titer: 350 Todd units/ml

By early evening Peter had been taken for a chest X-ray and an EKG was performed. Ms. Kang stayed with Peter. Dr. Eng visited and confirmed Peter's diagnosis as "acute glomerulonephritis immune complex disease" and left the following orders:

Vital signs and temperature qid—call M.D. if BP above 140 systolic

Stools for Guiac

Nasopharyngeal P throat culture for culture and sensitivity

Daily weights in A.M.

1 gram sodium diet—no citrus juices; add lactobacillus to milk

Strict intake and output (call M.D. if urinary output falls below 20 ml/hour); limit fluids to 300 cc/8 hours

Strict bedrest

Seizure precautions

After Dr. Eng left, the evening nurse took the opportunity to talk with Ms. Kang about Peter's condition. She suggested that some of Peter's bed toys as well as his pajamas be brought to the hospital. Sue was able to contact John by phone before he left for the hospital and instructed him to bring the articles suggested by the nurse.

Peter slept poorly that night and he appeared anxious when Judy Grass arrived on the unit the next morning. The results of Peter's EKG and chest X-ray were as follows:

• EKG: NSR

> rate: 88

> impression: within normal limits

• Chest X-ray—negative

• Peter's summary sheet read as follows:

Time	V.S.			BP	I	O	Comment
	T	P	R				
2:30	37.4	88	26	136/80	0	50 ml	lethargic
11 P.M.	37.6	94	28	138/82	190 ml	175 ml	concentrated urine
7 A.M.	37.0	86	24	130/78	250 ml	0	restless night
3 P.M.	37.8	92	30	132/80	210 ml	150 ml	anorexic

On the third hospital day, Peter had an increase in his urinary output to 830 ml/24 hrs. His blood pressure had dropped to 120/70–125/75. Peter was less lethargic and he was asking for more than juices to drink. Dr. Eng increased Peter's fluids to 400 ml/day plus the amount of his urinary output.

STUDY QUESTIONS

6-15. What is meant by an immune complex disease? Explain.

6-16. Complete the following laboratory grid:

Test	Normal range	Peter's value	Significance of deviation

6-17. What is the difference between oliguria and anuria? How do you know?

6-18. How might you explain the hemoglobin of 10 g %?

6-19. How does the kidney function to maintain the acid-base balance? How do the lungs function? (See Appendix F.)

6-20. What is Peter's acid-base imbalance? Explain.

6-21. What are his electrolyte disturbances? How might they affect his cardiac status in the future?

6-22. What physiological compensatory mechanism would the body use to attempt to correct metabolic acidosis? Explain.

6-23. Why were citrus juices omitted from Peter's diet?

6-24. Why were a chest X-ray and an EKG done on Peter? A Guiac test?

6-25. How do you allow for insensible water loss when calculating fluid replacement?

DISCUSSION QUESTIONS

D-14. Give two reasons a Foley catheter to straight closed drainage is not used for this client.

D-15. If Peter's acidosis and volume overload fail to correct themselves with conservative medical treatment, the physician will institute peritoneal- or hemo-dialysis. Discuss these treatment modalities and the implications for nursing care.

D-16. How might the fact that Peter is adopted affect the parents' reaction to his acute illness?

D-17. What is the (im)balance between Peter's intake and output? Explain.

D-18. What is the rationale for each of Peter's medical orders?

Order	Rationale

D-19. Create a nursing care plan for Peter. What are the nursing diagnoses, objectives, and actions? What is the rationale for care and how is the effectiveness of care evaluated?

Nursing diagnosis	Objectives	Rationale	Nursing actions	Rationale	Method and frequency of evaluating effectiveness

D-20. How can Peter's family be included in meeting the goals and objectives of Peter's care?

D-21. What topics should be discussed with Ms. Kang about Peter's condition and hospitalization? What should be explained about each?

Topic	Explanation

D-22. What health teaching problems should the nurse discuss with Peter's family prior to his discharge? Develop a discharge teaching plan for Peter; for his parents.

BIBLIOGRAPHY

Abraham, Rudolph. *Pediatrics.* 16th ed. New York: Appleton-Century-Crofts, 1977, pp. 1266–1271.

Barber, Janet; Stokes, Lillian; and Billings, Diane. *Adult and Child Care.* 2d ed. St. Louis: C. V. Mosby Co., 1977, pp. 744–745.

Benensen, Abram, ed. *Control of Communicable Diseases in Man.* 12th ed. New York: American Public Health Association, 1975.

Benson, Evelyn, and McDevitt, Joan. *Community Health and Nursing Practice.* Englewood Cliffs, N.J.: Prentice-Hall, Inc., 1975, pp. 59–70.

Bergersen, Betty. *Pharmacology in Nursing*. 13th ed. St. Louis: C. V. Mosby Co., 1976, pp. 483–487.

Chow, Effie. "Cultural Health Traditions: Asia· Perspectives." In *Providing Safe Nursing Care for Ethnic People of Color*, edited by Marie Branch and Phyllis Paxton. New York: Appleton-Century-Crofts, 1976.

Cohen, Stephen, et al. "Metabolic Acid-Base Disorders, Part I: Chemistry and Physiology." *American Journal of Nursing* 77 (October 1977): 1–32.

_____. "Metabolic Acid-Base Disorders, Part II: Physiological Abnormalities and Nursing Actions." *American Journal of Nursing* 78 (January 1978): 1–20.

_____. "Metabolic Acid-Base Disorders, Part III: Clinical and Laboratory Findings." *American Journal of Nursing* 78 (March 1978): 1–16.

Hammons, Chloe. "The Adoptive Family." *American Journal of Nursing* 76 (February 1976): 251–257.

Hymovich, Debra, and Barnard, Martha Underwood. *Family Health Care*. New York: McGraw-Hill, 1973, pp. 188–197, 234–247.

Juenker, Donna. "Child's Perception of His Illness." In *Nursing Care of the Child with Long-Term Illness*, edited by Shirley Steele. New York: Appleton-Century-Crofts, 1977.

Kempe, Henry, et al. *Current Pediatric Diagnosis*. 4th ed. Los Altos, California: Lange Publications, 1976, pp. 475–476.

Little, Dolores, and Carnevali, Doris. *Nursing Care Planning*. 2d ed. Philadelphia: J. B. Lippincott Company, 1976.

Malasanos, Lois, et al. *Health Assessment*. St. Louis: C. V. Mosby Co., 1978.

McCrory, W. W., and Shibuya, Madoka. "Post-Streptococcal Glomerulonephritis in Children." *Pediatric Nursing Clinics of North America* 11 (August 1964): 633–647.

Pendagast, Eileen G., and Sherman, Charles O. "A Guide to the Genogram Family Systems Training." *The Family* 5 (1977): 314.

Petrillo, Madeline, and Sanger, Sirgay. "A Working Knowledge of Childhood." In *Emotional Care of Hospitalized Children*. Philadelphia: J. B. Lippincott Co., 1972.

Pumphrey, John B. "Recognizing Your Patients' Spiritual Needs." *Nursing '77* 7 (December 1977): 64–70.

Robinson, Corinne, and Lawler, Marilyn R. *Normal and Therapeutic Nutrition*. 15th ed. New York: Macmillan, 1977.

Scipien, Gladys, et al. *Comprehensive Pediatric Nursing*. New York: McGraw-Hill, 1975.

Steele, Shirley, "Nursing Care of the Child with Kidney Problems." In *Nursing Care of the Child With Long Term Illness*. New York: Appleton-Century-Crofts, 1977.

Stroot, Violet R.; Lee, Carla A.; and Schaper, C. Ann. *Fluid and Electrolyte: A Practical Approach.* 2d ed. Philadelphia: F. A. Davis Co., 1977.

Vaughan, Victor, and McKay, James. *Nelson Textbook of Pediatrics.* 10th ed. Philadelphia: W. B. Saunders, 1976. pp. 1199–1205.

Wang, Rosalind. "Streptococcal Sore Throat." *American Journal of Nursing* 77 (November 1977): 1796–1798.

Widmann, Frances. *Goodale's Clinical Interpretation of Laboratory Tests.* 7th ed. Philadelphia: F. A. Davis Co., 1973.

CHAPTER SEVEN

Secondary Complication: Acute Otitis Media Following Measles

LINDA K. HARRISON

MARGARET A. MERVA

OVERVIEW

Boni Loussac is the nine-year-old child of a rural Eskimo family. Boni develops rubeola during an epidemic of the disease in her school. A public health nurse is sent to the area to assist the village in controlling the spread of the disease. Unfortunately, Boni develops acute otitis media and the public health nurse manages this complication of rubeola with the assistance of the village's health aide. The agency's approved protocol for acute otitis media is used, and since there is no means of contacting a physician, other health care problems are also managed by the nurse.

CONTENT EMPHASIS

- Environmental-community assessment—rural Eskimo village
- Epidemic of rubeola—assessment, management, and immunity
- Home management of acute otitis media
- Nutritional assessment—rural family

SETTING

- Rural home visit
- Public health nurse's temporary office

OBJECTIVES

Upon completing this chapter, the student will be able to:

1. Describe health problems of populations living in extreme environments.
2. Determine the socioeconomic and environmental factors affecting the epidemiological behavior of infectious diseases.
3. Appraise the health care provider's role in shortage areas.
4. Differentiate active, passive, and permanent immunity.
5. Describe the biomedical controls for infectious disease contagion.
6. Evaluate the pediatric client's response to viral infections.
7. Identify the possible secondary complications for clients experiencing viral infections with pulmonary complications.

DEFINITION OF TERMS

The following terms are used in this case study and should be defined before proceeding:

Active immunity	Koplik spots
Catarrhal	Maculopapular rash
Contagion	Passive immunity
Coryza	Permafrost
DPT series	Permanent immunity
Endemic	Photophobia
Epidemic	Prodromal phase
Exanthema	Protocols
Fomites	Rubeola (morbilli) (red measles)
Gamma globulin	TPV oral vaccine
Health service shortage area	Trained health aide
Incubation phase	Tundra
Infectious phase	Viraemia

COMMUNITY-ENVIRONMENTAL ASSESSMENT

Kuskokwim is a small town in southwestern Alaska. Its population of 1,500 is comprised mainly of native Eskimos. This area experiences severe winters with permafrost conditions that hinder the maintenance of sanitary water and waste disposal. Due to the isolation caused by the extreme winter weather the community is often without staple foods, supplies, and services for extended periods of time.

The principle industry is fishing, with some fruits and vegetables raised during the summer in the nearby tundra region. Consequently, the average income for this community is well below the established poverty level. The past year has been unusually difficult for the community as the fishing was poor and food became scarce in the midst of a hard winter. Eskimo dwellings in western Alaska are typically wood-framed and heated by oil- or wood-burning stoves located in the middle of one large room. Partitions separate the sleeping areas near the walls from the living areas.

The community's four-room schoolhouse is attended by approximately 100 students ranging in age from 7 to 14. Endemic diseases have frequently necessitated school closings during the winter and spring months. Presently, the school is closed due to an outbreak of rubeola. This crisis resulted in a nurse practitioner being flown to Kuskokwim from the Anchorage public health department to assist in the treatment and future prevention of this and other childhood diseases. The management of acute episodes of community health problems in rural or health service shortage areas of Alaska is regularly carried out by the public health nursing staff. Protocols officially approved by the public health department serve as the nurse's guide in field practice. It has been anticipated that the nurse would spend four weeks in Kuskokwim before returning to Anchorage. A trained village health aide from the community is assisting her.

STUDY QUESTIONS

7-1. What are some of the current beliefs of the Eskimo population on the following topics: family, children, health, illness, and health care providers?

7-2. What is the present system of health care delivery in rural Alaska? Why have the morbidity rates for tuberculosis, pneumonia, and other diseases decreased?

7-3. How do the following factors contribute to the epidemiology of disease: malnutrition, poor hygiene, housing, and scarce health services?

7-4. What is the responsibility of government (federal, state, and local) in the control of communicable diseases? How is this role carried out?

DISCUSSION QUESTIONS

D-1. What effect does the lack of a sanitary water supply and the lack of sewage treatment management have upon a community's health? Explain.

D-2. What is the rationale for closing schools when a disease becomes an epidemic? How is the time for reopening the school determined?

D-3. What functions might be assumed by a health aide in areas where there are few if any health services? Explain.

CLIENT ASSESSMENT

Boni Loussac is a nine-year-old Eskimo girl living with her parents Waino and Nenana Loussac and two siblings—Aleutia (seven years) and Joey (three years). Boni is a third-grade student at the Kuskokwim school.

Boni is one of the students who was directly affected by the rubeola epidemic that had recently spread through the school. Being a health-conscious mother, Nenana was quite concerned about whether she could prevent the occurrence of the "red measles" (as she referred to them) in her other children—particularly in her youngest, Joey. She had contracted rubeola herself during childhood. None of the children had been immunized against rubella, rubeola, or parotitis; although they had all received the DPT series, TPV oral vaccine, and a smallpox vaccination. She spoke with the village health aide, Milio, who discussed the problem with the visiting nurse practitioner, Ms. Westwick.

The nurse was able to make an unscheduled home visit that day, January 24. Nenana was pleasantly surprised to see the nurse, and she offered her a chair near the stove. During her visit, Ms. Westwick was careful to consider the cultural beliefs and attitudes that would have an effect upon health care. During the interview, Ms. Westwick directed her questions to both Nenana and Boni in an attempt to establish a positive rapport with both of them.

Nenana related that Boni stayed home from school with a slight fever (38.3°C) and malaise on January 20 (ten days after school had been closed). Following a day of sneezing, coughing, and nasal congestion, Boni broke out in a rash. Ms. Westwick noted the maculopapular rash on Boni's face and neck; it had spread to her legs. All these signs and symptoms seemed to be relatively mild, including a few Koplik spots on the oral mucosa.

Having reviewed Boni's disease course, Ms. Westwick gave both Joey and Aleutia 500 mg of rubeola gamma globulin. Nenana was informed about the course of the disease, including the early symptoms of rubeola. The nurse encouraged Nenana to contact her if either of the children demonstrated these symptoms or if she could be of further assistance to the Loussac family.

STUDY QUESTIONS

7-5. Complete a growth and development information card on a nine-year-old female, a seven-year-old female, and a three-year-old male.

7-6. What is the etiology of rubeola? mode of transmission? communicable phase? prodromal phase? clinical manifestations? prognosis?

7-7. Rubeola most frequently occurs in the late winter and in the spring. Outbreaks tend to occur in two-year-cycles. What are the reasons for these occurrences?

7-8. Can rubeola affect the pregnant woman or her fetus? Explain.

7-9. Why are the clinical manifestations of rubeola often more severe in adults than in children? in infants and toddlers as compared to school-aged children? Explain.

7-10. Are infants protected against rubeola at birth? If so, for what length of time? Explain.

7-11. Describe the pathological changes occurring to the skin and mucous membrane of the child with rubeola.

7-12. What are Koplik spots? Describe their appearance. Describe the spread and appearance of measles exanthema.

7-13. What other diseases resemble measles?

7-14. What measures can be taken to prevent rubeola?

7-15. What are the indications for the use of gamma globulin for rubeola? Does gamma globulin always prevent the occurrence of rubeola in the recipient? Explain.

7-16. What is the immunization schedule for children as recommended by the American Academy of Pediatrics?

7-17. When is a tuberculin test indicated? Should it be given before or after the rubeola vaccine? Explain.

7-18. What information should Ms. Loussac be given regarding the effects of gamma globulin on her two younger children?

7-19. What measures can be taken to reduce the transmission of rubeola?

7-20. Compare Boni's experience with rubeola to the textbook description of the same disease.

7-21. How does the person gain immunity from rubeola following administration of live vaccine? from an episode of the disease?

DISCUSSION QUESTIONS

D-4. Is it appropriate for Ms. Westwick to make an unscheduled home visit? Explain.

D-5. How might the Loussac's cultural beliefs and attitudes alter Ms. Westwick's approach to the family?

D-6. What kinds of questions might the nurse ask directly to Boni during her visit? What questions should be asked of Boni's mother?

D-7. Should children with measles be hospitalized? Explain.

ACUTE EARACHE

Nenana became quite concerned about Boni's health on January 29. Boni had slept very poorly the previous evening and had a fever. However, her rash was disappearing. Recalling that the nurse had encouraged her to contact her if she needed assistance, Nenana sent for Ms. Westwick that morning.

The following health history and physical assessment data were collected by the nurse when she visited the Loussac home at 12:00 P.M. that day:

CHIEF COMPLAINT: Pain in left ear

PRESENT ILLNESS: Mother states "Boni slept very little last night and had a fever. . . . " "This morning, she said her left ear hurts."

Client states "I feel sick again. Will I ever get better?" (Starts to cry while holding her left ear.)

Recuperating from rubeola, maculopapular rash first appeared January 22.

T—40°C orally.

Coryza, c/o pain in left ear.

PAST HISTORY: Has experienced 1–2 episodes of upper respiratory infections with occasional accompanying earaches yearly since three years of age. No childhood illnesses until recent rubeola. Immunized for smallpox, TPV, and DPT. No known allergies.

FAMILY HISTORY: (See genogram); noncontributory health history.

NUTRITIONALHISTORY/EATING HABITS: Mother states that client has been eating poorly the last two days, since the occurrence of rubeola. "She seems to have lost some weight." Boni's appetite is fair. Normally drinks two glasses milk per day. Refuses eggs and fish. Eats small amounts of other meats. Likes fruits and vegetables, cereals, and sweets.

SOCIAL HISTORY: Enjoys school and receives above-average grades. Occasionally stays overnight at a friend's house. Makes friends easily. Immediate family members participate together in many recreational events. Father is often away on commercial fishing trips for as long as two weeks at a time.

PHYSICAL ASSESSMENT (significant findings only):
  Height: 122 cm   Weight: 25 kg

Vital signs: T—40°C, P—100, R—28

Integument: Mild maculopapular (measles) rash on lower extremities

Head and neck: Slight lymph-adenopathy of mastoid, parotid and preauricular glands.

Eyes: PERRLA; wears glasses for myopia.

Ears: normal external ear; hearing testing deferred.

otoscopic examination:

left ear—landmarks barely distinguishable; bulging reddened tympanic membrane; no light reflex.

right ear—dense white plaque noted at 9 o-clock position; light reflex at 5 o'clock, landmarks are distinguishable.

Nose: reddened mucosa with moderate mucus drainage; narrowed nasal passages; slightly deviated nasal septum.

Throat: slightly swollen tonsillar tissue; bright pink with small amount drainage.

Lungs: clear breath sounds; percussion tones are resonant.

Heart: NSR; BP 94/62; good pulses.

Abdomen: no tenderness upon palpation; bowel sounds noted.

As a result of her special training and experience, the nurse diagnosed Boni as having acute otitis media. The following medications were prescribed for Boni according to the established public health protocol:

Ampicillin: 250 mg q 6 h × 10 days.

Auralgan solution: gtts iv in affected ear q 4 h prn for ear pain.

Ephedrine sulfate syrup: 20 mg q 6 h prn for nasal congestion.

ASA 300 mg q 4 h prn for temperature > 38.0° C.

Follow-up evaluation in 10 days.

The medical supplies were kept at the temporary nurse's post (the school). Arrangements were made for the village health aide to deliver the medicines to the Loussac home later that day. However, Ms. Westwick explained to Nenana the instructions for giving Boni the ampicillin (liquid), Auralgan (ear drops), and ephedrine sulfate (syrup). The nurse knew that the village health aide would again review the administration of the drugs with Ms. Loussac when she arrived with the medications. In the meantime, Ms. Westwick suggested ways that Boni's mother could make Boni more comfortable. If Boni did not show significant improvement in the next day Nenana was instructed to contact Ms. Westwick or the village health aide. Before leaving, the nurse planned a return visit with Ms. Loussac and Boni at the school on the morning of February 9.

The village health aide, Milio, arrived with the medications Boni needed at 3 P.M. that same day. Milio assisted Boni's mother in measuring and administering each of the medications. Milio promised to return the next day to check on Boni's progress.

STUDY QUESTIONS

7-22. What are the complications of rubeola? Why do they occur?

7-23. What are the classifications of otitis media? How do they differ?

7-24. What is the etiology of acute otitis media? What are the clinical features? List the possible complications.

7-25. What factors predispose one to a secondary disease following rubeola?

7-26. Evaluate the progress of rubeola in Boni at the home visit.

7-27. What is the significance of the otoscopic findings? Why was the hearing test deferred at this time?

7-28. Complete drug information cards on the following: gamma globulin, ampicillin, Auralgan, ephedrine sulfate, aspirin.

7-29. What specific instructions should Ms. Westwick give to Boni's mother about the administration of the following: ampicillin, Auralgan, ephedrine sulfate?

7-30. What ways can Ms. Westwick suggest to Boni's mother that might make Boni more comfortable? Explain the rationale for each.

Method	Rationale

DISCUSSION QUESTIONS

D-8. In light of the circumstances, was it a good idea for Ms. Westwick to have the health aide deliver the medications to the Loussac home? Discuss your reasoning.

D-9. Why is it a good idea to schedule the follow-up evaluation now rather than to wait a few days?

D-10. In this instance, what is "significant improvement within the next day?" How can Nenana evaluate her daughter?

D-11. In addition to the problems relating to Boni's middle-ear infection, what other present and potential nursing problems can you identify? What could be done by the nurse about each of these problems?

Problem	Nursing action	Rationale	Evaluation

FOLLOW-UP VISIT

On February 9, Nenana came to the school with Boni in the morning. Ms. Westwick was waiting for them at her temporary post. Boni gleefully announced to the nurse, "I'm finally well again and now I can go to school!" Ms. Loussac stated that she had given her daughter the ampicillin as prescribed from January 29 through February 7. In addition, she told Ms. Westwick that neither Aleutia nor Joey had shown any evidence of contracting the measles as yet.

Ms. Westwick did a follow-up evaluation of Boni in light of her past illnesses. The assessment findings were recorded in the client's health record as follows:

... Otoscopic examination demonstrates easily distinguishable landmarks and a light reflex in both ears. Tympanic membranes are pearly gray and intact; AC > BC; no evidence of mucus membrane irritability or drainage; afebrile; energetic. ...

Ms. Westwick praised the efforts of both Boni and her mother in successfully carrying out the prescribed regime. The nurse stressed how cooperative and thorough they had been in adhering to the treatment plan.

Ms. Westwick took advantage of this opportunity to carry out some health teaching—particularly related to Boni's nutritional status. At the conclusion of their visit, Boni hurried to her classroom and Ms. Loussac returned home to care for Joey.

DISCUSSION QUESTIONS

D-12. What should Ms. Loussac be instructed to do with any remaining ampicillin syrup once the prescription is discontinued?

D-13. At this point, is it appropriate for Boni to be attending school again? Explain.

D-14. What is the suggested daily food intake for children 6–9 years of age? Complete the table below. How should the nurse deal with this nutritional problem, considering the Eskimo culture and available dietary supplies?

Food group	Number of servings	Suggested foods
Milk, cheese		
Meat group		
Fruits, vegetables		
Fats/carbohydrates, Desserts/sweets		

D-15. How can the nurse foster discussion of Boni's diet with Boni and her mother?

SUGGESTED ACTIVITIES

1. Visit a rural health center.
2. Spend a day with a public health nurse who is seeing clients who live in rural settings.
3. Attend an immunization clinic.

BIBLIOGRAPHY

Benensen, Abram S., ed. *Control of Communicable Diseases in Man.* 12th ed. New York: American Public Health Association, 1975.

Benson, Evelyn, and McDevitt, Joan. *Community Health and Nursing Practice,* Englewood Cliffs, N.J.: Prentice-Hall, 1975, pp. 59–70.

———. "Epidemology." In *Community Health and Nursing Practice.* Englewood Cliffs, N.J.: Prentice-Hall, 1975.

Bergersen, Betty. *Pharmacology in Nursing.* 13th ed. St. Louis: C. V. Mosby Company, 1976.

———. "Serums and Vaccines." In *Pharmacology in Nursing.* 13th ed. St. Louis: C. V. Mosby Co., 1976.

Christakis, George, ed. "Nutritional Assessment in Health Programs." *American Journal of Public Health* 63 (November 1973): 18–52.

Christie, A. B. *Infectious Disease—Epidemiology and Clinical Practice.* 2d ed. London: Churchill Livingston Publishing Co., 1974, pp. 374–400.

Dansky, Kathryn. "Assessing Children's Nutrition." *American Journal of Nursing* 77 (October 1977): 1610–1611.

Freeman, G. "Middle Ear Disease." *Nursing Times* 73 (January 13, 1977): 56–57.

Garb, Solomon. *Laboratory Tests in Common Use.* 6th ed. New York: Springer Publishing Co., 1976.

Huber, C. J., et al. "The Boel Test as a Screening Device for Otitis Media in Infants." *Nursing Research* 27 (May/June 1978): 178–180.

Johnston, Maxene. "Folk Beliefs and Ethnocultural Behavior in Pediatrics." *Nursing Clinics of North America* 12 (March 1977): 77–86.

Juenker, Donna. "Child's Perception of His Illness." In *Nursing Care of the Child With Long Term Illness.* 2d ed. Edited by Shirley Steele. New York: Appleton-Century-Crofts, 1977.

Krugman, R. D., et al. "Combined Administration of Measles, Mumps, Rubella, and Trivalent Oral Poliovirus Vaccines." *Public Health Reports* 92 (May/June 1977): 220–222.

Little, Dolores E., and Carnevali, Doris L. *Nursing Care Planning.* 2d ed. Philadelphia: J. B. Lippincott Co., 1976.

Malasanos, Lois, et al. *Health Assessment.* St. Louis: C. V. Mosby Co., 1978.

Marcy, Michael, and Kibrick, Sydney. "Measles." In *Infectious Diseases.* 2d ed. Edited by Paul Hoepnich. Hagerstown, Md.: Harper and Row, 1977.

McInnes, Mary Elizabeth. *Essentials of Communicable Disease.* 2d ed. St. Louis: C. V. Mosby Co., 1975.

Mechner, Francis, et al. "Patient Assessment: Examination of the Ear." *American Journal of Nursing* 75 (March 1975): 1–24.

Mullen, John, et al. "Control of Measles Outbreak in an Elementary School." *Public Health Reports* 92 (May/June 1977), 217–219.

Nicholson, Wilma. "A Solo Practice in Rural Community Health." In *Innovations in Community Health Nursing.* Edited by Anne R. Warner. St. Louis: C. V. Mosby Co., 1978.

Nysather, John O.; Katz, Arnold E.; and Lenth, Janet L. "The Immune System—Its Development and Functions." *American Journal of Nursing* 76 (October 1976): 1614–1616.

Pasternack, Sarah B. "Annual Well-Child Visits." *American Journal of Nursing* 74 (August 1974): 1472–1475.

Paxton, Phyllis. "Epidemiology in Health and Disease." In *Providing Safe Nursing Care for Ethnic People of Color.* Edited by Marie Branch and Phyllis Paxton. New York: Appleton-Century-Crofts, 1976.

Petrillo, Madeline, and Sanger, Sirgay. "A Working Knowledge of Childhood." In *Emotional Care of Hospitalized Children.* Philadelphia: J. P. Lippincott Co., 1972.

Scipien, Gladys, et al. *Comprehensive Pediatric Nursing.* New York: McGraw-Hill, 1979.

Smart, Mollie S., and Smart, Russell C. *Children.* 3d ed. New York: Macmillan, 1977.

Stillner, Marianne. "Providing Mental Health Services in Rural Alaska." In *Innovations in Community Health Nursing.* Edited by Ann R. Warner. St. Louis: C. V. Mosby Co., 1978.

Thompson, Jacqueline. "Current Nutritional Considerations: Manipulation of the Internal Environment and the Role of the Nurse." In *Nursing Care of the Child With Long Term Illness.* 2d ed. Edited by Shirley Steele. New York: Appleton-Century-Crofts, 1977.

Top, Franklin, and Wehrle, Paul. *Communicable and Infectious Disease.* 8th ed. St. Louis: C. V. Mosby Co., 1976. pp. 425–434.

Westwick, Jennivieve. "On the Road in Alaska." *American Journal of Nursing* 74 (September 1974): 1674–1675.

CHAPTER EIGHT

A Dysfunctional Family System: School Phobia

ANDREA BRETZ SAVITZ

OVERVIEW

Thirteen-year-old Susan Alaire refuses to attend school. After having two psychiatric consults, one of which recommends Susan's separation from her family, Mrs. Alaire calls a family therapist for help in keeping her child at home. An extensive family history is obtained and the family's problems are identified by each family member. The family therapist notes that Susan has been negatively labeled and that there are several dysfunctional triangles within the family. The therapist begins the process of detriangulation.

CONTENT EMPHASIS

- Dysfunctional family system
- Labeling of a client—at school and at home
- Emotional triangulation
- Family therapy

SETTING

- Family therapist's office

OBJECTIVES

Upon completion of this chapter the student will be able to:

1. Comprehend the family as a system.
2. Describe the interactions between family members using a family systems framework.
3. Categorize dysfunctional family member interactions into emotional triangles.
4. Recognize family communication skills that are free of emotional triangles and negative labeling.
5. Recognize the effectiveness of family therapy as a treatment modality.

DEFINITION OF TERMS

The following terms are used in this case study and should be defined before proceeding:

Child study team
Detriangulation
Dysfunctional family system
Emotional cutoffs
Emotional triangle
Family
Family of origin
Family systems therapy
Labeling
Nodal events
Phobia
Third-party payments

FAMILY ASSESSMENT

A family therapist, Kathleen Werner, R.N., M.A., received a phone call at her office from a potential client, Josephine Alaire, on January 26. Josephine had been referred to Kathleen by one of her previous clients. Josephine stated that she needed immediate help for her thirteen-year-old daughter Susan, who was afraid to return to school. Josephine further explained that a member of the school's child study team had visited their home last week because Susan had not returned to school from Christmas vacation. In an emotional voice, Josephine then said, "The child study team met today and they recommended that Susan should receive residential treatment." After a brief silence, Mrs. Alaire emphatically stated that she and her husband did not want Susan living away from home. Kathleen Werner gave Josephine an appointment for the following evening. She encouraged Josephine to have all members of the Alaire household present for the appointment.

The first family therapy session was attended by Josephine, her husband William, and their two children, Susan, age 13, and Valerie, age 11. After the introductions, Kathleen gave the family the following information:

1. An explanation of the therapist's role.
2. A complete explanation of her professional fee.
3. The predicted length of the therapy sessions.
4. That questions would be asked about the family's history.
5. That a genogram and notes would be taken.
6. That questions would be directed to each family member. Everyone's opinion would be heard. No one was to interrupt another family member.
7. That everyone's opinion of the family problem(s) would be heard.
8. That in the future family members would be given assignments, such as a suggested behavioral change.

Kathleen then began the session by asking how Josephine and William met. She learned that they met shortly after high school while they were students at business school. They married after a year's courtship. Both were nineteen.

The Alaire's had geographically maintained their residence within a few miles from their respective families of origin. They frequently visited both families. At present, they live in a two-bedroom home on a small lot. However, they are constructing a third bedroom so that each child can have a separate room.

William described himself as basically quiet. When he feels stress he likes to be alone either to settle himself down or find a solution. In any case he does not like to talk to anyone when he feels upset. He is comfortable being the primary breadwinner of the family and he prefers to leave disciplining of the girls to his wife.

Josephine explained that she is verbal when she is upset. She stated that she usually wants to find someone who will listen to her. Disciplining is a major stress in her life. She knows that she shouts many empty threats at the girls, such as, "I'll kill you if you do that again." Josephine finds that talking with William is of little value in calming her, since talking either ends in an argument or William leaves the room.

Josephine felt she could not discuss problems with her own family of origin. When asked why, Josephine explained that her parents had recently gone through a stormy divorce after thirty years of marriage. Her father, Frank, had often commented to Josephine that she "could have done more" to keep her parents together. Josephine gradually developed the habit of avoiding the issue when she spoke with either parent. In fact she began to avoid issues altogether.

After a silence, Kathleen asked Josephine if there had ever been anyone in the family with whom she could talk. Josephine responded by saying that at one time she had talked with her mother-in-law. After a pause Josephine went on to say, "I haven't talked to Genevieve in about a year, though. But before that time I would frequently go to Genevieve with my problems. I really admired her."

Josephine then stated that she had attempted to put into practice all of Genevieve's suggestions. Josephine had found, however, that Genevieve's advice concerning the children did not always work, particularly after Susan had started to menstruate a year ago last Christmas. Josephine stated, "parenting a child is different from parenting an adolescent. Genevieve's advice on rearing stopped working altogether. But Genevieve would interfere anyway and I felt undermined by my own mother-in-law."

William was upset by the friction between his wife and his mother. However, he reported that he had never attempted to play "peacemaker." He admitted that secretly he had been hoping that the women would work out their differences. Although he agreed with Josephine's approach to parenting, he had not shared his opinion with his mother. He stated that he had learned early in life that the best way to disagree with his mother was to do it quietly.

Shortly after Josephine's relationship with Genevieve had deteriorated, arguments had become more frequent in the Alaire household. Genevieve's criticism of her daughter-in-law's parenting was reported to Josephine by way of Susan and Valerie. Josephine said that this was when she had started to actively seek her husband's support. But William would not speak with his mother about the friction. Then Josephine stated, "About that time, when I was under so much stress, Susan dropped out of school." After a long pause, Josephine quietly continued, "Then when I thought that nothing else could go wrong, Genevieve stopped speaking to me." The only communications Josephine received from Genevieve came through William, the children, or her father-in-law, Harold.

Kathleen then turned her attention to Valerie and Susan. Although their opinions varied slightly on some topics, Valerie and Susan agreed completely that Genevieve was their favorite grandparent. The other grandparents were described as loving, however they were not "special." When Kathleen asked about Genevieve's "specialness," she was told that Grandma Alaire listened and understood them. They regularly told Genevieve about their home life. Usually this meant that Genevieve heard about the times when Josephine had yelled at the girls, had restricted one of the girls' activities, or had denied one of the girls some desired object. When Josephine did not buy the girls what they wanted, Grandma Alaire would surely purchase it. Consequently, the girls competed with one another for Genevieve's attention. Through the years one way to get Grandma's attention had been to phone her and explain the gripe to her. Grandma Alaire would often come right over to tell Josephine just what to do.

STUDY QUESTIONS

8-1. What is a school child study team? What purpose does it serve?

8-2. What disciplines are usually represented on a child study team?

8-3. What is a family therapist? How are they trained? From what mental health disciplines do family therapists usually come?

8-4. Why did Kathleen Werner take a family history before asking about the problem(s) in the family?

8-5. What information is needed before the family therapist can design a plan of care?

8-6. Due to the complexity of families, family therapists often want to audiotape or videotape the family therapy sessions. If Kathleen had wanted to videotape or audiotape, what would she have required from the Alaire's? What explanation could she have given to the family?

8-7. Can a family therapist apply family systems theory to an individual entering into therapy alone? Explain.

8-8. How long should the first family therapy session take? What should be covered?

DISCUSSION QUESTIONS

D-1. Compare (1) family therapy systems theory, (2) psychoanalytical theory, and (3) behaviorist theory. How are they different?

D-2. What is the rationale for each of the items explained to the Alaire family before the therapy session started?

Item	Rationale
1. Fee	
2. Length of session	
3. Family history	
4. Notes—genogram	
5. Direction of questions	
6. Role of therapist	
7. All opinions heard	
8. Assignments	

CLIENT ASSESSMENT

When Kathleen believed she had gotten enough information on the family as a whole, she turned the Alaire's attention to their perception of the problem. All family members, including Susan, labeled Susan the "sick" one. Kathleen asked William how Susan had come to be labeled sick. William thought for a moment and then said, "My mother was the first person to call Susan 'sick'... Valerie has been calling Susan 'crazy'." Then Kathleen asked Susan how she had earned the labels "sick" and "crazy." Looking a bit startled, Susan said, "I am afraid to go to school."

"Josephine," Kathleen questioned, "what led up to Susan's present situation?" Josephine related that Susan's first prolonged school absence occurred after the Easter break at the local public school last year. "Oh," Kathleen said, "Was there anything unusual about the Easter holiday?" William interjected, "Things were terrible.... We had always been a close family.... My parents had always enjoyed spending holidays with us...." Josephine picked up on William's line of thinking, "Genevieve and I could not seem to find anything to talk about... You could have cut the tension with a knife."

"Then, you say, Susan dropped out of school?" questioned Kathleen. "Yes," said Josephine, "I could not understand it... I still don't... Susan is an excellent student." William stated that they tried everything to end Susan's absenteeism. Coaxing, bribing, and pushing Susan did not work. Susan would become "hysterical" and she would insist on going back to bed for most of the day.

"Finally," Josephine stated, "the child study team at the school referred Susan to Dr. Vega for a psychiatric evaluation." Josephine then handed copies of the reports to Kathleen. Josephine stated, "I signed for copies of these child study team reports this morning at the school. I hope they make sense to you... William and I could only understand parts of the reports."

Report 1 was based on four evaluation sessions conducted by Juan Vega, M.D. Three sessions were attended by Josephine, William, and Susan. The fourth session was also attended by Genevieve. The impression and recommendation section found in the report read as follows:

Consultant: Juan Vega, M.D. (Psychiatrist)

Identified Patient: Susan Alaire

Age: 12 years

Address: 39 Oak Road
                Merryheart, Ca. 09738

Date(s):   4/25; 4/26; 4/29; 5/1

Impression: Susan is a severe school-phobic adolescent. An intense emotional triangle exists in the family consisting of Susan's mother, father, and paternal grandmother.

Recommendation: Force is not to be used to facilitate Susan's return to school.

Based on Juan Vega's report, the school system provided Susan a home tutor for the remainder of the school year. Therefore, when Susan returned to school in September, she was allowed to enter the eighth grade.

Kathleen sought clarification from Josephine, "After you had been so unsuccessful last spring, how did you convince Susan to return to school last September?" Josephine answered. "I did not have to convince her... I just enrolled her in a new school at Susan's request. When Susan started school at St. Anne's Academy last fall, William and I thought that her problem was over." Josephine continued by saying that when Susan refused to reenter school after last month's Christmas break, William and she had felt helpless.

Kathleen asked if this past holiday was as upsetting as last Easter. William stated softly that this past Christmas had been the first major holiday without the traditional family gathering. Genevieve had refused to go to "Josephine's house." Josephine was having progressively more difficulty disciplining Susan and Valerie. Everyone in the house was screaming at each other. The holiday had been generally unpleasant.

St. Anne's Academy notified the public school system of Susan's absenteeism. After Susan's physical well being was established by the Alaire's pediatrician, the child study team started another evaluation. The team referred Susan to Joel Marcus, M.D., for a second psychiatric evaluation.

Kathleen noted that the impression and recommendation sections found in the second psychiatric opinion read as follows:

Consultant: Joel Marcus, M.D. (Psychiatrist)

Identified Patient: Susan Alaire

Age: 13 years

Address: 39 Oak Road
Merryheart, Ca. 09738

Date(s):   1/18

Impression: I believe Susan to have much deeper pathology than presented in a school phobia. However I reserve diagnostic classification of Susan pending a suggested comprehensive psychological workup.

Recommendation: Residential treatment should be considered.

Josephine was very upset by Joel Marcus's recommendation. Kathleen asked the other members of the family what they thought about the Joel Marcus report. William, Susan, and Valerie were also upset by the recommendation. It was obvious that the entire family was against residential treatment for Susan.

Before Kathleen ended the first session she gave the family some feedback. She started by asking a nondirected question, "With so many people in the family as tense as Susan, how did Susan become the only one called sick?" Without waiting for someone to think up an answer, Kathleen started to talk again. This time she asked each one of the Alaire's, "Who is the most sensitive to his/her immediate family member's emotions?" Each believed that Susan was very sensitive to everyone within the family.

STUDY QUESTIONS

8-9. Why did Kathleen ask each family member for his or her preception of the Alaire's family problem(s)?

8-10. Why is negative labeling of a family member dysfunctional?

8-11. What is the difference between a neurotic and a psychotic family system?

Family system characteristics	Neurotic	Psychotic
Roles of members Power structure Copying behaviors Functions of family Patterns of communications Support systems		

8-12. Is the Alaire family system neurotic or psychotic? How do you know?

DISCUSSION QUESTIONS

D-3. Why didn't Kathleen wait for an answer to the question: "With so many people in the family as tense as Susan, how did Susan become the only one called sick?".

D-4. Under what theoretical approach to therapy do you believe Juan Vega, M.D. practices? Why? Joel Marcus, M.D.? Why?

D-5. If Kathleen did not focus her attention on Susan, but spent an equal amount of time looking at the various family members, what would be her purpose?

D-6. What other forms of nonverbal behavior could be helpful when interacting with a dysfunctional family?

FAMILY SYSTEM ASSESSMENT

Kathleen explained during the first session that the behavior of one family member is influenced by the way other family members behave. For example, if a husband comes home and hugs his wife while saying, "Hello," her reaction to him will be quite different from times he has entered the house and immediately criticized the odor of the cooking dinner. Consequently, all members of a family system are participants in the development of their own behavior and other family members' behaviors. Therefore, if one family member has socially unacceptable behavior, the problem exists within the family system; the member of the family having the deviant behavior is only part of the problem. Behaviors are not seen as isolated events in one person's life.

Kathleen went on to relate that most family therapists believe that blame, guilt, and/or labeling are nonproductive. The important step is to recognize that, in order for any family member to change, family member interactions must also change. The change can be started by any individual in the family system. "In any case," Kathleen continued, "the largest challenge a person can face is making a change in oneself."

When the Alaire family left, Kathleen initiated a data base record and documented what had occurred. The record included a family genogram (see genogram), a list of the family's nodal events,[1] and a list of the family's emotional triangles. The nodal events were recorded in the order of their occurrence.

NODAL EVENTS

Susan and Valerie's Childhood: Over-closeness of paternal grandmother.
Four Years Ago: End of Josephine's parents' marriage.
Christmas Last School Year: Marked entry of Susan's adolescence (menses).
   Josephine ceased accepting parenting advice from Genevieve.
April Last School Year: Susan refused reentry to public school.
June Last School Year: Genevieve stopped speaking to Josephine.
Summer: Increased arguments between Josephine and William.
September This School Year: Susan reentered school (St. Anne's Academy).
Christmas This School Year: Absence of paternal grandparents at Christmas celebrations.
   Susan refused reentry to Catholic school.
January Present: Recommendation for consideration by the child study team for placement of Susan in residential treatment center. Entry of family into family therapy.

Kathleen then listed her impression of the most toxic emotional triangles in the Alaire family. Starting with the most important triangle, Kathleen drew the chart shown on page 115.
Kathleen then made her nursing diagnoses and planned for the next session.

STUDY QUESTIONS

8-13. Why do many family system therapists believe that blame, guilt and/or labeling are nonproductive in families and family therapy?

8-14. Why is it helpful for a therapist to list nodal events in their order of occurrence?

8-15. How does an emotional triangle work according to Thomas Fogarty? according to Murray Bowen? How are Fogarty's and Bowen's conceptualizations of the working of an emotional triangle alike? different?

8-16. Why is it helpful for a therapist to diagram a family's emotional triangles?

[1]Philip J. Guerin, Jr. *Family Therapy* (New York: Gardner Press, Inc. 1976). P. 455.

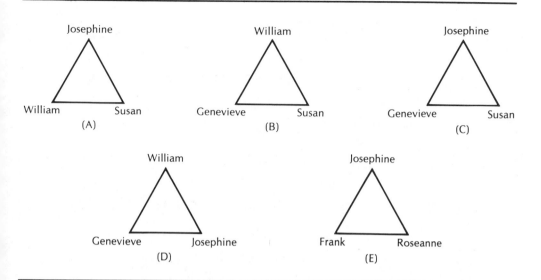

8-17. Why does Thomas Fogarty believe that all emotional triangles are dysfunctional?

8-18. What do you think was Kathleen's rationale for listing the triangles in the order that she used?

DISCUSSION QUESTIONS

D-7. What is the significance of the nodal events in the Alaire family?

D-8. What is the significance of the emotional triangles in the Alaire family?

D-9. Based on the data collected by Kathleen, list nursing diagnosis(es) she could have given the Alaire family. Why?

IDENTIFICATION AND TREATMENT OF DYSFUNCTION

Since triangulation is always a dysfunctional communication,[2] Kathleen explained emotional triangles to the Alaires during the second therapy session. Kathleen used data collected in the Alaire family's first therapy session to derive examples of triangles. She explained that almost every time that Susan was involved in an emotional triangle, Susan would behave in what the family called a "sensitive" or "sick" way. Susan often reacted to arguments or ill feelings between two other family members. When Susan's behavior drew the attention of two family members, their arguments were forgotten without being resolved. Susan would become the third angle of a triangle. The tension between the two arguing people would transfer to Susan, to a degree. The

[2]Thomas Fogarty, "Triangles." *The Family* 2 (February 1975): 11.

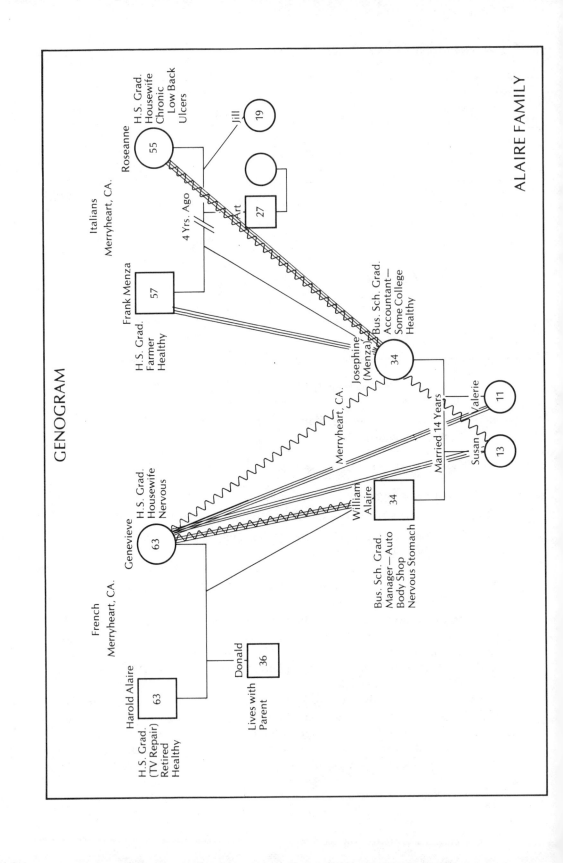

GENOGRAM

ALAIRE FAMILY

two family members who stopped the argument before they resolved their disagreement were and are ready to fight about the same issue another time.

With Susan and Valerie temporarily out of the session, Kathleen Werner mapped out a plan of action that was acceptable to Mr. and Mrs. Alaire. Kathleen then assigned behavioral changes that were designed to start de-triangulation of the William-Josephine-Susan triangle. William was put in complete charge of Valerie and Susan when he was at home. Josephine was instructed to pull out of her disciplinary role whenever William was present. Only William could ask Josephine for an opinion. Major decisions involving the girls were to be William's responsibility.

William and Josephine then remarked on the simplicity of their assignments. Kathleen responded by predicting that they would not have an easy time. Finally, she instructed William and Josephine that they could not criticize the progress of each other. Each was only to monitor his or her own success or failure. Then Kathleen gained written permission from William to contact the principal of St. Anne's Academy, and the therapy session ended.

Only William and Josephine attended the next family therapy session. With some basic guidelines on discipline given by Kathleen, William had progressed as disciplinarian. However he stated that he disliked the role. At the same time Josephine was feeling a bit lost without her old role as disciplinarian. However, she did remark that she did not miss the disciplinary fights she had had with her daughters. Both Josephine and William were avoiding the label of "sick," for Susan.

Kathleen, therefore, believed that they had progressed enough to discuss the next step in the plan of care. She told the Alaires that she had spoken to Sister Linda, the principal at St. Anne's Academy. The Alaire family case had been reviewed. The school was willing to accept Susan's return the following week, even if Susan was hysterical.

The Alaires looked shocked. They asked how they could get Susan back to school, since they had always failed in the past. At that point Kathleen reviewed with them everything that Susan had done in the past to keep from going to school. Susan had used crying spells, screaming sessions, refusals to get dressed, rolling on the floor, hanging on to the door jamb, and even fake convulsions. When these behaviors failed, Susan would phone Genevieve with physical complaints.

Kathleen worked out some alternative behaviors that the Alaires could use when Susan resisted reentry to school. Kathleen gently reminded William that he had successfully been in charge of Susan for two weeks, and that he was a physically strong man. She went on to say that William could carry Susan to the car if necessary. Sister Linda was fully aware that Susan might arrive at school in her pajamas. William would bring Susan's uniform to school as well. The only request that Sister Linda made was to know the exact date that Susan would reenter school.

William and Josephine agreed to the plan. They decided that Wednesday would be school reentry day and that they would take Susan early so that her classmates would not see her arrival, in case it was stormy.

STUDY QUESTIONS

8-19. What is detriangulation and how can a therapist assist a family to detriangulate?

8-20. Why was it necessary to obtain written parental permission to contact St. Anne's Academy?

8-21. Outline some disciplinary guidelines that could help William to deal with Susan and Valerie.

8-22. Why were the Alaire parents cautioned to monitor their own progress and not their spouse's progress?

DISCUSSION QUESTIONS

D-10. Susan is no longer frequently being labeled as sick. What bearing does this information have on the Josephine-William-Susan triangle?

D-11. Why did Kathleen choose to assist the family to detriangulate the William-Josephine-Susan triangle first?

D-12. Why did Kathleen wait until a later session to give the parents instruction about Susan's return to school?

FOLLOW-UP CARE

Josephine, William, Susan, and Valerie were present at the fifth family therapy session. Half of the session was given to the entire family, and the other half was held with only Josephine and William. Susan looked like a different person. She sat more erect, looked slimmer and prettier. She was back in school.

When alone with Kathleen, the parents reported on February 22, the day of Susan's reentry to school. William had needed help. He requested Josephine's assistance. Susan had tried every tactic that had worked in the past to prevent school reentry. However, when William stated that, if necessary, he would carry her to school screaming in her pajamas, Susan calmed down and got dressed. That evening, Susan told her parents that she was happy to be back in school.

Now Kathleen knew that the family members were ready for one of the major challenges in family therapy. She would teach them how to recognize emotional triangles without her assistance. Further, Kathleen would continue to assist the Alaire's to develop direct communications between family members. When two family members had an issue to discuss, Kathleen would encourage the members to discuss the issue alone. Another member of the family was not to interfere. In other words, Kathleen would support the detriangulation of all the emotional triangles within the family.

STUDY QUESTION

8-23. Prepare a teaching plan for the Alaires on the following items:

Item	Goals	Objectives	Content	Evaluation of learning (method and criteria)
Communications				
Triangulation				
Labeling				

CHAPTER STUDY QUESTIONS

1. What is the developmental task(s) of a young adolescent?
2. Can Kathleen collect third-party payment for her professional services in your home state?
3. Is there federal legislation on professional nursing in regard to collecting third-party payments?

CHAPTER DISCUSSION QUESTIONS

1. Why does Kathleen consider the development of one-to-one communication important in the Alaire family?
2. Is the diagnosis "school-phobic adolescent" compatible with family systems theory?
3. Josephine's family of origin is Italian and William's family of origin is French. From a cultural standpoint, how could Genevieve's and Josephine's basic beliefs on discipline differ?
4. If you were to choose to practice professional nursing privately, how would you go about setting your fee for service? Explain.

SUGGESTED ACTIVITIES

1. Visit a family therapy postgraduate training institute. Ask:
    a. From what disciplines do they accept trainees?
    b. How are trainees supervised?
    c. How long is the training program?
    d. What is the minimal educational degree(s) that a trainee must hold?
    e. Does the institute certify its trainees? If so, by what power?
    f. What mental health disciplines are represented on the faculty?

2. Interview a trained family therapist in any of the major mental health disciplines (that is, a psychiatrist, a social worker, a psychologist, a nurse, a clergyman).

   a. Where did he or she train?
   b. What are the characteristics of most of his or her clientele?
   c. What is the most frequent problem encountered?
   d. Does he or she receive third-party payment?
   e. How are clients referred to him or her?
   f. What is the therapist's conceptual frame of the family?

3. Interview the head of a child study team. Ask:

   a. What disciplines are represented on the team?
   b. What is the function of the team?
   c. What is the ratio of team members to students?
   d. From the time of referral, how long must a child wait before a work-up is begun?

4. Investigate the curriculum of your nursing program and a nearby graduate nursing program. What content is given on:

   a. Families   c. Family systems
   b. Family therapy   d. Family systems theory

BIBLIOGRAPHY

Fogarty, Thomas. "Triangles." *The Family* 2 (1975): 11–19.

Guerin, Philip J., Jr., ed. *Family Therapy.* New York: Gardner Press, Inc., 1976.

Haller, Linda Lacey. "Family Systems Theory in Psychiatric Intervention." *American Journal of Nursing* 74 (March 1974): 462–463.

Hymovich, Debra P., and Barnard, Martha Underwood. "The School-aged Child with His Family." In *Family Health Care.* New York: McGraw-Hill Book Company, 1973.

Kalkman, Marion E., and Davis, Anne J. *New Dimensions in Mental Health— Psychiatric Nursing.* 4th ed. New York: McGraw-Hill Book Company, 1974.

Murray, Ruth, and Zentner, Judith. "Assessment and Health Promotion for the School Child." In *Nursing Concepts for Health Promotion.* Englewood Cliffs, New Jersey: Prentice-Hall Inc., 1975.

Paul, Norman L., and Grosser, George H. "Operational Mourning and its Role in Conjoint Family Therapy." *Community Mental Health Journal* 1 (Winter 1965): 339–345.

Pendagast, Eileen G., and Sherman, Charles O. "A Guide to the Genogram Family Systems Training." *The Family* 5 (1978): 3–14.

Smoyak, Shirley, ed. *The Psychiatric Nurse as a Family Therapist.* New York: John Wiley & Sons, Inc., 1975, pp. 1–10, 141–148.

CHAPTER NINE

The Sexually Assaulted Adolescent: Rape

CYNTHIA DEGAZON

OVERVIEW

Letticia Almond, a fourteen-year-old junior high school student, is sexually assaulted in the park near her home. Her outraged mother notifies the police and drives Letticia to the local hospital. Besides the usual physical emergency room care, Letticia's immediate emotional trauma is treated and her follow-up care is planned by a sex counselor. The necessary legal specimens are collected by the police department's rape investigator.

CONTENT EMPHASIS

- Assessing and treating the physical and emotional trauma of rape
- Legal implications—recording data and collecting specimens
- Prevention of sexual assault

SETTING

- Emergency room

OBJECTIVES

Upon completion of this chapter the student will be able to:

1. Analyze the physical and psychological trauma experienced by rape victims.

2. Comprehend the legal ramifications of accurate specimen collection and documentation of data.

3. Create a plan of intervention based upon expected health outcomes.

4. Explain the function of emergency rooms in the delivery of health care to rape victims and their families.

5. Analyze society's approach to rape as a community health problem.

DEFINITION OF TERMS

The following terms are used in this case study and should be defined before proceeding:

ABO grouping	Serology tests
Complete blood count (CBC)	Sex counsellor
Gonorrhea culture (G.C.)	Sexual assault
Pedophilia	Statutory rape
Rape	Triage nurse
	Woods lamp

FAMILY ASSESSMENT

Letticia Almond is an attractive, fourteen-year-old black girl. She is 143 cm tall, of medium build, and weighs 54.4 kg. She has already reached puberty. She has maturing physical development and she has had a regular menstrual cycle for one year. She attends a coeducational Orange County public school and is in the eighth grade. Her teacher states that she is well liked by her classmates and that she is a serious student who performs well academically.

Letticia lives in a small frame house with three bedrooms, one bath, a living room and a family-size kitchen owned by her maternal grandmother, Rosa Peters. The houses in this section of Orange County are built on less than a quarter acre of land. The home is shared by Letticia, her mother Margaret, an older sister Sarah, a younger brother James, and her grandmother. Her father died four years ago in an automobile accident. Prior to his death, Mr. William Almond was in the process of establishing his own electrical repair shop. Financially, he was just managing the day-to-day family expenses and could not afford the minimum insurance coverage for his family's protection. Consequently, he had no life insurance.

The Almonds were married soon after they graduated from high school. They had their first daughter, Sarah, before their first anniversary. Mrs. Almond was a busy homemaker; she was ill prepared for employment following her husband's death. When he died, Mrs. Almond was faced with the

GENOGRAM

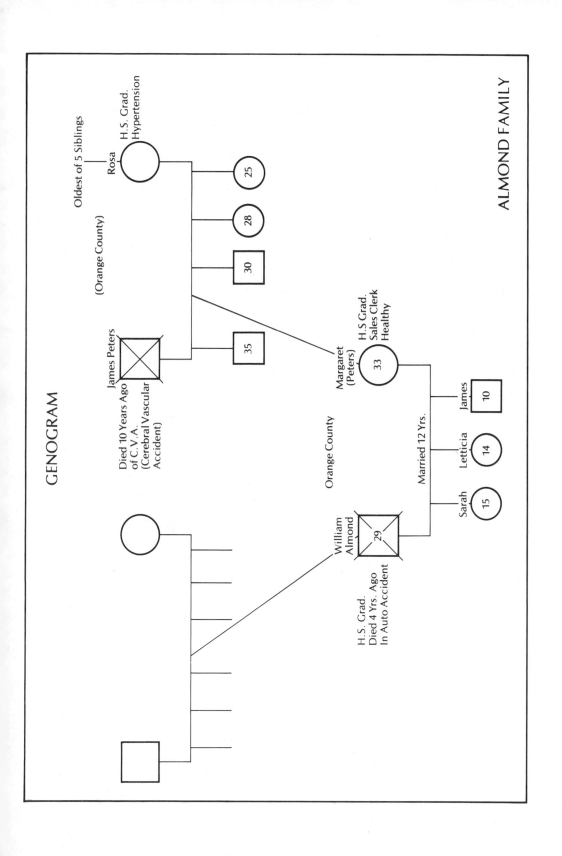

Oldest of 5 Siblings

Rosa
H.S. Grad.
Hypertension

(Orange County)

James Peters

Died 10 Years Ago
of C.V.A.
(Cerebral Vascular
Accident)

25

28

30

35

Margaret
(Peters)
H.S Grad.
Sales Clerk
Healthy

33

William
Almond

Orange County

H.S. Grad.
Died 4 Yrs. Ago
In Auto Accident

29

Married 12 Yrs.

Sarah
15

Letticia
14

James
10

ALMOND FAMILY

total responsibility for the care and financial support of her family. She decided to decrease expenses by accepting Rosa's invitation to combine households. Margaret moved her entire family to her mother's house and found a job as a sales clerk in a nearby department store. After three months of service Margaret was given the company paid benefit of Blue Cross and Blue Shield health insurance for herself and her family.

Letticia's school was a fifteen-minute walk from home and there was a beautiful floral park on the way. During the fall, when the afternoon was warm, Letticia would stop in the park after school to admire the colorful foliage. Frequently she would sit on her favorite bench and begin her homework assignment. Occasionally she would just sit and enjoy the beauty around her before going home. Since most of her classmates lived closer to school, she often had to walk through the park alone.

STUDY QUESTION

9-1. What is the normal development of a fourteen-year-old girl? How does Letticia compare to the normal fourteen-year-old?

DEVELOPMENT

Type	Normal 14-year-old girl	Letticia
Physical characteristics		
Secondary sex characteristics		
Psychological-emotional		
Sociologic a: with peers b: with family		

DISCUSSION QUESTION

D-1. In the event of stress, what support systems are available to Letticia?

SEXUAL ASSAULT

At 3:15 P.M. on October 7, Letticia arrived in the park and sat on her favorite bench. After spending a few minutes admiring the beauty around her, she opened her books and began her studies. Suddenly an assailant's hands were around her throat. The man was throttling her neck and Letticia found herself unable to scream and barely able to gasp for air. She groped toward the hands around her neck to loosen their grip, but to no avail.

"I'm not going to hurt you, if you do what I tell you," uttered her assailant threateningly. No one was in sight. The man commanded her to walk toward a cluster of trees a few yards away. Letticia moved hesitatingly. Her assailant pushed her forward roughly. When his grip loosened, Letticia asked in a quiet, fearful voice, "Who are you and what do you want?" He responded, "I ask the questions, you do as you are told." At this time Letticia turned around and saw that her assailant was a white man of medium height and average build, in his middle twenties. Letticia did not recognize him.

Suddenly the man screamed, "What is your name, girl?"

"Letticia," she mumbled.

"Letticia, honey, you're an awfully pretty girl with a nice, round bottom. I mean to have you. . . . "

She cringed, pulling her coat closer to her body and searching for a way to escape. She trembled and could not believe this was happening. She saw no way to escape from him. The attacker continued to push Letticia until they reached the center of a wooded area.

"Take your clothes off!" he exclaimed.

She began to slowly unbutton her coat. He ripped off her coat and slapped her across the face, yelling, "I told you to take off your clothes, woman!" Still not complying with his command, Letticia was slapped again and tears began to stream down her face as he threw her to the ground and pulled up her skirt. He quickly opened his pants with one hand while he tore off her underpants with the other hand. Letticia bit her lips as she uttered, "Dear God, please let me live." She struggled to cross her legs, but was overpowered by her attacker.

When he had finished with her, he slapped her across the face. "You'd be wise not to talk, lady. I know more about you than you think and I'll get you." He hurriedly pulled his clothes about him as he ran off into the woods. Letticia lay on the ground, crying as she tried to think of what to do. Finally, she wrapped her coat around her, picked up her underwear, and ran blindly toward home.

STUDY QUESTIONS

9-2. What are some of the common characteristics of rape victims?

9-3. What are some of the psychosocial theories concerning rape?

9-4. Describe the environment that a rapist often selects for a sexual assault.

9-5. What age groups are most prone to being raped? Why?

9-6. How does a rapist select his victim?

9-7. What are some characteristics of a rapist who would select an adolescent, such as Letticia, for a victim?

DISCUSSION QUESTION

D-2. What preventive measures could Letticia have taken to protect herself from rape?

LETTICIA'S AND HER FAMILY'S REACTION

As Letticia reached home, in a state of shock, she ran past her grandmother Rosa, who was in the yard, and dashed into the house looking for her mother. Mrs. Peters suspected something was wrong and followed Letticia through the house. Mrs. Peters kept questioning Letticia but her granddaughter would not respond.

Mrs. Almond had felt closer to her children since her husband's death, and the children felt closer to their only surviving parent. Communication had always been open and truthful. Mrs. Almond had shared the information she had about menstruation with her daughters and Letticia knew her mother to be a person from whom she could obtain help and support.

It was Mrs. Almond's day off from work and she was sitting on the bed sewing when Letticia came into the room. She noticed the expression of fear on her daughter's face, her swollen eyes, the perspiration rolling down from her face and her disheveled appearance. She was also breathing hard. Mrs. Almond dropped her sewing and exclaimed, "My God, what happened to you?" Letticia ran into her mother's arms and began to sob. Her grandmother, observing the scene from the doorway, asked in an anxious but caring voice, "Are you hurt?" Letticia did not respond, but continued crying. With her arm still around Letticia, her mother asked, "Did you fall? You must tell me what happened."

"He hurt me," Letticia responded.

"What do you mean? Were you in a fight?"

Mrs. Peters remained in the room, looking very tense with her hands grasping her face. Letticia replied, "No. He pushed me on the ground and climbed on top of me."

After a short silence, Mrs. Almond screamed, "Oh, my God. No! No! No!" Feeling her daughter's hurt, the stunned Mrs. Almond, began to explode with rage.

With tears running down her face, Mrs. Peters stretched her hands to the ceiling and shouted, "I'll kill him if I catch him, I'll kill him." After a brief silence she turned to Margaret and said, "Call the police. Tell them to arrest him."

Mrs. Almond was so intent on her daughter's condition that she did not hear her mother's direction. Mrs. Almond began to wipe the tears away from Letticia's face and led Letticia on to the bed where she wrapped her daughter in clean warm blankets. Mrs. Almond kept repeating to Letticia, "It will be alright, everything will be alright."

Still under stress, Letticia related the incident to her mother and grandmother. Both Mrs. Almond and her grandmother listened to what Letticia told them with tears in their eyes. Mrs. Almond told Letticia that she was going to take her to the doctor. Letticia said that she did not want to leave the house, nor did she want to see anyone. She just wanted to take a shower, take some aspirin, and go to bed. Mrs. Almond persisted. Letticia agreed to see a doctor. Mrs. Almond dissuaded her daughter from taking a shower because she remembered hearing something on TV about not bathing in rape cases.

Mrs. Almond called Letticia's pediatrician. His answering service informed her that the doctor was on vacation, but that another physician was covering. Unfortunately, the covering physician could not be reached. In disgust, she called the local police department. Within fifteen minutes a policeman responded to the call. At the Almond's home the policeman called the emergency room at the community hospital to notify them that he was bringing an "alleged rape victim" to the hospital. He also notified the investigator working in the Sex Crime Analysis Unit (SCAU). The policeman suggested to Mrs. Almond that she bring a change of clothing to the hospital for Letticia.

STUDY QUESTIONS

9-8.   Would Letticia's reaction to the rape differ if she had known her rapist? Why?

9-9.   What are the most common physical complaints of sexual assault victims?

9-10. Why was it an appropriate response when Mrs. Almond told her daughter not to shower?

9-11. Why did the police say "alleged rape victim?"

9-12. Why should Letticia wear the clothes that she wore during the rape to the hospital? Why should she take a change of clothes with her?

9-13. Why didn't Letticia want to leave the house?

9-14. Why would Mrs. Almond call the pediatrician before calling the police?

DISCUSSION QUESTIONS

D-3.   What is the difference between the reaction of an adult and the reaction of a child to rape? Explain.

D-4. What impact could rape have on the psychological development of an adolescent girl? How could it affect her social development?

D-5. Discuss Mrs. Almond's reaction to the knowledge that her daughter was raped. What other types of reaction could be displayed by family members of rape victims?

EMERGENCY ROOM

Letticia was taken to the emergency room of a large voluntary hospital nearby. Upon arrival, the police officer took the family to the triage nurse. Ms. Elsie Benson, R.N. escorted the family to a private room where she performed a cursory physical assessment on Letticia. Her findings included the following:

BP: 130/80

Pulse: 90

Resp.:   25

Temp.:   36°C (99°F)

HEENT: swollen face and lips.

Skin: Bruises on the thighs, chest, elbows, and neck.

The hospital's sex counselor, Ms. Goodhart, R.N., was notified of the family's arrival and came to the ER. She worked with sexually assaulted victims and their families. Her role was to ensure that the physical and emotional needs of sexual assault victims were identified and provided for in a therapeutic manner.

Ms. Goodhart introduced herself and described her role to the family. She then escorted Letticia to a private room while Mrs. Almond remained in the triage area to give identifying data and permission for Letticia's care. When Mrs. Almond finished, she requested to join Letticia. By this time, Letticia's anxiety was less visible. She had been informed of the hospital's protocol for handling rape victims and what would be happening to her in the emergency room.

The police investigator arrived and joined the group. Ms. Goodhart began her interview by asking both Letticia and her mother how they were feeling. Letticia said that she was afraid and had pain "in the belly." The nurse responded by saying "Do you know why you are afraid?" Letticia replied, "Yes."

Ms. Goodhart said, "Can you tell me why?"

Letticia held her head down, looking very embarrassed. After a pause, Mrs. Almond suggested that she tell the nurse what had happened, so that the nurse could help her.

Letticia told her story from the time she arrived in the park until she reached home. When Letticia neglected to give details, Mrs. Almond would encourage her to think harder. Letticia was able to give a brief description of her assailant to the investigator.

For legal reasons the counselor carefully documented all verbal and non-verbal observations. Ms. Goodhart learned that Letticia had not been sexually active before the incident. (Refer to Assessment Guide, Appendix G).

Patricia Brown, M.D., an obstetrical/gynecological resident, arrived in the ER to complete the physical assessment, prescribe laboratory tests, and implement a medical plan for treatment. Mrs. Almond was allowed to remain with her daughter during the physical examination. Dr. Brown explained to Letticia and her mother what the examination would entail. She explained that she would be gentle and would explain each step. Letticia began to relax somewhat.

Dr. Brown prescribed the following work-up:

G.C. culture

Vaginal smear and washing

Two additional vaginal smears for police

Serology

Pregnancy test

CBC

Sperm—ABO grouping

Obtain pubic hair combings and fingernail scrapings

The following specimens were given directly to the police investigator, who remained outside the room during the physical examination:

Pubic hair combings and fingernail scrapings

Client's clothes

Vaginal smear studies

Dr. Brown noted that Letticia had much tenderness during the vaginal examination. The vulva was swollen and a 2 cm vaginal laceration was noted and repaired. A prescription for Darvon 65 mg po STAT and q 4 h PRN was written for Letticia.

Ms. Goodhart gave the Almonds her telephone number and told them they were welcome to call should they need to talk, or if there were any problems. The telephone number and address of the local crisis center were also given to them. Ms. Goodhart also stated that she would telephone the family. Before the Almonds left the emergency room, Letticia's mother decided to sign the necessary papers to institute court proceedings.

STUDY QUESTIONS

9-15. Why did the triage nurse perform only a brief physical assessment?

9-16. Who can give consent for treatment of an adolescent rape victim in your state? Why?

9-17. What documents did Mrs. Almond have to sign?

9-18. What are the nursing care objectives for Letticia in the ER? List them in order of priority. What is the rationale for each and how are the objectives achieved?

Objective	Rationale	Nursing actions

9-19. What are the normal results of the following tests and why did Letticia have each test? (see Appendix G)

Test	Normal results	Reason for test being performed on Letticia
G. C. culture		
Vaginal smear and washing		
Oral smear		
Rectal smear		
Serology		
Pregnancy test (specify)		
CBC		
ABO grouping and Rh		
Pubic hair comb		
Fingernail scrapings		

9-20. Why were the specimens given to the sex crime police investigator?

9-21. Why was the investigator permitted in the room with the counselor?

9-22. If the investigator was not present in the ER, whose responsibility would it be to transport the specimens to the pathologist? Why?

9-23. Complete a drug information card on Darvon.

9-24. Why is it important for the nurse to record all verbal and nonverbal observations during the interview?

DISCUSSION QUESTIONS

D-6. What support could the sex counselor offer Letticia? Letticia's mother?

D-7. Penicillin was not prescribed for Letticia. State possible reasons for this decision. What specific information should be given to Letticia and Mrs. Almond regarding this decision?

D-8. Why should Letticia be more carefully prepared for a vaginal exam than most clients?

CHAPTER STUDY QUESTIONS

1. Develop a nursing care plan for the Almond family that would include:
   a. Agency referrals
   b. Frequency of telephone and home visit follow-up
   c. Assessment of psychological adjustment
   d. A plan to meet the client's needs for emotional support
   e. Family adjustment.

2. Letticia's family is headed by a female. What are the possible implications for the nurse who is counseling this victim?

3. What predictable postrape patterns could Letticia show? What adjustment period would one expect Letticia to have? Why?

4. What is the rationale for keeping statistics on rape victims?

5. On what should the nurse counsel rape victims in regard to reporting the crime. Why?

CHAPTER DISCUSSION QUESTIONS

1. What are some of the physical and psychobiological sequelae that can develop in postrape clients? why? How can they be treated?

Sequelae	Possible reasons	Treatment

2. How can rape be prevented? What should potential rape victims be told?
3. How can a nurse assist society in preventing rape?
4. To what agencies in your community could a victim of sexual assault be referred?

SUGGESTED ACTIVITIES

1. Develop a plan on rape prevention appropriate for a school nurse to discuss with high-school students.
2. Visit a crisis center. Discuss the role of the counselor. Discuss the follow-up protocol.
3. Complete an assessment on a rape victim. (See Appendix G for assessment form.)
4. Visit the prosecutor's office and find out the legalities of rape prosecution in your state.
5. Attend a court hearing on rape.
6. Visit a police rape squad. What functions do they perform?

BIBLIOGRAPHY

Bergersen, Betty. *Pharmacology in Nursing.* 13th ed. St. Louis: C. V. Mosby Co., 1976.

Burgess, Ann C., and Holmstrom, Lynda L. "The Rape Victim in the Emergency Ward." *American Journal of Nursing* 73 (October 1973): 1740–1745.

––––––. "Assessing Trauma in the Rape Victim." *American Journal of Nursing* 75 (August 1975): 1288–1291.

––––––. *Rape: Victims of Crisis.* Bowie, Maryland: Robert J. Brady Co., 1974, pp. 37–66, 120–151.

Burgess, Ann W., and Laszlo, Anna T. "Courtroom Use of Hospital Records in Sexual Assault Cases." *American Journal of Nursing* 77 (January 1977): 64–68.

Clark, Terri Patrice. "Primary Health Care: Counseling Victims of Rape." *American Journal of Nursing* 76 (December 1976): 1964–1966.

Garb, Solomon. *Laboratory Tests in Common Use.* 6th ed. New York: Springer Publishing Co., 1976.

Goldstein, Bernard. *Human Sexuality.* New York: McGraw Hill, 1976, pp. 252–258.

Jacques, G. "Cultural Health Traditions: A Black Perspective." In *Providing Safe Nursing Care for Ethnic People of Color.* Edited by Marie Foster Branch and Phyllis Perry Paxton. New York: Appleton-Century-Crofts, 1976.

Little, Dolores E., and Carnevali, Doris L. *Nursing Care Planning,* 2d. ed. Philadelphia: J. B. Lippincott Co., 1976.

Malasanos, Lois et al. *Health Assessment.* St. Louis: C. V. Mosby Co., 1978.

Pendagast, Eileen G., and Sherman, Charles O. "A Guide to the Genogram Family Systems Training." *The Family* 5 (1978): 3–14.

Petrillo, Madeline, and Sanger, Sirgay. "A Working Knowledge of Childhood." In *Emotional Care of Hospitalized Children.* Philadelphia: J. B. Lippincott Co., 1972, pp. 19–33.

Roach, Lora B. "Assessment: Color Changes in Dark Skin." *Nursing '77* 7 (January 1977): 48–51.

Scipien, Gladys. *Comprehensive Pediatric Nursing.* New York: McGraw-Hill, 1975, pp. 705–711.

Woods, Nancy Fugate. *Human Sexuality in Health and Illness.* St. Louis: C. V. Mosby Co., 1975, pp. 95–107.

CHAPTER TEN

High Risk Adolescent Pregnancy: Preeclampsia

LINDA K. HARRISON

OVERVIEW

Theresa Paradour is a fifteen-year-old daughter of a Mexican-American migrant family. While in her second trimester of pregnancy, this unmarried adolescent seeks medical assistance at a clinic for migrant workers. Theresa's pregnancy is complicated by preeclampsia during her last trimester. Her labor and delivery require specialized management in order to prevent further complications to the mother and possible fetal death.

CONTENT EMPHASIS

- Migrant health problems
- High-risk pregnancy in an adolescent
- Assessment and management of preeclampsia—antepartum
- Prevention and treatment of complications during labor and delivery

SETTING

- Migrant health clinic
- Hospital labor and delivery unit

OBJECTIVES

Upon completing this chapter, the student will be able to:

1. Describe the characteristics of migrant farm workers that influence their health care practices.

2. Comprehend the normal events of pregnancy and childbirth.

3. Identify the unwed adolescent's physical and psychological response to a complicated pregnancy and childbirth.

4. Design expected health outcomes for a preeclamptic adolescent.

5. Select appropriate interventions for a preeclamptic adolescent that will minimize the potential complications of delivery to the mother and the neonate.

6. Analyze the preeclamptic client's response to selected intervention techniques.

DEFINITION OF TERMS

The following terms are used in this case study and should be defined before proceeding:

Amniotic membranes
Amniotomy (AROM)
Antepartum
Apgar score
Diagonal conjugate
Effacement
Episiotomy
Expected date of confinement (EDC)
External conjugate
Fetal distress
Fetal heart monitor
Floating cephalic position
Forceps delivery
Forceps operation
Intercristal

Interspinous
Last menstrual period (LMP)
Left occiput anterior position (LOA)
Left occiput posterior position (LOP)
Left/right lower quadrant (RLQ)
Left/right upper quadrant (LUQ)
Menarche
Otitis media
Poverty level (U.S. official)
Public health nurse (PHN)
Quickening
Spinal anesthesia
Transverse diameter

FAMILY ASSESSMENT

Maria and José Paradour are natives of Mexico who moved to Texas. Since they did not speak English or have a special skill, the Paradours were forced to seek jobs as migrant farm workers. While living in Texas, Mrs. Paradour gave birth to five children. The family's financial resources were minimal and they lived below the official level of poverty in the United States. Both Maria and José worked on the farms from sunup to sundown in order to supply their family with the basic necessities of life. The children worked next to their parents in the fields as soon as they were old enough.

The Paradours' diet consists mainly of corn and beans. Poultry and beef, usually in the form of ground meat, is eaten about twice a week. Occasionally fish is bought from the traveling fish salesman. A small amount of evaporated milk is purchased, but it is usually reserved for the younger children.

The children's health histories are characterized by incomplete immunizations, innumerable incidences of respiratory infections, otitis media, and sore throats. Academically, the children are not performing well. Their schooling has been sporadic as a result of the family's need to follow the harvest seasons.

The Paradour family forms a closely knit group. Their few material belongings are shared freely as is their love and affection for each other. José and Maria are permissive parents who allow the children independence, encourage them to be responsible, but frown upon disrespectfulness. Recently, the Paradour family relocated from Texas to begin seasonal migrant work in the fruit belt of Michigan. Theresa's mother had noticed a change in her daughter's behavior, as well as in her physical appearance. Upon questioning her, Mrs. Paradour's suspicion of Theresa's pregnancy was confirmed. With hesitancy, Theresa related that the baby's father was back in Texas and was unaware of her pregnancy. Although Mrs. Paradour was upset about the event, she insisted that Theresa go to the migrant health clinic the following week.

STUDY QUESTIONS

10-1. What are the beliefs of the Mexican-American migrant family on the following topics: superstitions and supernatural healers, ailments and their remedies, pain, infant health problems, marriage, family structure, health care providers (that is, nurses, physicians)?

10-2. What is the socioeconomic status of most first generation Mexican-Americans? Explain.

10-3. What is the current "official poverty level" in the United States?

10-4. How can a Mexican citizen obtain United States citizenship?

10-5. What are the common health care problems affecting the migrant worker?

10-6. Describe the typical diet of a Mexican migrant worker. When do they eat?

10-7. Complete a growth-and-development information card on a fifteen-year-old female.

DISCUSSION QUESTIONS

D-1. Why do the migrant workers often have a higher incidence of certain health care problems? Explain.

D-2. What does the government (federal, state, and local) do for the migrant workers? for their health care problems?

D-3. Analyze the Mexican migrant workers' diet. Are there inadequacies? How can a professional nurse assist the workers to prevent these inadequacies?

Food group	Inadequacies	Suggested change
Dairy products Meats Eggs Vegetables/fruits Breads and cereals Butter and margarine		

D-4. Complete the following nutrition table on a fifteen-year-old female:

Food group	15-year-old female	Pregnant 15-Year-Old Trimester			Rationale for alteration in diet
		1	2	3	
Dairy products Meats Eggs Vegetables/fruits Breads and cereals Butter or margarine					

D-5. What nutrients are probably missing from Theresa's diet and what nursing measures can be instituted to increase the adequacy of her diet?

Nutrient	(In)adequacy of Theresa's diet	Nursing measure to increase adequacy

Protein
Fat
Carbohydrate
Vitamins
    (A, B, C, and D)
Minerals
    (calcium and iron)		

D-6. What are some of the ways that a Mexican American individual might express his or her emotions or feelings?

CLIENT ANTEPARTUM ASSESSMENT

Theresa was seen at the Wednesday evening clinic session by Ms. Lawson, the public health/clinic nurse, and Dr. Robson. The following data was obtained by the health team:

May 15
15-year-old Mexican-American single female seen by clinic staff for confirmation of pregnancy and subsequent antepartal care. Client is accompanied by her mother. Client complains of no menstrual period since "early in November," has constipation and frequent backaches.
Allergies: Penicillin

PAST HEALTH HISTORY: Rubella and rubeola contracted during early childhood. No immunization record. States she has had DPT and polio shots. Pelvic injury at age ten years due to auto accident. Recurrent respiratory infections with sore throats and occasional otitis media throughout life.

OB/GYN HISTORY: Client denies previous pregnancies or abortions.
Menarche occurred at about twelve years old.
Menstrual cycle: Usually 30 days with 3–4 days of light to moderate menstrual flow for the last 1–1½ years.
LMP: "Early in November" according to client
EDC: (by dates) August 7–14
Weight: (prior to pregnancy) 54.5 kg (client estimated)
Height: 147.5 cm

PHYSICAL ASSESSMENT:
General: Client is fidgety and is very guarded with her verbal communication.
Weight: 62 kg
Height: 147.5 cm
HEENT: Five dental caries noted in bicuspids; nasal mucosa is grayish pink; thyroid not palpable
Cardiac: NSR; AP: 82, regular; BP: 128/86
Pulmonary: Clear breath sounds upon auscultation; R: 18/minute, regular.
Breasts: Tender upon palpation; no palpable masses noted; clean everted nipples; well developed, symmetrical breasts

Abdomen: Slight protrusion; soft; no complaint of tenderness when palpated. Fundal height at 25 cm. Fetal palpation is noncontributory

FHT: 126 in LLQ. Patient states that she has felt fetal movement every day for the past three weeks

Musculoskeletal: Nonedematous extremities; stands c̄ lordosis posture and shoulders slumped forward.

Neurological: (refer to diagram)

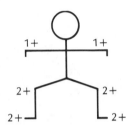

GENITOURINARY: External genitalia: No evidence of discoloration or lesions; Bartholin's glands and Skene's glands are nonpalpable; scant amount of clear vaginal discharge present. Internal examination: nulliparous cervix free of nodules or erosion; ovaries are nonpalpable; vaginal mucosa is purplish in color with moderate amount of clear secretions.

PELVIC MEASUREMENTS:
Diagonal conjugate: internal—12 cm; external—11.0 cm
Transverse diameter: 8 cm
Interspinous diameter: 25.5 cm
Intercristal diameter: 28.5 cm
External conjugate: 19 cm
Average pubic arch and sacral curve
Moveable coccyx; blunt spines

LABORATORY RESULTS:
Hgb: 9.7 g/100 ml
Hct.: 35 mg %
Blood Type: A positive
VDRL: neg.
GC smear: neg.
Pap smear: normal cells
Urinalysis: Sp. gr.—1.020; glucose—negative; albumin—trace
Rubella titer: 110

ANTEPARTAL FLOW SHEET

Date	Weight (in Kg)	B.P.	Urine			FHT*	Fundal height	Comments
			Albumin	Glucose	Edema			
5/15	62.3	128/86 nervous	Neg.	Neg.	—	126	25 cm	prenatal vitas. Rx: Constipation, backac
5/29	63.0	110/72	Trace	Neg.	—	130	26 cm	nutrition counseling
6/12	63.0	110/76	Trace	Neg.	—	136	29 cm	floating cephalic position
6/26	64.5	114/78	Trace	1+	—	136	32 cm	
7/10								Missed Appt.; PHN referral
7/17	66.3	120/84	1+	Neg.	+	132	34 cm	Social worker referral
7/24	68.0	130/92	1+	1+	++	132	35 cm	neuro reflexes (2+ –3+); Low Na die encouraged
7/31	68.2	138/100	2+	1+	++	136	38 cm	c/o headaches; reflexes 3+ (knee an elbow); placed on bedrest at home Rx: Diuril 250 mgm b.i.d. phenobarb 30 mgm b.i.d.
8/7	68.2	130/90	1+	1+	+/++	140	37 cm	Pelvic measurements repeated; findir indicate a borderline adequate ou

*Placement of rate indicates the location of the fetal heart sound on Theresa's abdomen RUQ | LUQ / RLQ | LLQ

Following the initial clinic examination, Ms. Lawson discussed the routine schedule for antepartal clinic visits and their importance with Mrs. Paradour. The nurse also suggested ways to minimize Theresa's problems of constipation and backache. Ms. Lawson attempted to help Theresa examine her dietary habits and the importance of improving the quality of her diet. Theresa appeared interested in the discussion and agreed to all the changes.

Fortunately, the same nurse saw Theresa at almost every clinic visit. Eventually, Theresa began to share some of her feelings with Ms. Lawson. Theresa continued to express a growing determination to "make things better for this baby."

Theresa Paradour's antepartal flow sheet (above) summarizes the course of her pregnancy.

STUDY QUESTIONS

10-8.　Explain the neurological diagram in the assessment.

10-9.   At what stage of pregnancy does quickening occur?

10-10. How is the measurement of fundal height used to assess pregnancy?

10-11. What is the psychological impact of the first pregnancy on an adult single woman?

10-12. Why are pelvic measurements taken? What is the normal range for each? Compare these measurements with Theresa's measurements in the table below.

Measurement	Normal range	Theresa's measurements	Significance of deviation

Diagonal conjugate
  Internal
  External			

Transverse			
Interspinous			
Intercostal			
External conjugate			

10-13. What is considered a significant change in blood pressure, urine albumin and glucose, and edema during pregnancy?

10-14. What are the signs and symptoms of preeclampsia? What is considered to be the possible cause of this disorder?

10-15. Complete a drug information card on chlorothiazide and phenobarbital.

10-16. Why would chlorothiazide and phenobarbital be the preferred medications under these circumstances? How do these drugs affect the fetus?

10-17. What is the reason(s) for Theresa's Hgb of 9.7 g? What specific foods should the nurse recommend to Theresa?

DISCUSSION QUESTIONS

D-7.   What is the psychological impact of the first pregnancy on a single adolescent? What emotional support systems are available to Theresa?

D-8.   In addition to the professional nurse and the physician, who might provide the health team with useful input as to Theresa's needs?

D-9.   What suggestions would you make to Theresa in light of her problems with constipation and backaches?

D-10. In addition to the social worker referral, what other referral(s) might be useful to the client?

D-11. Based on Theresa's history and physical assessment, what are her nursing diagnoses? What are the nursing care objectives and the nursing actions for each? How should the effectiveness of care be evaluated?

Nursing diagnosis	Nursing care objective	Rationale	Nursing action	Rationale	Method and frequency of evaluating effectiveness

D-12. What changes (if any) should be made in the above nursing care plan for Theresa after each visit to the clinic?

LABOR

On August 9, Theresa awoke with abdominal cramping. She had noticed occasional cramping during the night. Regular contractions became evident by 9:00 A.M. and Theresa was taken to the hospital by her parents. In the emergency room, a pelvic examination was performed by Edwin Geisberg, M.D., the physician on call at the hospital that day. The exam revealed that the client's cervix was dilated 3 cm and was 50% effaced. The fetus was in L.O.P. position at −1 station. Amniotic membranes were intact. Theresa was admitted to the labor and delivery unit by Dr. Geisberg. A summary copy of Theresa's antepartum record had been forwarded to the hospital during July.

Ms. Buehler, R.N., admitted Theresa to the unit. She was accompanied by her mother, Mrs. Paradour. After reviewing the antepartum record, Ms. Buehler performed her nursing assessment. It revealed the following:

August 9, 11:00 A.M.: Fifteen-year-old Mexican-American single female admitted through ER accompanied to unit by her mother. States that "pain started about 9:00 A.M.". Appears very tense with contractions and speaks only when spoken to.

Edema + +; no c/o visual disturbance or headaches. Fundoscopic exam reveals segmented arteriolar spasms.
Neuro reflexes: 3 + knee; 2+ for all other reflexes.

The remaining assessment findings were placed on the Labor/Delivery flow sheet used by the unit. Mrs. Buehler briefly and calmly explained to Theresa and her mother that she was to rest as much as possible. Ms. Buehler covered Theresa with blankets, padded and placed the side rails up, and dimmed the room lights. While doing this, she also told Theresa the frequency with which she would be checked and explained to her the use of the call bell.

LABOR/DELIVERY FLOW SHEET

Date: August 9
EDC: August 7–14

Name: Theresa Paradour
Gi Po   15 y.o.

Time	BP	P	FHT	Contractions			Cervical Dil. and Eff.	Station	Urine Alb/Gluc	Other
				Freq. (min.)	Duration (sec)	Strength				
11 A.M.	130/100	100	136	7–9	45–60	mod.	3 cm/60%	−1	2+/neg	LOP; 3+ knee jerk
12 P.M.	136/98	92	132	7	45–60	mod.			2+/neg	Valium 10 mg IM
1 P.M.	136/100	92	136	7	60	mod.				
2 P.M.	134/98	94	136	5–6	60	mod.			2+/neg	3+ knee jerk 3+ Achilles reflex
3 P.M.	138/100	100	140	5–6	60–70	mod.				Valium 10 mg IM
3:30 P.M.	132/100	100	136	6	60–70	mod.	5 cm/80%	−1	1+/neg	AROM; LOP; 3+ knee/Achilles
4:00 P.M.	132/108	94	136	6–7	60–70	mod.				Dozing periodi- cally; alert
6:00 P.M.	144/114	96	136	4–5	60–80	mod.	6 cm/100%	0	2+/1+	C/O headache; scotoma; Mag- nesium sulfate 4 mg iv; variable fetal decelerations
6:30 P.M.	128/88	90	140	5	60	mod.				Headache subsid- ing; 2+ neuro reflexes
7:30 P.M.	126/90	86	132	4–5	70–90	strong	7 cm/100%	2+	1+/neg	LOT; normal neuro. findings
9:00 P.M.	128/90	88	132	2–3	70–90	strong	9 cm/100%	2+	1+/neg	LOA
9:30 P.M.	128/94	90	132	1–2	90	strong	10 cm/100%			pushing

Transferred to Delivery Room

Theresa's mother began crying audibly as she proclaimed, "Oh, my poor baby Theresa!" Mrs. Paradour's anxiety was hardly what Theresa needed right now, thought the nurse. In a tactful manner, Ms. Buehler encouraged Mrs. Paradour to wait outside the unit. The nurse reassured Mrs. Paradour that Theresa would be closely watched.

Ms. Buehler returned to her activities, making certain that the items needed in the event of eclamptic convulsions were readily available. An external fetal heart monitor was applied to Theresa's abdomen. As Ms. Buehler was explaining to Theresa what she might expect to occur during labor, Dr. Geisberg entered the room. Ms. Buehler then shared her assessment findings with Dr. Geisberg. Based upon this information, his physical examination, and Theresa's history, the following medical orders were written:

Maintain bedrest with minimal stimulation

Convulsive precautions

Magnesium sulfate, 10 g available near the patient's bedside

VS, BP, FHR, reflexes q 1 h then q 30 min. as the active phase of labor is presenting

Valium 10 mg IM now

Hematocrit and hemoglobin stat

Serum electrolytes stat

Type and crossmatch for two units packed cells

IV of 5% D/W at 100 ml/hr

Monitor urine output; protein and glucose at each voiding

Theresa needed reassurance to get through the seemingly endless pain-producing procedures—blood specimens drawn, getting the IV started, the Valium injection. To Ms. Buehler, Theresa appeared almost panic stricken—a state that could easily compound her medical problems. Supportive nursing care would be particularly important with this client.

At 3 P.M., Ms. Buehler noted that Theresa was growing quite uncomfortable as her contractions became more frequent. Her back pain was only partially relieved by repositioning and counter-pressure. The nurse notified Dr. Geisberg of Theresa's progress. A vaginal examination and amniotomy were performed. Ms. Buehler carefully noted the characteristics of the amniotic fluid. An order for "morphine sulfate 10 mg IV for pain stat" was written and promptly administered.

Around 6:00 P.M. that evening, Theresa complained of a headache and occasional spots before her eyes. Ms. Buehler checked the client carefully (see flow sheet) before notifying Dr. Geisberg. Magnesium sulfate 4 g over 20 minutes via the intravenous route was administered to Theresa by the physician. Fortunately, Theresa responded well to the magnesium sulfate. She experienced no toxic effects. There was no evidence of prolonged fetal distress noted except for a few variable decelerations.

STUDY QUESTIONS

10-18. What are the implications of the LOP fetal position in labor?

10-19. What are the significant findings in Ms. Buehler's initial nursing assessment of Theresa? Explain.

10-20. What are the symptoms that indicate eclampsia is imminent? What is the nurse's responsibility in this instance?

10-21. Differentiate between mild, moderate, and severe preeclampsia and eclampsia in terms of etiology, clinical manifestations, treatment, and prognosis.

	Mild	Moderate	Severe
Etiology			
Clinical manifestations			
Treatment			
Prognosis			

10-22. What is the reason for each of the initial actions by the nurse?

Action	Rationale
Covered with blankets	
Padded and placed side rails up	
Dimmed the lights	
Encouraged to rest	
External fetal heart monitor	

10-23. What are the possible causes of the variable deceleration pattern noted on the fetal heart monitor? What is the significance of early and late fetal heart decelerations?

10-24. What is the rationale for each of the medical orders?

10-25. What items should be made readily available in the labor room of a preeclamptic client?

10-26. What characteristics should the nurse note and record when an amniotomy (AROM) is performed?

10-27. Complete a drug information card on the following medications: Valium, morphine, magnesium sulfate.

10-28. How do the above drugs affect the fetus?

10-29. What are the precipitating factors that cause seizures among pregnant women? What nursing action can be used to prevent a seizure?

10-30. What are the signs and symptoms of a seizure and what are the nursing implications of each?

Signs and symptoms	Scientific rationale of signs and symptoms	Nursing objective and action	Method and frequency of evaluating response

DISCUSSION QUESTIONS

D-13. How does Theresa's condition compare to the classical clinical picture of preeclampsia?

D-14. What topics should be discussed with Mrs. Paradour? Outline the topics in the order in which they should be presented. What would you explain about each?

Topic	Explanation

D-15. Graph the progress of Theresa's labor and delivery and compare with the classic Friedman curve.

D-16. What do headaches and scotoma indicate in a laboring client? What other symptoms might be observed that indicate the same problem?

D-17. What are the specific nursing care implications when clients are treated with magnesium sulfate? What are the manifestations of toxicity? What should be closely observed? What is the nurse's responsibility for documentation?

D-18. What other treatments for preeclampsia can be used besides magnesium sulfate? Explain each.

D-19. Prepare a nursing care plan for Theresa during labor. What is the rationale for each objective and nursing action? How can the effectiveness of care be evaluated?

Objective	Nursing Action	Rationale	Method and Frequency of Evaluating Response

D-20. What revisions should be made as Theresa's labor progresses?

DELIVERY

With the supportive direction of Ms. Buehler, Theresa progressed through her labor and was taken to the delivery room. Regional anesthesia was administered. An RML episiotomy and outlet forceps were used to facilitate the delivery of a 6½ pound girl. (Apgar scores were 8 at one minute and 9 at five minutes.) Mrs. Paradour visited her daughter in the recovery room before she left that evening. Theresa remained in the obstetric recovery unit until the next morning. Then she was transferred to the postpartum unit.

The nursing staff continued to monitor her closely for signs of eclampsia for an additional two days. On the fifth day postpartum, Theresa and her newborn daughter were discharged. According to her mother, they would both return to the migrant family clinic for follow-up. A hospitalization summary report was completed and sent to the clinic.

CHAPTER DISCUSSION QUESTIONS

1. Discuss Theresa's interaction with Ms. Lawson. Why was a referral made to the clinic's social worker?
2. What are the purposes of monitoring the fetal heart sounds with the equipment?

FETAL MONITORS

Equipment	How does equipment work?	Precautions in using equipment
Bell fetoscope		
Head fetoscope		
Doppler probe		
Fetal phonocardiography		
Electronic maternal-fetal monitor internal external		

3. What would you explain to a client before applying an external fetal heart monitor? How would you answer questions about the fetal heart sounds?
4. As the postpartum nurse, what referrals would you make upon Theresa's discharge? For what services? Explain.

SUGGESTED ACTIVITIES

1. Visit a farm that employs migrant farm workers. Observe their living environment and ask about their daily life style. Do the children of the migrants attend school? Where do they go if they need health care? After they have completed work at their present location, where do they go?

2. Observe the activities in a migrant health clinic. What kinds of care do the clients need, in their opinion?

3. Observe a laboring patient who is being electronically monitored for uterine contractions and fetal heart rate. Identify the parts of the electronic maternal-fetal monitor. Analyze the read-out tracing.

4. Attend a prenatal health clinic. What are the major characteristics of the clients attending the clinic? What specific services are offered to the clients? What is the regular schedule for prenatal visits?

BIBLIOGRAPHY

Abril, Irene F. "Mexican-American Folk Beliefs: How They Affect Health Care." *The American Journal of Maternal Child Nursing* 2 (May/June 1977): 168–173.

Bergersen, Betty. *Pharmacology in Nursing.* 13th ed. St. Louis: C. V. Mosby Co., 1976.

Branch, Maria Foster, and Paxton, Phyllis Perry, eds. *Providing Safe Care for Ethnic People of Color.* New York: Appleton-Century-Crofts, 1976, pp. 41–80.

Brunner, Lillian Sholtis, and Suddarth, Doris Smith. *The Lippincott Manual of Nursing Practice.* Philadelphia: J. B. Lippincott Co., 1974, pp. 1007–1011.

Butts, Priscilla. "Magnesium Sulfate in the Treatment of Toxemia." *American Journal of Nursing* 77 (August 1977), 1294–1298.

Clark, Ann L., ed. *Culture Childbearing Health Professionals.* Philadelphia: F. A. Davis Co., 1978.

Clark, Ann L., and Affonso, Dyanne D. *Childbearing: A Nursing Perspective.* Philadelphia: F. A. Davis Co., 1976.

Galloway, Karen G. "The Uncertainty and Stress of High Risk Pregnancy." *The American Journal of Maternal Child Nursing* 1 (September/October 1976): 294–299.

Garb, Solomon. *Laboratory Tests in Common Use.* 6th ed. New York: Springer Publishing Co., 1976.

Hall, Joanne E., and Weaver, Barbara R., eds. *A Systems Approach to Community Health.* Philadelphia: J. B. Lippincott Co., 1977, pp. 519–528.

Holey, Elizabeth S. "Promoting Adequate Weight Gain in Pregnant Women." *The American Journal of Maternal Child Nursing* 2 (March/April 1977): 86–89.

Jensen, Margaret Duncan; Benson, Ralph C.; and Bobak, Irene M. *Maternity Care—The Nurse and the Family.* St. Louis: C. V. Mosby Co., 1977.

Little, Dolores E., and Carnevali, Doris. *Nursing Care Planning.* 2d ed. Philadelphia: J. B. Lippincott Co., 1976.

Malasanos, Lois, et al. *Health Assessment.* St. Louis: C. V. Mosby Co., 1978.

Martinez, Ricardo Arguijo, ed. *Hispanic Culture and Health Care.* Saint Louis: C. V. Mosby Co., 1978.

Oxorn, Harry, and Foote, William R. *Human Labor and Birth.* 3d ed. New York: Appleton-Century-Crofts, 1975.

Robinson, Corinne H., and Lawler, Marilyn R. *Normal and Therapeutic Nutrition.* 15th ed. New York: Macmillan, 1977.

Sonstegard, L. J. "Magnesium Sulfate Treatment of Toxemia." *Perinatal Press* 2 (January 1978): 8.

Torre, Carolyn T. "Nutritional Needs of Adolescents." *The American Journal of Maternal Child Nursing* 2 (March/April 1977): 118–127.

CHAPTER ELEVEN

Emotional Adolescent Crisis: Attempted Suicide

ANDREA B. SAVITZ

JEAN FISHER

OVERVIEW

Timothy is the nineteen-year-old son of John and Ruth Baker. The Bakers practice the Bahai faith and are influential members of their community. Tim was labeled as an "underachiever" in high school and was seen as a behavior problem at home, particularly when compared to his siblings. Tim is mechanically oriented and would prefer to attend mechanical courses in a local community college, however his parents "pressure" him to attend a baccalaureate program. When he begins to fail his freshman courses, he attempts suicide during final exams. He is initially assessed by a nurse in the college's counseling service and is then hospitalized.

CONTENT EMPHASIS

- Stress factors—freshman college student
- Suicidal risk-assessment
- Crisis intervention—attempted suicide
- Prevention of suicide

SETTINGS

- Roof of dorm
- College infirmary

- Psychiatric unit
- Private therapy

OBJECTIVES

Upon completing this chapter the student will be able to:

1. Evaluate the psychological characteristics operating within a client and his or her family that predispose the client to attempt suicide.
2. Analyze the characteristics of a client/family in order to assess a client's suicide risk.
3. Determine the therapeutic role of the nurse in crisis intervention for a suicidal client.
4. Promote behaviors in clients that are conducive to the prevention of suicide.

DEFINITION OF TERMS

The following terms are used in this case study and should be defined before proceeding:

Bahai faith	Fantasies
Crisis intervention	Frost-bite
Emotional isolation	Stress
Emotional triangle	Stress pattern
Family system	Suicide

FAMILY ASSESSMENT

The Baker family lives in Flint, Michigan, in a spacious private home outside the Detroit area. They have practiced the Bahai faith for twenty years. John Baker is a highly successful Vice President of Technical Design for one of the major auto manufacturers. Ruth, John's wife of twenty-five years, is a part-time children's librarian. Since the early days of their marriage, the Bakers have been financially secure, due to John's advancement in the company. The Bakers give credit for John's success to the fact that they have lived most of their marital life as Bahai members.

Both John and Ruth have gained community respect and recognition. John is on the town council, and Ruth sits on the boards of a number of charitable organizations. In fact, both of the Bakers are so busy doing for others that

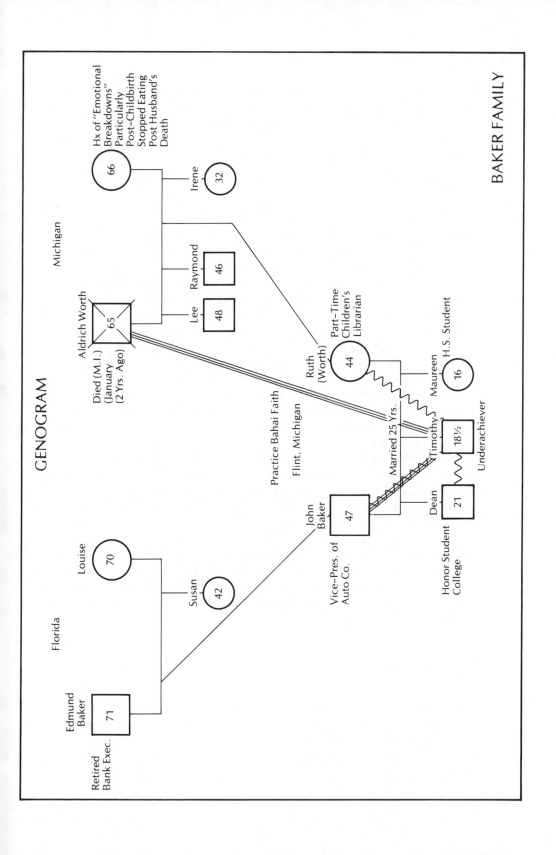

they often see one another only late in the evening. Nevertheless, John and Ruth have reared three children. Their children are Dean, age 21, Timothy, age 18½, and Maureen, age 16 (see genogram).

Dean is an honor student at Princeton University. His parents frequently comment to one another about how pleased they are with Dean's progress. Tim is in his first year of collegiate study at Michigan State. Tim struggles with academics. The Baker's only daughter, Maureen, is a hard worker. Good grades do not come easily to Maureen. However, she will probably enter her senior year as the potential salutatorian of her class. Maureen is pert and pretty, and leads an active social life.

Ruth's parents, Aldrich and Mary Worth, were truck farmers in Michigan. They had four children. The Worths rarely left the farm during their marital life. While the Worths' homebound life style was not often talked about by the family, it was assumed to be in direct relationship to Mary's mental health. Mary had had a number of "breakdowns" in her early adulthood. Two breakdowns were related to childbirth, but the facts were unclear. At one point, Mary was hospitalized for a "breakdown" when she was in her late forties. Subsequently, Aldrich or his children made most of the major family decisions throughout the years without consulting Mary.

After Aldrich died, two years ago last January, the farm was taken over by Lee, their oldest child. Lee drastically modernized the operations of the farm and the farmhouse. Little could be recognized of the old Worth homestead when he finished.

During the readjustment period following Aldrich's death, Mary stopped eating and lost almost 30 pounds. Lee once commented to the family that he feared that his mother was slowly committing suicide. But in the end, Mary finally began to eat. No one sought professional help for Mary during the time that she refused nourishment.

John Baker's parents, Edmund and Louise, have been residing in Florida for six years. Edmund had been a bank executive and his wife Louise had always stayed at home to manage the house. They come to visit their son's family at Christmas and once each summer. Edmund and Louise take an active interest in their grandchildren's progress. They often mention concern over Tim.

STUDY QUESTIONS

11-1. What are the basic beliefs of the Bahai faith on the following topics: family, marriage, children, health/illness, health care providers, maintenance of one's body, healing.

11-2. Who was Bahaullah? Explain.

11-3. What are the characteristics of a suicide-prone client?

D-1. What behavior profile characterizes the infant, preschooler, and school-age child who later might become suicidal?

CLIENT ASSESSMENT

Tim Baker is the middle child of John and Ruth Baker. Tim is rarely praised by his relatives. If the family's relatives do ask about Timothy, they usually start with, "How is Timothy doing in school now?" He was labeled early in his school career by the school system as an "underachiever." He never got through a school year without tutoring. He was the only Baker child who had to be asked by his parents for his report card.

John Baker, Tim's father, has difficulty being sympathetic toward Tim. At times John has gone into a rage over Tim's school record. Ruth, Tim's mother, also considers Tim to be difficult. She never seems to forget his temper tamtrums or accident-proneness in early childhood. While in his teens, when Tim complained of boredom, his parents believed it was because he made no effort to acquire friends and because he was losing interest in the Bahai faith. John and Ruth Baker have discussed how at times their attitude toward Tim is not the attitude of a good Bahai. Then they rationalize that Tim is a very trying son.

Tim did, however, ask to spend part of his summers on the farm with his maternal grandparents, Aldrich and Mary Worth. On the farm grades were not important. His aloneness was not talked about either. There were no other young people near the farm. Aldrich would often ask when Tim could visit; he particularly enjoyed Tim's quiet company, and besides, Tim was very helpful. He liked working the farm equipment and was good on the tractor and knew how to repair the separator that was always breaking down.

As Tim's high school days proceeded, he disliked each year a little more. He would tell his sister Maureen about his feelings. However, as Maureen entered her own adolescence, she became less and less available to Tim. As it became more obvious that Maureen was going to be another success story like her brother Dean, Tim stopped talking to her altogether. Besides, Maureen had begun to criticize Tim for his attitude toward school. In fact, on the last occasion Tim had tried to confide in Maureen about his life, she was short with him. Maureen said, "Why don't you just try loving school for a change, join a team . . . do *something* . . . anything!!" Tim did not look for her understanding anymore.

When Aldrich, Tim's grandfather, suddenly died in the January when Tim was a junior in high school, Tim mourned alone. No one knew that he spent time crying in his room. Tim kept his grief to himself. He did not even share it with his grandmother, Mary. Tim learned that seeing Mary only served to bring on a new wave of grief. His academic marks dropped significantly the spring following Aldrich's death.

Because of his grades and his general underachiever label, Tim was surprised when he got accepted to Michigan State. However, he was not particularly happy at the prospect of attending. Tim had only submitted an application because of his family's encouragement. He had wanted to go to the local community college for a technical background in machinery. But his father said, "A son of mine should develop his mind." Tim saw himself as a future heavy machinery operator and mechanic. He did not want to seek a degree. Tim only wanted to study things that related specifically to his interest in heavy equipment.

STUDY QUESTIONS

11-4. What is the development task(s) of the adolescent?

11-5. What factors included in Tim's history place him in the category of persons-at-risk for developing suicidal tendencies? Explain.

11-6. How does an emotional triangle function? Explain.

11-7. Can an individual be in more than one emotional triangle? Explain.

DISCUSSION QUESTIONS

D-2. Timothy Baker is a participant of what emotional triangles?

D-3. What family member behaviors do you believe relate directly to Aldrich Worth's death? Explain.

D-4. What events closely coincided in Tim's family history that added to his degree of isolation within the family system?

D-5. Given the Bakers' family history, is the family living the life prescribed by the Bahai faith? Explain.

THE SUICIDE ATTEMPT

Tim had just returned to college after the Christmas break for his exams. His memory of the visit home was upsetting. He had mentioned that he believed he might be failing to his father. John had exploded, saying, "You flunk and you can just forget you are a Baker." The rest of the family blamed Tim for a ruined mini-family reunion. Dean, who was also home from college, had said that he could see that college had not *changed* Tim. Maureen had stated that she was sure Tim could "mess up a free lunch."

At school Tim felt he could talk to no one. He had a room on the eighth floor. His roommate Paul was a sophomore majoring in French. Paul's grade point average was excellent. Tim and Paul shared few interests, and they knew it. Yet, Paul extended friendship to Tim. It was Tim who was standoffish. Tim never took Paul up on an invitation.

It appeared to Tim that most students seemed to be doing fairly well studying something that they liked. Tim kept his failures to himself. During the first semester when he was not studying, he had developed the habit of staying alone in his room reading *Popular Mechanics* or sitting up on the recreation deck roof that he called "the clouds." After a while even the escape of reading got him down. He tried dating, but the experience felt empty, too. When one girl turned him down for their third date, he just did not call again. Tim never wrote home, and only thought of his family in terms of their possible reaction to his grades.

At exam times during the first semester, Tim had often developed a stomachache. When the college nurse observed a pattern to his upsets, she discussed the availability of the school's walk-in counseling center with Tim. Tim never went.

On the evening of January 16, Tim returned to his room after having sat for an exam. He had answered only half of the questions. Yet, Tim was the last to leave the examination. He sat down and wrote a short letter to his parents explaining that he would not be causing them any further embarrassment. He addressed and affixed a stamp to an envelope. He stuffed the note in the unsealed envelope and propped it on his desk. Then Tim gathered all his things together and packed them neatly into his suitcase. He piled his tablets, pens, pencils, and *Popular Mechanics* in orderly groups on Paul's desk. On the top page of Paul's memo pad he wrote, "Make good use of this stuff, obviously I didn't. See you in the clouds, Frenchie. P.S. Mail the letter on my desk, please."

Then Tim walked out of his room and started down the elevator to sign out the key to the rooftop recreation deck.

In the meantime, Paul entered the room. He had been in a friend's room on the seventh floor. The appearance of the room struck him as very strange. He laid on his bed for a moment looking at the memo Tim had left. Then, holding the unsealed enveloped addressed to Tim's parents, Paul decided to read it.

After reading the letter, Paul got a gut reaction that something was wrong. He walked to the hall intercom. Over the intercom Paul asked if anyone had checked out the deck key, remembering that Tim called the deck the "clouds." The dorm monitor said, "Yes."

"By any chance is Tim Baker's name on the sign out sheet?" Paul asked.

The monitor said, "Yes, that's right... God only knows why he wanted the deck key, it's freezing..."

Paul did not hear the end of the sentence, he just ran. He triple-stepped the staircase one level up to the deck. When he opened the deck door he saw

Tim's back. Tim was sitting precariously on top of the retaining fence. Paul backed into the stairwell and grabbed the deck intercom. He said to the dorm monitor, "Tim's up here on the deck thinking of jumping—get help. He's already on top of the fence."

STUDY QUESTIONS

11-8.   What characteristics are demonstrated in most high-risk suicidal persons?

11-9.   Statistically (for the United States): Which age groups have the highest percentage of persons at suicidal risk? which sex? which occupation? What sex has the highest percentage of persons who attempt suicide and succeed?

11-10. What factors are considered when making a suicidal assessment of a client?

11-11. Using the principle that "all behavior has meaning," what are some of the theories regarding the meaning of suicide and suicidal behavior?

11-12. What factors should be considered in planning a treatment plan for a client who has suicidal ideas or who has made a suicide attempt?

11-13. What attitudes are essential for health personnel working with a suicidal client?

11-14. Is there a difference in approach when working with a client who has made a less serious suicide attempt as compared with a serious attempt? Explain.

11-15. Discuss the family system as it is presented and describe its possible contribution to Timothy's current emotional state.

DISCUSSION QUESTIONS

D-6.   What nodal event in Tim's history do you believe was responsible for the change in his mental status from a person with suicidal potential to one of high suicidal risk? Explain.

D-7.   Did the college nurse use the nursing process after she recognized a pattern in the episodes of Tim's GI upsets? Explain.

D-8.   Could the college nurse have done more in an effort to prevent Tim's suicide attempt after having recognized his stress pattern?

D-9.   Of the many factors mentioned by various authors for the assessment of suicidal potential, which characteristics do you believe hold the most value as predictors of suicidal risk? Explain your choice.

D-10. Tim's grandfather had been a significant figure in his life. Could there be a connection between Tim's mental state and the anniversary of his grandfather's death? Explain.

FOLLOW-UP CARE

The dorm monitor immediately notified the college security guard about Tim. The security guard dispatch unit notified the security guard on patrol in Tim's dorm. Then the dispatcher arranged a back-up for the security guard and alerted the campus walk-in counseling center. The center sent Ms. Linda Degan, R.N., a member of the crisis team. By the time Ms. Degan arrived, Paul was already talking to Tim.

Tears were streaming down Paul's face as he said, "Please, Buddy, don't do this thing... I had no idea things were so bad."

The security guard was off in the background. His advice to Paul was to try to keep Tim talking. The guard was trying to figure out how to get Tim down if he would not come down on his own. Floors below Tim, the security unit stood watch with a net.

Ms. Degan slowly walked up to join Paul. After an hour, an exhausted, sobbing Tim came down off the deck fence. Ms. Degan traveled with Tim in a security guard squad car to the counseling center, an affiliate of the medical center.

After taking care of Tim's immediate physical needs, Ms. Degan pulled up a chair next to Tim's bed. He was still shivering occasionally. There was a possibility of mild frostbite of his fingers, nose, and ear lobes. That was the only positive finding on Ms. Degan's brief initial physical assessment. Tim was encouraged to drink coffee and soup as Ms. Degan talked with him.

Ms. Degan filled out a Suicidal Risk Assessment Sheet on Tim (see Appendix H) for his historical record. He was given the suicidal high-risk rating of 13 from the following data:

Family suicidal history	1 (based on Tim's maternal grandmother's history)
Degree of family isolation	4 (based on Tim's subjective report)
Presence of maturational crisis	4 (based on Tim being an adolescent)
Extent of suicidal plan and outcome fantasies	4 (based on Tim's subjective report and objective data—the suicidal note and letter left in his dorm room, and the actual attempt)
Total	13 (high risk)

Ms. Degan started Tim's family genogram while taking the suicidal assessment. During this period of time Tim started to sob again. He reported on his grandfather Aldrich, "I guess that was really it for me when Granddad died. He's the only one in the family who gave a damn about me. You and Paul really should not have talked me out of it... You really shouldn't have..."

Later, Ms. Degan consulted with Fred Gordon, M.D., the psychiatric attending physician at the medical center, to arrange a referral for Tim. Dr. Gordon accepted Ms. Degan's assessment. Consequently, Dr. Gordon believed admission would be the best course of action for Tim. The physician then requested that a copy of Ms. Degan's initial assessment, including her nursing diagnoses, be sent with Tim to the hospital. He also asked for Ms. Degan's feedback on her earlier phone call to Tim's parents and took down the Baker family's Blue Cross/Blue Shield number. Then Dr. Gordon arranged for Tim's admission. Tim was admitted to the medical center via stretcher later that evening. He was still physically and emotionally exhausted.

Ms. Rosalinda Ross, R.N., M.A., a primary care mental health nurse, admitted Tim to the psychiatric unit at the medical center. She reviewed Ms. Degan's assessment and referral, and then designed her nursing care plan. Shortly thereafter, she was notified that Tim's parents had arrived. After securing coverage for Tim, Ms. Ross met with the Bakers. Following introductions, the Bakers immediately wanted to know if Tim was physically well. Ms. Ross assured them that their son had no physical injuries. Then, after a brief silence, John Baker suddenly stood up, saying, "It's just like him to do something like this. He never thinks what his behavior is doing to the family."

Ruth Baker started to cry, saying, "Sit down, John."

Ms. Ross decided that the time was right to show Tim's suicidal letter to them. When John read the letter indicating that Tim had planned suicide to end the family embarrassment due to his failures, Mr. Baker was speechless. At last, as tears filled his eyes, John said, "I had no idea that we had been so hard on him.... Some Bahai I am."

Ms. Ross continued to see the Bakers and Tim for regular therapy sessions during Tim's three-week hospital stay. Timothy was then discharged to home. Therapy was continued privately for approximately a year in the private sector at weekly intervals. Then therapy sessions were scheduled less and less frequently and Tim was eventually discharged.

Today, at 24, Timothy is a successful heavy machinery operator. He maintains an apartment in the same county as his parents, and he has a satisfying social life, as well.

STUDY QUESTIONS

11-16. What is the goal of crisis intervention?

11-17. What are the steps of crisis intervention?

11-18. Is suicide, or its attempt, a legal offense in your state? Explain.

11-19. What nursing diagnosis(es) would you use to design a treatment plan for Tim?

11-20. Will your state's Blue Cross/Blue Shield pay for the following expenses for a suicidal patient: hospitalization—how long? out-patient therapy? clinic therapy?

11-21. What is the cause of frostbite? Describe the pathophysiology involved. How is frostbite assessed? treated?

11-22. Outline the major points of the following approaches to therapy for a suicidal client: behaviorist, psychoanalytical, psychotherapeutic, family.

CHAPTER DISCUSSION QUESTIONS

1. Was the taking of a genogram by Ms. Degan therapeutic for Tim at the time? Explain.

2. Given Timothy's history in this case study, do you agree with Ms. Degan's suicidal risk index score of 13? Explain.

3. Was Ms. Degan's approach: the generic method of crisis intervention, the individual approach method of crisis intervention, or the systems approach method of crisis intervention? Defend your opinion.

4. From what field of therapy (behaviorist, psychoanalytical, psychotherapeutic, or family system) do you believe Tim could gain the most as a long-term intervention process after crisis resolution? Explain.

5. Discuss current attitudes in this country toward suicide, taking into consideration different cultural and religious beliefs.

6. Considering Tim's age, what instruction should be given to him and his family concerning his Blue Cross/Blue Shield Health Insurance coverage?

7. When high suicidal risk is a factor, do you believe that a referral to a psychiatrist for a second opinion and/or treatment is always indicated? Explain and document.

8. Is suicide a private matter? a family matter? and/or a community matter? Explain.

SUGGESTED ACTIVITIES

1. Interview a Hot-Line volunteer. Suggested questions:
   a. What procedure do you follow if someone phones in threatening suicide?
   b. What question do you ask first of the potential suicide victim?
   c. What directive do you give first to the potential suicide victim?

    d. How do you assess the potential for suicide over the phone?

2. Visit your clergyman and ask for the religious interpretation of suicide in your denomination.

3. Assess the availability of a crisis center on your campus.

    a. What are the disciplines of the personnel manning the center?

    b. What procedures do the staff members follow when a client has a high suicidal index?

4. Interview a mental health professional and ask what parameters he or she uses to make a judgment of the client's potential for suicide?

BIBLIOGRAPHY

Aguilera, Donna C., and Messick, Janice M. *Crisis Intervention: Theory and Methodology.* 3d ed. St. Louis: C. V. Mosby Co., 1978.

Archer, Sarah, and Fleshman, Ruth. "Health Insurance: How We Pay for Health Care." In *Community Health Nursing,* Mass.: Duxbury Press, 1975.

Burgess, Anne J., and Lazarre, Aron. *Psychiatric Nursing in the Hospital and the Community.* 2d ed. Englewood Cliffs, N.J.: Prentice-Hall, Inc., 1976.

Esslemont, J. E. *Baha'u'llah and the New Era.* Wilmette, Ill.: Bahai Publishing Trust, 1976.

Faigel, Harris. "A Developmental Approach to Adolescence." *Pediatric Clinics of North America* 21 (May 1974): 353–359.

Guerin, Philip J., Jr., ed. *Family Therapy.* New York: Gardner Press, Inc., 1976.

———. "Suicide." Lecture given at The Center for Family Learning, New Rochelle, New York, January 30, 1978.

Guyton, Arthur C. *Textbook of Medical Physiology.* 5th ed. Philadelphia: W. B. Saunders Co., 1976.

Hall, Joanne E., and Weaver, Barbara R. *Nursing of Families in Crisis.* Philadelphia: J. B. Lippincott Co., 1974.

Hatton, Corrine Loing et al. *Suicide: Assessment and Intervention.* New York: Appleton-Century-Crofts, 1977.

Kalkman, Marion E., and Davis, Anne J. *New Dimensions in Mental Health– Psychiatric Nursing.* 4th ed. New York: McGraw-Hill, 1974.

Little, Dolores E., and Carnevali, Doris L. *Nursing Care Planning.* 2d ed. Philadelphia: J. B. Lippincott Co., 1976.

Mitchell, Martha. "Suicide as a Family Nursing Problem." In *Family Health Care.* Edited by Debra P. Hymovich and Martha Underwood Barnard. New York: McGraw-Hill, 1973.

Pendagast, Eileen G., and Sherman, Charles O. "A Guide to the Genogram Family Systems Training." *The Family* 5 (1977): 3–14.

Petrillo, Madeline, and Sanger, Sirgay. "A Working Knowledge of Childhood." In *Emotional Care of Hospitalized Children*. Philadelphia: J. B. Lippincott Co., 1972.

Pumphrey, John B. "Recognizing Your Patients' Spiritual Needs." *Nursing '77* 7 (December 1977): 64–70.

Sedgervick, Rae. "The Family as a System: A Network of Relationships." In *Psychiatric and Mental Health Nursing*, Barbara A. Backer, Patricia M. Dubbert, and Elaine J. P. Eisenman. New York: D. Van Nostrand Co., 1978.

Snyder, Joyce, and Wilson, Margo. "Elements of a Psychological Assessment." *American Journal of Nursing* 77 (February 1977): 235–239.

Westercamp, Twilla M. "Suicide." *American Journal of Nursing* 75 (February 1975): 260–262.

CHAPTER TWELVE

Surgical Assault: Hysterectomy

FANG-LAN WANG KUO

OVERVIEW

Joan Washington is a twenty-two-year-old black woman who has been married to Carson Washington for three years. They are Jehovah's Witnesses. They have been attending a family-planning clinic. After experiencing dysmenorrhea and periodic vaginal bleeding for two years, Joan undergoes an examination and several diagnostic tests, which reveal a pelvic mass. When the mass is removed surgically, a hysterectomy is also necessary. Since their religion prohibits the intravenous administration of blood products, special consent forms must be signed. The nursing staff works to prevent physiological and psychological complications.

CONTENT EMPHASIS

- Prevention of conception—diaphragm
- Preoperative assessment and diagnostic tests—pelvic mass
- Religious restriction on health care—Jehovah's Witness
- Prevention of postoperative complications—physiological and psychological

SETTINGS

- Family-planning clinic
- GYN clinic
- Surgical unit

OBJECTIVES

Upon completing this chapter the student will be able to:

1. Identify various techniques to assist couples in family planning.
2. Create a teaching plan specific to the preparation of clients for diagnostic examinations.
3. Comprehend the religious beliefs of members of the Jehovah's Witness faith as it affects a client/family's health care.
4. Develop health care goals that prepare a client/family for an abdominal hysterectomy.
5. Design health outcomes for the prevention of physiological and psychological complications of a client experiencing a hysterectomy.

DEFINITIONS

The following terms are used in this case study and should be defined before proceeding:

Anesthesia induction agent
Anesthesia maintenance agent
Artificial menopause
Dysmenorrhea
Endometriosis
Exploratory laporatomy
Fibroid uterus
Gynecology
Hysterectomy
Incentive spirometry

Intravenous pyelogram (IVP)
Intermittent positive-pressure
  breathing (IPPB)
Jehovah's Witnesses
Laporatomy
Nasogastric (N/G) tube
Oophorectomy
Ovarian cyst
Retention suture
Subtotal hysterectomy

FAMILY ASSESSMENT

Ms. Joan Washington is a twenty-two-year-old black woman from West Virginia. Her financially struggling family still lives there. When Joan could not find work after graduating from high school, she reluctantly moved to New York City to join an employed female friend. She hoped to be as fortunate as her friend had in finding work. When Joan talked about the day she left home, she always mentioned how she did not stop crying until her arrival at the Port Authority Bus Terminal in New York City. Joan maintains contact with her family by weekly letters.

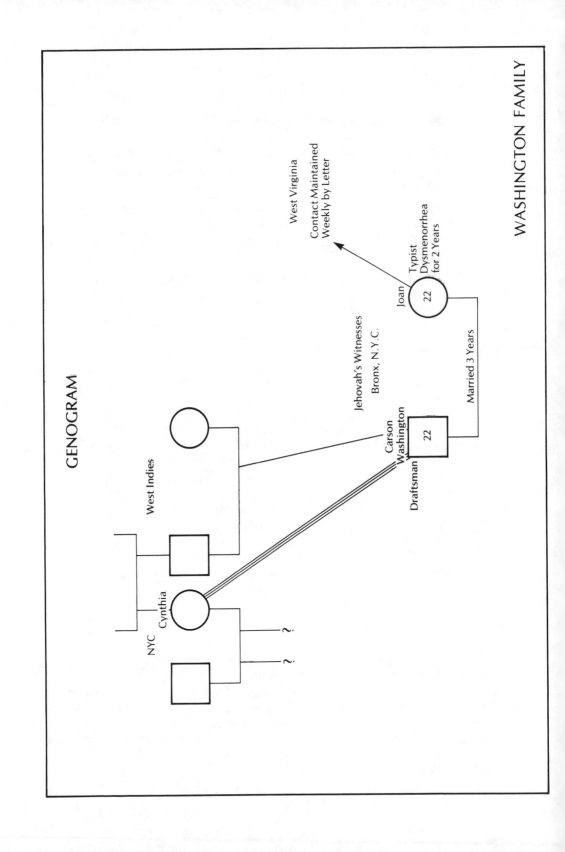

After a month of job hunting, Joan secured a position as a typist with a large legal firm. Shortly thereafter she met Carson Washington, who later became her husband. At present they have been married for three years. (See genogram.)

Carson Washington, a twenty-two-year-old black man, came from the West Indies six years ago. He lived with his maternal aunt Cynthia's family until he married. Carson works as a draftsman.

The Washington's combined net income of $980 a month just covers their $900 monthly expenses. In fact, the only financial protection the Washingtons have is their Prudential Health Insurance through Carson's employment. Without this, the Washingtons would have no health insurance. They reside in a one-bedroom walk-up in the Bronx. They hope that within three years they will be able to scrape together enough money to be able to start a family. At present Joan prevents pregnancy by using the diaphragm she was fitted for at the time of her marriage. In the meantime, they devote all of their free time to converting others to their beliefs as Jehovah's Witnesses.

STUDY QUESTIONS

12-1. In what developmental stage is the Carson Washington family?

12-2. What are the religious beliefs of Jehovah's Witnesses about the following topics: family, marriage, children, health care, blood products, techniques of contraception?

12-3. What are the benefits of a Prudential Health Insurance Policy in your area?

12-4. Who is best qualified to fit a woman for a diaphragm? Why?

12-5. How does the diaphragm method of birth control prevent pregnancy? Explain.

12-6. How is a diaphragm maintained when not in use? How is it cleaned?

12-7. How often should a diaphragm be replaced? Explain.

12-8. How often should a diaphragm fitting be checked? Explain.

12-9. How effective is a diaphragm in preventing conception?

DISCUSSION QUESTIONS

D-1. What are some philosophical beliefs of Jehovah's Witnesses about the following topics: birth control, health, medical plans, and woman?

D-2. Prepare a teaching plan to instruct a female client in the use and care of a diaphragm. What is the context for each objective? How can the client's learning be evaluated?

Objective	Content	Method of Teaching	Method of Evaluating Learning Effectiveness
1. To explain the mechanism by which the diaphragm prevents conception.			
2. To explain the technique for checking for possible defects in the diaphragm before use.			
3. To identify the advantages and disadvantages of using the diaphragm from the female and male's point of view.			
4. To explain how to select the proper size of diaphragm.			
5. To explain how to prepare the female and her sexual partner prior to sexual intercourse.			
6. To identify the possible complications from using the diaphragm.			
7. To explain how to care for the diaphragm after use.			

D-3. What are the beliefs of West Indians about the following topics: birth control, children, family, health, marriage, medical plans, woman, blood transfusion?

D-4. What are some of the difficulties experienced by couples who are raised in different cultures? Explain each.

CLIENT ASSESSMENT

During the last two years, Joan's menstrual flow has been accompanied by progressively more discomfort. Recently she has noted midcycle vaginal bleeding. The extra bleeding upset her more than the dysmenorrhea. Consequently, she decided to obtain the opinion of a health professional. Joan made an appointment at the neighborhood family-planning clinic.

After doing a complete assessment on Joan, Ms. Frances, the nurse-midwife employed at the family planning clinic, recorded the following:

HISTORY: Menstrual flow progressively more uncomfortable over the last 2 years, characterized by low back pain, abdominal cramping, rectal spasms, and lower abdominal pressure.

CHIEF COMPLAINT: Dysmenorrhea, profuse midcycle bleeding, fatigue, general malaise.

IMPRESSION: a firm, well-defined, nonmovable abdominal mass in the right lower quadrant. Irritable uterus which is 8×5 cm^2.

RECOMMENDATION: Referred to GYN clinic.

When Joan had redressed, she was invited back to Ms. Frances's office. Ms. Frances explained her findings to Joan. Joan began to twist her hair and repeatedly repositioned herself in the chair. Ms. Frances moved closer to Joan and rested her hand on Joan's hand. Then Ms. Frances said softly, "I believe that you should see a doctor. The GYN clinic on Loren Street is nearest to where you live."

After Joan had been given time to digest what the nurse-midwife had said, Ms. Frances arranged for an appointment at the GYN clinic for Joan.

The following week, James Smith, M.D., the GYN clinic's attending physician, reviewed the first-year GYN resident's findings on Joan. Dr. Smith confirmed Ms. Frances's impression. He also added the following to Joan's record:

RECOMMENDATION: Schedule for IVP
                 R/O endometriosis
                 R/O fibroid uterus

Ms. Andrews, R.N., the GYN clinic nurse, watched Joan's eyes fill with tears as Dr. Smith explained his recommendation. He spoke softly and slowly. However, his description remained quite technical. After Dr. Smith and the resident had left the room, Joan turned to Ms. Andrews. She encouraged the client to ask questions. Joan said in a tense voice, "What does all this mean?"

Ms. Andrews patiently explained in lay terms the impression that Dr. Smith had of Joan's physical state. She pointed out that the exam revealed that some extra tissue was present in Joan's lower abdomen. Ms. Andrews explained further that no one could be sure what the extra tissue was until more tests were taken. Then she told Joan about the intravenous pyelogram.

When Carson arrived home that night, Joan burst into tears. He knew Joan to be a very steady person, so her behavior alarmed him. Carson remembered that Joan said that she had an appointment at the clinic. He put all the information together and came up with the worst. Carson thought Joan had been told she had cancer. He picked up the phone and called his Aunt Cynthia. Carson asked Cynthia to come right over... that Joan was very upset. Then he held Joan in his arms as he sat next to her on the couch. Joan started to calm down.

By the time Cynthia had arrived, Joan had explained her condition to Carson. With Carson and Cynthia's support, Joan decided to go and have the recommended IVP.

Aunt Cynthia put it this way, "Honey, you've got to know what something is before you can do anything about it. But, from now on you're not going to face this alone. I'm going with you to those doctors!"

Carson thanked Cynthia for the kindness and understanding she was showing. He remarked to Cynthia, "I just cannot get off from work to be with Joan. But she sure does need somebody with her."

Two days after the IVP was done, Cynthia was waiting with Joan in Dr. Smith's office. Dr. Smith looked over the IVP report that read as follows:

IMPRESSION: Abdominal mass pressing on right ureter—size 4×8 cm^2

The women held each other's hands as they searched Dr. Smith's face.

Dr. Smith sensed Joan's tension. He too felt uneasy, because the news for Joan was not good. Dr. Smith started by explaining the findings on the intravenous pyelogram. He told Joan that the mass could be on the right ovary or an extension of the uterus. At any rate, the mass was not normal. His opinion was that it should be removed. Because he feared kidney damage due to pressure, Dr. Smith recommended surgery at an early date.

Joan whispered, "I wish you hadn't had to tell me this." When Joan said nothing more, Cynthia added, "Joan will want time to discuss this with her husband."

Dr. Smith continued, "I can understand that. If Mr. Washington has any questions, please have him phone me. At any rate, Joan, I would like you to get back to me within the week."

That evening Carson called Dr. Smith. He decided that Dr. Smith's judgment sounded rational. He did not like the idea of Joan undergoing surgery, but something had to be done to help end his wife's pain. Also, the possibility of cancer still upset him. Therefore, Carson said, "The doctor must know best. Phone him tomorrow and tell him to go ahead and schedule you for surgery." Carson's voice was trembling as he finished the sentence.

STUDY QUESTIONS

12-10. What services are provided by a family planning clinic? Explain each.

12-11. What services are provided by a GYN clinic? Explain each.

12-12. What did Ms. Frances mean by an irritable uterus?

12-13. Is midcycle vaginal bleeding always an indication of illness?

12-14. What history is absolutely necessary before a client undergoes an IVP? Why?

12-15. Why was the intravenous pyelogram report nonspecific for the exact foci of Joan's abdominal mass?

12-16. What kidney problems can be caused by pressure on a ureter?

DISCUSSION QUESTIONS

D-5. Where are the family-planning clinics in your area? What forms of transportation pass by the clinic? Who is allowed to attend the clinic? Who pays for the clinic's operation?

D-6. How would you explain the need for an IVP to Joan Washington?

D-7. Design a teaching plan for preparing Ms. Washington for an IVP:

Objective	Content	Method of Teaching	Method of Evaluating Learning

PREOPERATIVE PHASE

Three days after phoning Dr. Smith, Joan was admitted to the hospital. Since it was a working day, Cynthia, rather than Carson, came with Joan. After a short time, the primary care nurse, Ms. Mary Young, R.N., came into Joan's semiprivate room. Cynthia said her good-byes to Joan and left for home.

Mary Young collected the following data:

VITAL SIGNS: T: 36.8 C   P:80   R:18   BP:130/80

GENERAL APPEARANCE: 80 kg, 160 cm, 22-year-old black female.

MENTAL STATUS: High-school graduate; presently employed as a typist; denies history of loss of consciousness, syncope, disorientation, or memory lapses.

EMOTIONAL STATUS: Fidgety; alert; reactivity increased; verbalized concern over scheduled surgery.

SENSES: Denies remarkable history.

BODY TEMPERATURE: Normal range 36.5–36.8°C; denies temperature exceeding 39.5°C during present illness.

MORTOR STATUS: Left-handed; denies history of limited range of motion or muscle masses; good muscle tone and movement.

RESPIRATORY STATUS: Denies smoking and history of respiratory problems; no adventitious sounds; breathing sounds are normal; equal movement of both sides of chest, respiratory rate 18/ minute and regular in rhythm. (Her mother had TB when the client was two years old—treatment unknown)

CIRCULATORY STATUS: Denies history of chest pain, palpatations or hypertension; heart sounds normal; no adventitious sounds; pulse rate 80 per minute, strong and regular in rhythm.

NUTRITIONAL STATUS: Good appetite; irregular meal times; diet reportedly high in carbohydrate; denies history of alterations in buccal cavity, mastication, or swallowing.

ELIMINATION STATUS: Denies history of alteration in bowel or bladder functioning; voids 5–6 times per day, requires no cathartics.

REPRODUCTIVE STATUS: Menarche age 12; 29-day menstrual cycle with 4–5 days moderate vaginal flow; dysmenorrhea for last two years; midcycle bleed last 3 months; last menstrual period (LMP) Monday last week; denies history of VD; negative pap smear; denies sexual relationship difficulties; breasts normal by inspection and palpation. (Client does not do self-examination of the breast—lacks knowledge of method.)

SKIN AND APPENDAGES: Light coffee-colored skin; good skin turgor; denies history of skin rashes or lesions. Short, coarse, black, naturally curly hair; nail integrity good.

REST AND COMFORT: Sleeps from 11 P.M. to 6 A.M.; denies insomnia or drug-dependent sleep.

When Ms. Young had completed the collection of data, she oriented Joan to the surgical floor. Then the second-year GYN resident entered Joan's room. The young physician did a medical history and physical examination. Ms. Young stayed with Joan throughout the examination.

After the resident had left, Ms. Young sat down next to Joan. The conversation started slowly. Ms. Young made it clear that "all" of Joan's questions were worthy of an answer. Soon Joan asked for definitions of some of the technical terms she had heard health professionals use when talking about her condition. After Ms. Young had defined all the medical terminology that Joan could recall, Joan looked blank. Ms. Young decided to wait for some feedback. Joan said, "I might not be able to have babies after tomorrow."

Ms. Young said softly, "That could happen."

A long silence followed. Then Joan sighed a deep sigh and said, "Thank you for telling me . . . I've been wanting to get that question answered by Dr. Smith . . . but I just couldn't ask. He kind of said it, but I just wasn't sure."

A little later, Dr. Smith brought in the surgical consent. He found that Joan had a good understanding of the terms listed. The consent was for the following:

Exploratory laporotomy
Possible bilateral oophorectomy
Possible hysterectomy

After Joan had signed the surgical consent, Dr. Smith left the following orders:

CBC
Blood chemistry profile
Type and cross-match for 2 units whole blood
Prothrombin time and clotting time
Urinalysis
EKG
AP chest X-ray
Surgical prep
Regular diet
NPO after midnight
Fleets enema in A.M. followed by a vaginal douche with Betadine in A.M.
Indwelling catheter in A.M. before OR

Later, the anesthetist arrived and left the following preoperative orders:

Dalmane 30 mg po hs
Phenergan 30 mg IM at 8:00 A.M. tomorrow
Demerol 50 mg IM at 9:00 A.M. tomorrow
Atropine sulfate 0.4 mg IM at 9:00 A.M. tomorrow

Well into the evening shift one problem concerning the medical plan was picked up. Lucy Farrel, R.N., Joan's evening nurse, noted Joan's religion. She recalled that Joan was scheduled for blood on call to the OR. Ms. Farrel immediately went to Joan's room and asked Joan for her personal belief concerning blood transfusions. Joan explained that she would not knowingly allow herself to receive blood . . . that it was against her religion.

Lucy Farrel notified Dr. Smith. Then she brought a form to Joan for her client's signature. The form stated that the client disallowed acceptance of blood or any blood products transfused. A medical alert stating the disallowance of blood and blood products was taped to the front of Joan's chart and marked on her presurgical sheet by Ms. Farrel. Then she returned to Joan and gave her postoperative instruction.

In the morning, Carson and Joan said a quiet prayer together before Joan's 9:00 A.M. preoperative medications were given. Joan was calm as she left for surgery.

STUDY QUESTIONS

12-17. The following are the results of Joan's presurgical tests. Complete the following laboratory grid:

Test	Joan's Test Result	Normal Range for Female Adult	Possible Cause for Alteration
Erythrocyte	3.7×10^6 mm^3		
Hemoglobin	10 g/100 ml		
Hematocrit	32%		
Mean corpuscular hemoglobin (MCH)	23 pg		
Mean corpuscular volume (MCV)	78 cu. μ		
Mean corpuscular hemoglobin concentration (MCHC)	29%		
Reticulocytes	1.2% of RBC		
Platelet	320,000		
Leukocyte	13,000 mm^3		
Neutrophile	60%		
Lymphocytes	28%		
Eosinophils	3%		
Prothrombin time	patient 14 sec. control 13 sec.		
Clotting time	8 minutes		
Rh	(+)		
Type	0		

Test	Joan's Test Result	Normal Range for Female Adult	Possible Cause for Alteration
Urinalysis Specific gravity	1.016		
Acetone	negative		
Glucose	negative		
RBC	negative		
WBC	negative		
Protein	negative		
pH	6.5		
EKG (12 leads) P-R interval	0.16 second		
QRS	0.08 second		
QT	0.36 second		
Interpretation	normal sinus rhythm		
Chest X-ray:	unremarkable		

12-18. What is the normal blood volume for a female adult?

12-19. What are the functions of blood? What will be the risk of not having blood transfusions when Joan is undergoing surgery?

12-20. Identify some of the major blood expanders. What are their limitations?

12-21. Does your state have a Patient's Bill of Rights? If yes, what is included? Explain.

12-22. What constitutes an "informed surgical consent"? Explain.

12-23. What is the correct way to secure a surgical consent? Was Joan's consent secured properly? Explain.

12-24. What are the pros and cons for giving a blood transfusion to someone who is religiously opposed to this during an episode of severe blood loss? Who should make the decision to give or not to give blood?

12-25. Complete a drug information card on the following medications: Phenergan, Demerol, atropine, Dalmane.

12-26. What is the effect of administering Demerol and atropine together preoperatively? What precautions should be taken?

12-27. Explain the purpose and nursing actions for each of the following medical orders. What is the rationale for each of the nursing actions? How is the procedure's effectiveness evaluated?

Order	Purpose	Procedure	Nursing Action	Rationale	Evaluation
Surgical prep					
Fleet's enema					
Vaginal douche with Betadine					
Indwelling catheter					

DISCUSSION QUESTIONS

D-8.   Based on the framework of the three psychodynamic dimensions, what is your assessment of Joan and Carson:

　　a. Intrapersonal dimension: inner experience of oneself as a person, the meaning of all that happens to her (him).

　　b. Interpersonal dimension: refers to those encounters between client and family, client and caretakers, client and agency.

　　c. Impersonal dimension: the nature of an operation and illness forces one in a direction that is contrary to client's established routine.

D-9.   Since Joan was admitted with an already documented illness, do you believe Ms. Young used her time wisely by taking a nursing assessment? Explain.

D-10. Could the incident concerning blood transfusions have been avoided? How?

D-11. Design a preoperative teaching plan for Joan on the following topics:

Topic	Goal	Objective	Content	Method of Teaching	Method of Evaluating Learning
Deep breathing					
Coughing					
Turning					
Ambulation					
Surgical dressing					
Bathing					

THE HYSTERECTOMY

Joan Washington's OR record read as follows:

GIVEN: Thiopental 2.5% IV as induction agent

GIVEN: N_2O via mask

SURGICAL INCISION: Lower midline of abdomen

CONFIRMED: Fibroid uterus, Rt. Ovarian Cyst and Endometriosis

SURGICAL PROCEDURE: Subtotal hysterectomy and Rt. Oophorectomy

Joan's vital signs stabilized (T: 36.5°C   P: 86   R: 20   BP: 110/70) while in the recovery room. A 1000 ml bottle of 5% D in ½ NS infused into her left cephalic vein via a number 18 gauge needle (angiocatheter). The Foley catheter inserted before surgery remained. An N/G tube was attached to low Gomco suction.

Carson was sitting in the surgical suite waiting area when Dr. Smith located him. Carson had called in sick at work so that he could get the day off. Carson looked gray. His hands were damp.

Dr. Smith informed Carson that he was sorry but he could save only Joan's left ovary due to the extent of her disease. Carson asked, "Are you telling me that Joan has cancer?"

"No," said Dr. Smith, "but she will never be able to bear children."

Carson dropped his face into his hands, saying, "Oh, Jehovah! Oh, my God!"

Dr. Smith asked for a nurse to stay with Carson until he was over the initial shock of the news. By 1:20 P.M. Joan was returned to her room by stretcher from the recovery room. She was conscious and oriented to person, place, and date. However, she felt tired. Her skin color was pale, warm, and without cyanosis; airway was clear without adventitious breathing sounds; abdominal dressing was clean, dry, and intact; scanty rubra vaginal discharge was observed; IV fluid with 5% dextrose in water was in progress; Foley catheter was in place. Vital signs: T: 36.4°C   P: 82   R: 18   BP: 110/68. The head of her bed was elevated to 15°, and her head was resting on one pillow.

Carson had had a long discussion with Dr. Smith. Carson's color was improved and his palms were no longer damp.

When Joan was able to focus on Carson, she asked him about her condition. Carson told her that God had heard their prayers. God had seen fit to protect her from cancer.

Then Joan asked, "Then I still have my womb?"

While squeezing Joan's hand, Carson said, "No, honey, you don't have your womb. What it all means is that we have each other, and you are going to be well."

Joan's tears stained her pillow before she lapsed back into sleep.

In the meantime Dr. Smith wrote the following orders:

NPO

N/G tube to low Gomco suction

Indwelling catheter to straight drainage

I&O

Bed rest; Dangle in A.M.

1,000 cc 5% D/W in ½ NS with 15 mEq KCL and 2 cc Berocca-C q 8 h

Demerol 75 mg IM q 4 h prn

IPPB with 10 cc normal saline t i d

Incentive spirometry q 2 h × 10

Hgb and Hct this P.M. and tomorrow A.M.

Joan physically progressed well (see postoperative flow sheets). However, emotionally Joan had some difficulty. She grieved over the loss of her womb. Ms. Smith continually helped Joan by giving her opportunities to talk. During the evening shift the nurse encouraged Carson's continued efforts to help Joan verbalize her feelings.

POSTOPERATIVE FLOW SHEET

Functional Areas / Days of the Surgery	Time	Vital Signs	Respiratory Status	Circulatory Status	Mental and Conscious Status	Vaginal Discharge	Surgical Wound Status
	1:20 to 3:00	118/78 36.4 82 18 / 118/80 36.4 82 18	Airway clear No adventitious breathing sounds	Blanching signs on nails Skin pale, warm to touch No cyanosis Pulse strong & regular	Orientated to person, place, and date Fatigued Sleeping most of time	Rubra vaginal spotting	Dressing clean, dry, and intact
Day of Surgery	3:00 to 11:00	130/82 36.8 82 18 / 130/80 36.8 80 18	No alteration	No alteration	Informed the outcome of surgery by husband and tearing quietly	Moderate rubra discharge V-Pad × 2	No alteration
	11:00 to 7:00	128/78 36.5 78 16	No alteration	No alteration	Good night's sleep	Moderate rubra discharge V-Pad × 1	No alteration
	7:00 to 3:00	128/80 37 78 18 / 130/80 37.2 80 18	No alteration	No alteration	Crying intermittently expressing feeling about not being able to bear children	Rubra vaginal spotting V-Pad × 1	Dressing changed Incision clean and dry Retention sutures intact
Day 1	3:00 to 11:00	130/82 37 80 18 / 128/80 37 80 16	No alteration	No alteration	Talked with husband about childless marriage	Rubra vaginal spotting V-Pad × 1	Dressing clean, dry, and intact

POSTOPERATIVE FLOW SHEET (*continued*)

Day of the Surgery	Time	Vital Signs	Respiratory Status	Circulatory Status	Mental and Conscious Status	Vaginal Discharge	Surgical Wound Status
	11:00 to 7:00	126/78 36.5 78 16	No alteration	No alteration	Restless night Fidgety	Rubra vaginal spotting V-Pad × 1	No alteration
	7:00 to 3:00	126/78 36.4 78 16	No alteration	No alteration	Stayed alone—told nurse that she was trying to see self as career girl	No spotting	No alteration
Day 2	3:00 to 11:00	126/74 36.6 80 16	No alteration	No alteration	Talked with husband again about childless marriage	No alteration	No alteration
	11:00 to 7:00	126/76 36.4 80 16	No alteration	No alteration	Slept soundly	No alteration	No alteration

POSTOPERATIVE FLOW SHEET

Day of the Surgery	Time	Fluid and Nutritional Status	Gastrointestinal Status	Physical Activity and Comfort	Medication	Therapy	Remarks
	1:20 / 3:00	NPO D5W m ½ NS 15 m Eq KCl & 2 c.c. Berocca C 300 c.c. N/G tube: 100 c.c. Foley: 600 c.c.	No bowel sound No nausea or vomiting	Bed rest & comfort No pain Turn & R.O.M.	IV: 15 m Eq. KCl Berocca-C 2 cc	IPPB: 10 c.c. NS × 1 Breathing exercise × 1 Ted stockings Peri-care × 1 Incentive spirometry × 1	V.S. q 4 hrs Dr. Smith informed Carson of Joan's surgery
Day of Surgery	3:00 / 11:00	NPO IV: 1000 c.c. N/G: 120 c.c. Foley: 700 c.c.	Weak bowel sound	Refused to sit up c/o "surgical pain" relieved by Demerol in 45 min. TUR & R.O.M. q 2-3 hours	IV: 15 m Eq KCl Berocca-C 2 c.c. Demerol 75 mg IM 11 am	IPPB: 10 c.c. NS × 2 Breathing exercise q 2 hrs Ted stockings Peri-Care; Foley Care; IV Care Incentive spirometry × 3	V.S. q 4 hrs Husband stayed till 10 pm Therapeutic support to Joan & Carson
	11:00 / 7:00	NPO IV: 1000 c.c. N/G: 80 c.c. Foley: 800 c.c.	Weak bowel sound	Comfort night TUR & R.O.M.	IV: 15 m Eq KCl Berocca-C 2 c.c.	As above	Hgb: 9.6 g; Hct: 30 24°: 1:2300 c.c. 30% 0:2400 c.c.
	7:00 / 3:00	Clear liquid diet: 660 c.c. IV: 900 c.c. N/G: 20 c.c. Voided: q.s.	Bowel sound strong Tolerated well to clear liquid	OOB in chair × 30' × 2 Surgical pain relieved by Demerol in 40 min.	IV: 15 m Eq KCl Berocca-C 2 c.c. Demerol 75 mg IM 1 pm	As above	Dr. Smith visited Husband stayed bedside since 9 am

POSTOPERATIVE FLOW SHEET (*continued*)

Functional Areas / Days of the Surgery	Time	Fluid and Nutritional Status	Gastrointestinal Status	Physical Activity and Comfort	Medication	Therapy	Remarks
Day 1	3:00 / 11:00	Oral: 100 c.c. IV: 800 c.c. Voided: q.s.	Expelling gas Tolerated soft diet well	OOB to BR with assistance; voided —dysuria	FeSO÷tab p.o. bid Multivitamin÷tab. p.o. o.d. Vitamin C 100 mg p.o. tid Colace 100 mg p.o. tid	As above	Hgb: 9.5 g. Hct: 30% D.C.: NPO Foley Catheter (tip for c/s)
	11:00 / 7:00	Oral: 100 c.c. IV: 800 c.c. Voided: q.s.	No alteration	Good night's sleep	None	Incentive spirometry × 2 Breathing exercise × 2 IPPB × 1 Ted stockings Peri-Care; IV care	
	7:00 / 3:00	Oral: 650 c.c. IV: 300 c.c. Voided: q.s.	Tolerated regular diet well c/o Constipation	Independent on ADL	FeSO÷tab Multivitamin÷tab. Vitamin C 100 mg × 2 Colace 100 mg × 2	As above	Weight: 76 Kg D.C.: I.V. Nutritional teaching by the dietician to be followed by nurse
Day 2	3:00 / 11:00	Oral: 450 c.c. Voided: q.s.	No alteration 1/Fleet enema	No alteration	FeSO÷tab Vitamin C 100 mg Colace 100 mg	Incentive spirometry Breathing exercise × 2 IPPB × 1 Peri Care	Encourage oral fluids
	11:00 / 7:00	Oral: 250 c.c. Voided: q.s.	No alteration	No alteration	None	None	

STUDY QUESTIONS

12-28. What is a fibroid uterus? endometriosis? an ovarian cyst? What medical-surgical (if any) treatments may be used for each of these conditions?

12-29. What are the various forms of hysterectomies? What is removed for each and what are the nursing implications for each?

Type(s) Hysterectomy	Tissue Removed	Nursing Implications

12-30. What are the physiologic functions of the uterus? the ovaries? What hormones are secreted by the ovary? What are physiologic effects of hysterectomy? Does Joan need to take oral female hormones? Explain.

12-31. What are the four stages of anesthesia? Explain each.

12-32. What is the difference between a local anesthetic and a general anesthetic?

12-33. What is the rationale for each of the postoperative medical orders?

Order	Rationale

12-34. How does a Gomco suction and an IPPB machine work?

12-35. How are a Gomco suction and an IPPB machine tested before being used? What nursing interventions are necessary and what is the rationale of each? What is the expected response of the client and how is the effectiveness evaluated?

Operational Principle	Testing Technique	Nursing Intervention	Rationale	Client's Response	Evaluation of Effectiveness

12-36. How might Joan's surgery affect her sexuality? Explain.

DISCUSSION QUESTIONS

D-12. What are the potential complications that can occur after a hysterectomy? What nursing actions can be done to prevent each? What is the rationale for each nursing action?

Potential Complication	Nursing Actions	Rationale

D-13. What are the nursing care objectives during Joan's immediate postoperative phase? What is the rationale for each? What are the nursing actions and what is the rationale for each action? How is the effectiveness evaluated?

Objective	Rationale	Nursing Action	Rationale	Method and Frequency of Evaluation

D-14. Revise the above care plan for the first postoperative day (review postoperative flow sheet).

D-15. Revise the above care plan for the second postoperative day (review postoperative flow sheet).

D-16. What is the major function of retention sutures? Why does Joan need retention sutures?

PROGRESS

Joan's recovery progressed without complications. She attributed this to her faith in Jehovah and Carson's support. In fact, by postoperative day 1 Joan was able to talk with Carson about their childless marriage, and the idea of adoption was initiated by Carson. By postoperative day 2 Joan had already verbalized interest in going back to her job as a typist. The nursing staff had answered all of Joan's questions about her sexuality and the possibility of adopting a child. Then by postoperative day 10 the retention sutures were removed, and the post-hysterectomy medical follow-up by Dr. Smith at the GYN clinic was scheduled before Joan was ready for discharge.

CHAPTER DISCUSSION QUESTIONS

1. What are the various types of family planning? What is the role of the nurse in each?

Type	Nurse's Role

2. What are the stages of grieving? How is a client in each stage assessed? How can the nurse assist the client as he or she is experiencing each stage?

Stage of Grieving	Assessment	Nursing Action	Rationale

3. How would the various stages of grieving be explained to Carson?
4. What are some of the psychological effects of hysterectomy? How can the nursing staff assist Joan to prevent undue anxiety and depression?
5. How can the professional nurse mobilize Joan's emotional support systems during each phase of care?

SUGGESTED ACTIVITIES

1. Take care of someone undergoing hysterectomy pre- and post-operatively.
2. Interview a client who has had recent major surgery. Review the following:
   a. How was the surgical consent presented to them?
   b. Who presented the surgical consent to them?
   c. How clear was her or his understanding of the surgery before signing the consent?

d. Was the actual surgical procedure consistent with what the client had believed was about to be done before surgery?

e. What is the client's understanding of the Patient's Bill of Rights?

BIBLIOGRAPHY

Barnard, Martha Underwood; Clancy, Barbara J.; and Krantz, Kermit E. *Human Sexuality for Health Professionals*. Philadelphia: W. B. Saunders Co., 1978.

Bergersen, Betty. *Pharmacology in Nursing*. 13th ed. St. Louis: C. V. Mosby Co., 1976.

Breu, Christine, and Dracup, Kathleen. "Helping the Spouses of Critically Ill Patients." *American Journal of Nursing* 78 (January 1978): 50–53.

Cohen, Stephen. "Helping Depressed Patients in General Nursing Practice." *American Journal of Nursing* 77 (June 1977): 1–32.

Cornish, Joan. "Psychodynamics of the Hysterectomy Experience." In *Current Practice in Obstetric and Gynecological Nursing*. Edited by L. K. McNall, et al. St. Louis: C. V. Mosby Co., 1976.

Garb, Solomon. *Laboratory Tests in Common Use*. 6th ed. New York: Springer Publishing Inc., 1976.

Hymovich, Debra P., and Barnard, Martha Underwood. *Family Health Care*. New York: McGraw-Hill, 1973, 169–179.

James, Sybil M. "When Your Patient Is Black West Indian." *American Journal of Nursing* 78 (November 1978): 1908–1909.

Little, Dolores E., and Carnevali, Doris L. *Nursing Care Planning* 2d ed. Philadelphia: J. B. Lippincott Co., 1976.

Luckmann, Joan, and Sorensen, Karen Creason. "Reproductive System." In *Medical–Surgical Nursing*. Philadelphia: W. B. Saunders Co., 1974, 1389–1453.

Marcinek, Margaret Boyle. "Stress in the Surgical Patient.' *American Journal of Nursing* 77 (November 1977): 1809–1811.

Martin, Leonide. "Menopause" and "Vaginal Discharge and Itching." In *Health Care of Women*. Philadelphia: J. B. Lippincott Co., 1978, 201–238.

Murray, Ruth, and Murphy, J. "Religious Influences cn The Person." In *Nursing Concepts for Health Promotion*. Englewood Cliffs, N.J.: Prentice-Hall, Inc., 1975, 303–328.

Pendagast, Eileen G., and Sherman, Charles O. "A Guide to the Genogram Family Systems Training." *The Family* 5 (1977): 3–14

Porter, Anne L. et al. "Patient Needs on Admission." *American Journal of Nursing* 77 (January 1977): 112–113.

Pumphrey, John B. "Recognizing Your Patient's Spiritual Needs." *Nursing '77* 7 (December 1977): 64–70.

Robinson, Corinne, and Lawler, Marilyn R. *Normal and Therapeutic Nutrition* 15th ed. New York: MacMillan, 1977.

Ryan, Rosemary. "Thrombophlebitis: Assessment and Prevention." *American Journal of Nursing* 76 (October 1976): 1634–1636.

Stephenson, Carol A. "Stress in Critically Ill Patients." *American Journal of Nursing* 77 (November 1977): 1806–1808.

Stroot, Violet R.; Lee Carla A.; and Schaper, C. Ann. *Fluid and Electrolytes: A Practical Approach.* 2d ed. Philadelphia: F. A. Davis Co., 1977.

Sweetwood, Hannelore. "Acute Respiratory Insufficiency: How to Recognize this Emergency—How to Treat it." *Nursing '77* 7 (December 1977): 24–31.

Williams, Margaret Aasterud. "Easier Convalescence from Hysterectomy." *American Journal of Nursing* 76 (March 1976): 438–440.

Woods, Nancy Fugate, and Woods, James. "Hysterectomy." In *Human Sexuality in Health and Illness*, St. Louis. C. V. Mosby Co., 1975, pp. 151–154.

CHAPTER THIRTEEN

Acute Alteration in Liver Function: Hepatitis A

CYNTHIA DEGAZON

OVERVIEW

Peter Albert is a twenty-eight-year-old electrical engineer from London, England. After divorcing his wife, he received custody of their three children and he invited his unmarried sister Emily to live with them and care for the children. He developed hepatitis A shortly after being transferred to the United States. After ignoring his initial symptoms, Peter is later treated in the emergency room. Peter and Emily are given specific directions for home care because Peter refuses hospitalization. A public health nurse follows Peter's care at home and she works to protect the other family members (and society) from contracting hepatitis A.

CONTENT EMPHASIS

- Assessment and treatment of a communicable disease—hepatitis
- Protection of society against communicable disease
- Divorced client—effect on family

SETTINGS

- Emergency room
- Home

OBJECTIVES

Upon completion of his chapter the student will be able to:

1. Analyze the effects of divorce on a family system.
2. Analyze the etiology and diagnostic tests for infectious hepatitis A.
3. Design a health teaching plan that will assist a client and his or her family to promote recovery, prevent complications, and prevent the spread of hepatitis A.
4. Develop the expected health outcomes for a client with hepatitis A.
5. Evalute the on-going health care plan designed for a client with infectious hepatitis A and his or her family.

DEFINITION OF TERMS

The following terms are used in this case study and should be defined before proceeding:

Anorexia   Jaundice
Coryza   Liver profile tests
Epidemiology (report)   Nonnegotiable demands
Sulminating   Pharyngitis
General certificate of education   Preicteric
  (GCE)   Prodromal symptoms
Hb$_s$Ag test   Workaholic
Health care provider

FAMILY ASSESSMENT

Peter and Mona Albert formerly lived in London, England. Although Peter had qualified on the General Certificate of Education (GCE) for entry into Oxford University, Peter and Mona were "forced" to be married by their parents immediately after graduating from secondary school because the young couple were to be the parents of a baby in less than six months. Both Peter's and Mona's families were practicing Episcopalians. Upon graduation, Peter sought employment as a technical assistant with the Tel-Air Company of London. He recognized the need for developing a vocation and shortly after his first son was born Peter enrolled in a one-year electronics program at the Royal Institute of Technology.

Peter enjoyed electronics and quickly learned the technical aspects of his job. His boss recommended him for the company's tuition assistance program so that Peter could pursue the program in electronics. His boss also permitted him to arrange his work schedule so that Peter would not have a conflict with his classes. All this made it possible for him to receive a diploma in electrical engineering.

Following the completion of his education, Peter started to advance very quickly in the organizational hierarchy. He continued to be a very energetic and aggressive individual throughout his years with the company. He often worked late evenings and had to be reminded to take his vacation.

Within four years of marriage, the Albert family had three children: Jean, Michael, and Deirdre. Peter was so preoccupied with his occupation that he was seldom home when the children were awake. Consequently, Mona carried the burden of disciplining the children. Peter's decision to pursue additional education was shared by his wife, Mona, but his continued efforts to place his job above all other matters forced many nonnegotiable demands upon his marriage and family. As a result, friction was produced that led to continuous conflict among the family members. An additional conflict developed when Mona revived her interest in pursuing a modeling career. After several small modeling jobs, Mona received an opportunity to sign a two-year contract with a large advertising firm. However, the contract required traveling to Paris, Rome, and other large cities in Europe. Peter was against the contract, but Mona hired a live-in maid and signed the contract anyway.

One year and six maids later, Peter asked his sister, Emily, to live with him and the children. When the initial modeling contract expired, Mona signed another contract. This time it was for five years. Peter and Mona's relationship became strained and unhappy.

Peter and Mona decided to dissolve the marriage. The divorce was finalized when Deirdre was five years old. Mona agreed to give custody of the children to Peter.

One year after the divorce, Peter was promoted to a senior technician for the research division. This division of the firm was located in Stoughton, Massachusetts, U.S.A. Peter was delighted with this transfer. He looked forward to the stimulation that would be provided by his colleagues in America and the opportunity to gain recognition for his creative efforts in circuit design. Peter's two sons, Jean and Michael, looked forward to exploring many places that they had learned about by watching movies and television. However, Deirdre was saddened by the thought of leaving her friends behind. Peter felt fortunate to have his unmarried sister Emily agree to relocate and continue to care for his children. This allowed him to continue his hectic schedule and still have the flexibility to travel on business when necessary.

Peter was always attentive to details, including matters pertaining to health. He always insisted on yearly check-ups for himself and the family. After his arrival in America, Peter used the Employee's Health Service as his

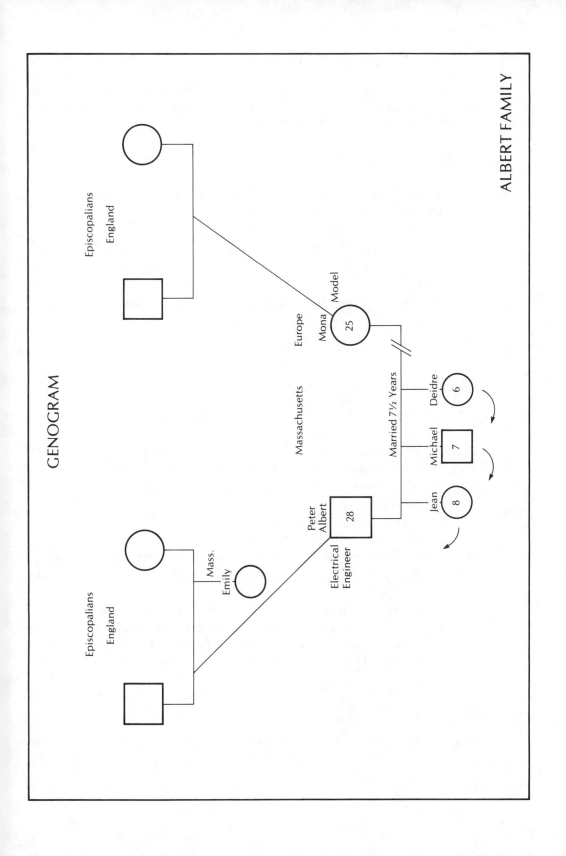

primary health care provider. He once consulted a family practitioner in an effort to select a physician, but was not satisfied with the outcome. However, he did select a pediatrician for his children.

STUDY QUESTIONS

13-1. What are the religious views of the Episcopalian church on the following topics: marriage, family, children, contraception, health, illness, divorce?

13-2. What are the two tracks of compulsory education in Great Britain? Explain.

13-3. How do the GCE's qualify a British student to enter a university? Explain.

13-4. What are the characteristics of a "workaholic?" Is Peter a workaholic? Explain.

13-5. Complete a growth and development information card on Jean (age 8), Michael (age 7), and Deirdre (age 5).

13-6. What are the current stresses for Dierdre?

DISCUSSION QUESTIONS

D-1. Compare the British educational system with the American educational system. How do they differ?

D-2. Are the individuals who pursue a technical occupation less intelligent than those who pursue a profession (college graduates)? Explain.

D-3. When preparing a health care teaching plan for Peter, what factors would you consider? Explain each.

D-4. What are the grounds for divorce in your state? What procedure is followed to receive a divorce? How is custody of the children decided?

D-5. What are the potential effects of divorce on the children of a divorced couple? on Peter's children (consider the developmental stages of Jean, Michael, and Deirdre)?

D-6. What are the problems of single parenting? Is Peter a single parent? Explain.

D-7. What information would you give to an individual who asks for a method of selecting a physician when the individual moves to a new area? selecting a health care provider? selecting a health care facility? Explain each.

CLIENT ASSESSMENT

It was a Friday afternoon in the fall when Peter realized that he had been plagued with a vague feeling of tiredness throughout the week. Peter also recalled that his appetite had diminished. He thought that the lack of nutrients might be the reason for his lassitude and tiredness. However he ignored his fatigue and continued to prepare for a meeting that he was planning to have with his superiors Monday morning. But Peter did decide that he was going to take it easy and relax with the children that weekend.

The next morning Peter was awakened by chills and a terrible headache. He had coryza, pharyngitis, and nausea. Peter was alarmed and found his complaints unexplainable and puzzling. While in the bathroom that morning, Peter tried to remember his activities of the previous week in an attempt to explain his sickly condition. He realized that his urine had gotten progressively darker and that this morning's urine was so dark that it was brown.

He became increasingly anxious as he thought of what might be his problem and of the possibility of being unable to work for a lengthy period of time. Peter awakened his sister and discussed his problem with her. Emily called for a taxi to take Peter to the Stoughton General Hospital; she remained with the children.

EMERGENCY ROOM

On arriving in the emergency room, Peter was relieved to find a staff nurse who appeared pleasant and efficient. Linda Taylor, R.N., greeted Peter and ushered him into a wheelchair. Peter was shivering and seemed too weak to walk. He described the sequence of events leading to his present condition. He denied past and present history of similar attacks. In addition, he denied any known allergies. Linda noticed Peter's jaundiced sclera, so she wheeled him into the single room as an isolation precaution.

The physical assessment done by Dr. Theodore Palmer, M.D. (medical resident) revealed the following:

> Chief Complaint: voiding brown urine.
>
> History of illness: weakness and anorexia for 1 week, chills, nausea, headache this A.M.; no change in diet; no medication taken.
>
> Vital Signs: T: 38.4°C   P: 96   R: 26   BP: 150/80
>
> Weight: 77 kg   Height: 168 cm
>
> HEENT: Eyes: PERLA, Sclera: Jaundiced
>
> Skin: pale, no rash or hives
>
> Lymphatics: enlarged and tender cervical nodes
>
> Lungs: clear breath sounds—rate 24/min

Heart: apical 96/min   regular rhythm

Abdomen: tenderness of RUQ aggravated by exertion.

Liver: Palpable and tender 1 finger below costal margin; total size—12 cm.

GU: no renal colic, no discharge, no frequency; voiding brown urine.

CNS: negative

Rectal: negative for Guaiac. Denied constipation or diarrhea; light-colored stool.

Peter's history revealed a denial of drug abuse, blood transfusions, ingestion of shellfish, or contact with a jaundiced person within the past six weeks. Peter also denied any recent travel. Dr. Palmer wrote the following orders on the emergency room record:

Liver function studies

Electrolytes

CBC

Urinalysis

Prothrombin time

Hb_sAg

Chest X-ray

1000 cc D_5W to KVO

Hepatitis precautions

Dramamine 50 mg IM q 6 h prn

Impressions: Jaundice of unknown origin; rule out: (1) hepatitis (2) gall bladder disease (3) neoplastic process.

Peter questioned Dr. Palmer as to his findings and the significance of the tests he ordered. Dr. Palmer answered all of Peter's questions.

Upset by the possibility of hospitalization and the long wait for laboratory results, Peter threatened to walk out of the emergency room against medical advice. Linda remained with Peter and allowed him to verbalize his feelings and fears. Peter asked Linda to call his sister and let her know that he was waiting for the test results.

While Peter was waiting for the laboratory results, he recalled that some four weeks ago he had purchased two dozen clams from a truck along the roadside. Emily had prepared the clams for the whole family, but the children had refused to eat them. Peter shared this information with Linda. He later asked Linda, "Do you think the clams I ate four weeks ago could be causing the problem now?"

The following are the results of Peter's laboratory tests:

Blood:
LDH: 290 units
SGOT: 700 units
SGOT 654 units
Alkaline phosphatase: 7.7
  units/100 ml
Albumin: 2.5 gms/100 ml
Globulin: 3.4 gms/100 ml
Bilirubin (total): 8 mg/100 ml
Cholesterol: 392 mg/100 ml
Glucose: 91 mg/100 ml
BUN: 6 mg/100 ml
K^+: 3.9 mEq/L
CO_2: 21 mEq/L
Na^+: 140 mEq/L
Cl^-: 100 mEq/L
Ca^+: 5.6 mEq/L
Mag^+: 2.0 mEq/L
P^-: 2.2 mEq/L

RBC: 7,000,000
WBC: 11,700
Hgb: 12.5 gm/100 ml
Hct: 40%

Platelets: 200,000
Neutrophils: 60%
Eosinophils: 5%
Basophils: <1%
Lymphocytes: 30%
Monocytes: 4%

Prothrombin time: 13.3/11.9 sec.
HB_sAg: negative
EKG: normal
X-ray (chest): negative

Urinalysis:
  Specific gravity: 1.024
  pH: 7.20
  Sugar: negative
  Protein: 2+
  Sediment: scant
  RBC: few
  WBC: 0
  Casts: 0
  Bilirubin: +

A diagnosis of hepatitis A was confirmed by Dr. Palmer. The decision was made to allow Peter to return home since an uncomplicated convalescence was expected.

STUDY QUESTIONS

13-7. What are the possible causes for dark urine? What is the physiologic basis of each cause?

13-8. What are the general causes of jaundiced sclera? What is the physiologic basis?

13-9. Why did Linda use isolation precautions for Peter in the ER? Explain.

13-10. Describe the anatomical location of the liver.

13-11. Name possible liver dysfunctions.

13-12. What are the physical abnormalities that were found when assessing Peter?

13-13. What are the prodromal signs and symptoms of hepatitis A? Discuss the physiological reason(s) for each. Identify those experienced by Peter.

13-14. Identify the common modes of transmission of hepatitis A. How did Peter get hepatitis A? Can he transmit the disease to others? Explain.

13-15. What information should be communicated by the nurse to the laboratory personnel? Give the rationale.

13-16. Complete a laboratory grid for Peter:

Test	Normal Range	Peter's Values	Amount of Deviation From Normal	Possible Cause for Alteration

13-17. Which laboratory tests are the most significant in diagnosing hepatitis A?

13-18. Complete a drug information card on dimenhydrinate.

13-19. What is the rationale for each of the medical orders? Explain.

13-20. Is hepatitis A a reportable disease? If so, who is responsible for reporting it? How is the report done?

13-21. Why did Dr. Palmer consider gall bladder disease and neoplastic process? Compare the differences and similarities with hepatitis.

13-22. Develop a nursing care plan for Peter while in the emergency room.

Problem	Goal	Interventions	Content	Evaluation of Learning

DISCUSSION QUESTIONS

D-8. How are the hepatitis precautions implemented in an emergency room in your area? What is the role of the nurse?

D-9. What is the potential impact on the family of the breadwinner becoming ill?

D-10. What can the nurse say to a client who is threatening to leave the emergency room before treatment is completed?

D-11. Should a client leave the hospital without signing a release? Discuss the legal responsibilities of the ER staff and the hospital in such a situation.

D-12. Discuss possible reasons that Dr. Palmer did not hospitalize Peter.

D-13. Discuss the treatment modalities for infectious hepatitis in your state.

DISCHARGE

Peter's discharge orders were as follows:

D/C IV

Theragram 1 cap. q d

Low fat diet

Bed rest

Teach client hepatitis precautions

Avoid all alcoholic intake

Return for further laboratory tests on Tuesday and Thursday

Clinic appointment in one week

Refer family for gamma globulin

Public health nurse referral

Dr. Palmer then completed the Department of Health notification form. Linda proceeded to review with Peter the precautions that must be strictly adhered to in order to prevent cross-contamination of his loved ones. The precautions consisted of:

1. The disposal or care of the dishes to prevent cross contamination.
2. Meticulous personal hygiene, especially handwashing after defecating.
3. Keeping of all personal belongings, such as toothbrush, eating utensils, and so on, away from those of his family.
4. Refraining from sexual contact, including the kissing of his children.
5. Careful disposal of all secretions and elimination.

Peter listened attentively to what Linda had to say. Linda encouraged Peter to ask as many questions as he wanted. She was careful that Peter understood

the instructions and allowed him to apply the information to his home setting.

Emily came to the emergency room to take Peter home. Linda took the
opportunity to have a conference with Emily so that she would be better
prepared to help Peter and the family.

STUDY QUESTIONS

13-23. Peter is expected to return for laboratory tests. Name the tests that would
be appropriate.

13-24. Identify two reasons why the ER physician referred Peter's sister and children to their private doctor.

13-25. What other classification of people should be referred to a physician for
preventive care if they were in contact with Peter?

13-26. How is the dosage of gamma globulin calculated? When is the drug given?
What is the rationale for giving it?

13-27. Complete a drug information card on the following medications: gamma
globulin, Theragram capsule.

13-28. Why was it necessary for Dr. Palmer to notify the Department of Health?

13-29. Treatment for hepatitis A consists of adequate rest, high caloric diet, and
plenty of fluids. Give the rationale for each.

13-30. Develop a sample diet to satisfy Peter's nutritional needs.

13-31. Why should the person with hepatitis refrain from alcohol?

DISCUSSION QUESTIONS

D-14. What are the major complications of hepatitis A? How can each be prevented? What information should be given to Peter about each?

Complication	Prevention	Explained to Peter

D-15. Prepare a teaching plan for Peter:

Topic	Goal	Interventions	Content	Evaluation of Learning
Diet/vitamin Rest/activities Fluids Isolation precautions Clinic appointments				

D-16. Prepare a teaching plan for Emily:

Topic	Goal	Interventions	Content	Evaluation of Learning
Isolation precautions Diet preparations Preventive care for self, children Peter's need for rest and quiet				

PUBLIC HEALTH NURSE VISIT

On Tuesday afternoon of the following week, the local health department's public health nurse, Sylvia Hess, R.N., visited the Albert family. Peter was delighted to see Sylvia, since he had remained in his room without social contact throughout the weekend.

Sylvia outlined the purpose of her visit and her role. She reviewed Peter's diet, his activities, the precautions that were being taken to prevent cross-contamination, and his plans for continued medical care. Sylvia was immediately told by Emily that she and the children had already received their "shots."

Although satisfied with the family's management of the situation, Sylvia reemphasized the importance of hand washing, particularly after defecation. Separate toilet facilities were being utilized. Peter was using the upstairs bathroom while Emily and the children were using the bathroom downstairs. Emily had purchased disposable dishes and utensils for Peter's meals and his dirty sheets and clothing were being kept apart from those of other household members and were laundered separately.

Emily expressed concern about Peter's poor appetite and intolerance of his meals. Sylvia recommended that Emily serve Peter six small meals per day instead of three large ones. When Sylvia inquired about the amount of bed-rest Peter was receiving, Emily indicated that she was answering all incoming phone calls. Sylvia then reminded Peter of the importance of avoiding fatigue.

Peter commented that the children were pleased to have "their Dad" at home. They were very cooperative in Peter's plan of care.

After completing the epidemiological report, Sylvia learned that the children's immunizations were up to date and that they had adjusted well to their new school and their new surroundings. Sylvia found Emily's blood pressure to be 150/100, and gave her a referral note to revisit her doctor. Before leaving, Sylvia made an appointment to see Emily in two weeks.

STUDY QUESTIONS

13-32. What kind of immunity, if any, is acquired by an individual after having hepatitis A?

13-33. What criteria should be used to determine when Peter may return to work?

13-34. How is the hepatitis virus destroyed? What methods can be used within the home?

13-35. Describe the responsibilities of the public health nurse in making a visit to Peter's home.

DISCUSSION QUESTIONS

D-17. How could the public health nurse assist Peter in decreasing his social isolation?

D-18. Discuss the pros and cons of alcohol restriction in the treatment of hepatitis.

D-19. What advice could the public health nurse give to Peter that would help him to meet his nutritional needs?

CHAPTER DISCUSSION QUESTIONS

1. What are the major differences between hepatitis A and hepatitis B?

Item	Hepatitis A	Hepatitis B
Identification Occurrence Causative agent Source of infection Transmission Incubation period Period of communicability Methods of control		

2. What is the prognosis for Peter's full recovery?

3. Discuss the preventive methods used by governmental agencies in the control of hepatitis A. What methods are utilized in your local area?

4. What is an epidemiological investigation? Why is this conducted? By whom?

5. Which agency(s) in your community make follow-up visits for communicable diseases?

SUGGESTED ACTIVITIES

1. Take care of someone with hepatitis.

2. Make a home visit with a public health nurse to a patient with hepatitis.

3. Interview a patient who has had infectious hepatitis.

4. At a local hospital review the nursing responsibilities for communicable disease control in the Nursing Manual.

BIBLIOGRAPHY

Archer, Sarah Ellen, and Fleshman, Ruth. *Community Health Nursing*. North Scituate, Mass.: Duxbury Press, 1975, pp. 8–11, 333–344.

Baer, Ellen D.; McGowan, Madeline N.; and McGivern, Diane O. "Taking a Health History." *American Journal of Nursing* 77 (July 1977): 1190–1193.

Baranowski, Karen; Greene, Harry L., II; and Lamont, J. Thomas. "Viral Hepatitis." *Nursing '76* 6 (May 1976): 31–38.

Beland, Irene L. *Clinical Nursing: Physiological and Psychosocial Approaches*. 3d ed. New York: Macmillan, 1975.

Benensen, Abram S., ed. *Control of Communicable Diseases in Man.* 12th ed. New York: American Public Health Association, 1975.

Benson, Evelyn, and McDevitt, Joan. "Epidemiology." In *Community Health and Nursing Practice.* Englewood Cliffs, N.J.: Prentice-Hall, 1975, pp. 59–70.

Bergersen, Betty. *Pharmacology in Nursing.* 13th ed. St. Louis: C. V. Mosby Co., 1976.

Brunner, Lillian Sholtis, and Suddarth, Doris S. *Textbook of Medical Surgical Nursing.* 3rd ed. Philadelphia: J. P. Lippincott Co., 1975.

Garb, Solomon. *Laboratory Tests in Common Use.* 6th ed. New York: Springer Publishing Company, Inc., 1976.

"Great Britain and Ireland: Education." *Encyclopedia Americana* 13 (1965): 262–69.

Guyton, Arthur. *Textbook of Medical Physiology.* Philadelphia: W. B. Saunders Co., 1976, pp. 936–944.

Harrison, T. R. *Principles of Internal Medicine.* 8th ed. New York: McGraw-Hill, 1977, pp. 1590–1600.

Hymovich, Debra P., and Barnard, Martha Underwood. *Family Health Care.* New York: McGraw-Hill, 1973, pp. 66–69.

Little, Dolores E., and Carnevali, Doris L. *Nursing Care Planning.* 2d ed. Philadelphia: J. B. Lippincott Co., 1976.

Luckmann, Joan, and Sorensen, Karen. *Medical-Surgical Nursing.* Philadelphia: W. B. Saunders Co., 1974, pp. 1131–1133.

Malasanos, Lois, et al. *Health Assessment.* St. Louis: C. V. Mosby Co., 1978.

McElroy, Diane Barnes. "Nursing Care of Patients with Viral Hepatitis." *Nursing Clinics of North America* 12 (June 1977): 305–315.

Melnick, J. L.; Dreesman, G. R.; and Hollinger, F. B. "Viral Hepatitis." *Scientific American* 237 (July 1977): 44–52.

Pendagast, Eileen G., and Sherman, Charles O. "A Guide to the Genogram Family Systems Training." *The Family* 5 (1978): 3–14.

Pumphrey, John B. "Recognizing Your Patient's Spiritual Needs." *Nursing '77* 7 (December 1977): 64–70.

Robinson, Corinne H., and Lawler, Marilyn R. *Normal and Therapeutic Nutrition.* 15th ed. New York: Macmillan, 1977.

Selye, Hans. *Stress without Distress.* New York: Signet Mentor Books, 1974.

CHAPTER FOURTEEN

Hemorrhage: Placenta Previa

LINDA K. HARRISON

OVERVIEW

Maria Sanchez is a twenty-nine-year-old woman of Puerto Rican descent. She has three young children and is pregnant with a fourth. Since her husband's unexpected departure, Maria obtained a job as a maid and moved in with her sister to decrease expenses. Maria began to bleed vaginally during her eighth month of pregnancy. After an unsuccessful attempt to treat the hemorrhage conservatively, a Cesarean section was performed. Several Catholic sacraments were administered during the course of Maria's difficulty. Enhancing mother-infant bonding as well as assisting Maria to accept the loss of a normal pregnancy were additional responsibilities with which the nursing staff had to deal.

CONTENT EMPHASIS

- Management of a hemorrhaging client
- Cesarean section—nursing management
- Roman Catholic beliefs and practices
- Situational crisis—marital conflict; threatened pregnancy

SETTINGS

- Labor room
- Delivery room
- Postpartum unit

OBJECTIVES

Upon completing this chapter the student will be able to:

1. Assess the circulatory status of a hemorrhaging client (placenta previa).
2. Analyze the nursing management of a hemorrhaging client in both the antepartum and postpartum phases of pregnancy.
3. Comprehend the religious implications related to the care of a hemorrhaging mother and her premature infant.
4. Design client care objectives to enhance the level of well-being for a mother and infant during and following a cesarean section.
5. Create intervention techniques that enhance mother-infant bonding.

DEFINITION OF TERMS

The following terms are used in this chapter and should be defined before proceeding:

Abortion
Abruptio placenta
Aggressive management
Apgar score
Appropriate size for gestational age (AGA)
Classical Cesarean section
Conservative management
Expected date of confinement (EDC)
External fetal monitoring
Forceps operation

Gravida
High-risk infant
High-risk mother
Last menstrual period (LMP)
Parity
Placenta previa
Right upper quadrant of abdomen (RUQ)
Regional anesthesia
Spinal anesthesia
Ultrasound scan

FAMILY ASSESSMENT

Maria Lopez had just completed high school and was working as a file clerk when she was introduced to Juan Sanchez. Both the Lopez and Sanchez families lived in the Puerto Rican section of a large industrial city. Maria was the middle of seven children, and Juan was the second oldest boy of eight siblings. Since her parents were still keeping a close watch on her comings and goings, Maria had to meet Juan secretly for almost a year. They were

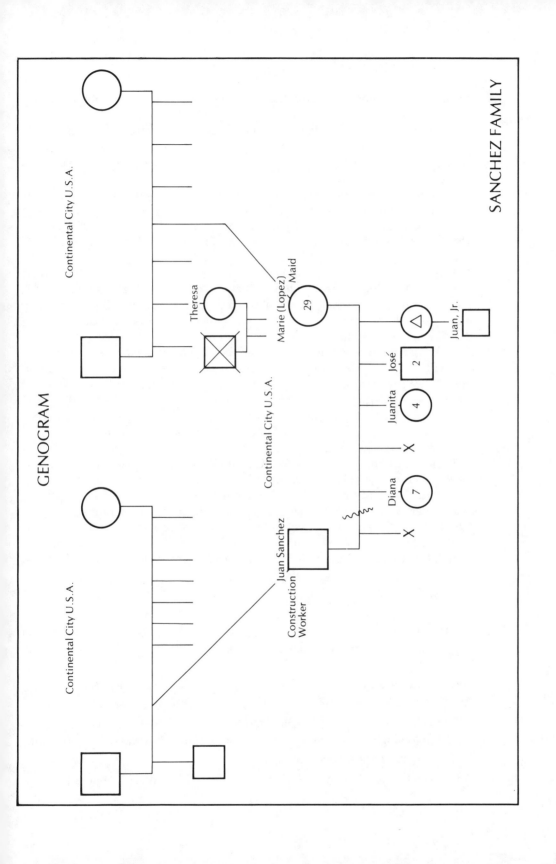

GENOGRAM

SANCHEZ FAMILY

Continental City U.S.A.

Continental City U.S.A.

Continental City U.S.A.

Juan Sanchez
Construction
Worker

Marie (Lopez)
Maid
29

Theresa

Diana
7

Juanita
4

José
2

Juan, Jr.

eventually married in a traditional Catholic ceremony two years after they met.

After nine years of marriage, their family consisted of three children, Diana (age 7), Juanita (age 4), and José (age 2). Two of Maria's five previous pregnancies resulted in spontaneous abortions during the second and third months of pregnancy, respectively.

Juan Sanchez is a construction worker with a small company. His job tends to be seasonal and occasionally it has taken him away from home for one or two weeks at a time. Lately, Juan has had frequent "run-ins" with his boss about his responsibilities and Juan's dissatisfaction over his wages and benefits.

Maria is now pregnant for the sixth time. Before she told Juan, she wanted to see Dr. Martinez. She wanted to make sure everything was normal this time since Juan was upset by the aborted pregnancies. Two days before she was to see Dr. Martinez, Juan left Maria and the children without knowing that Maria was pregnant. Since Juan was not even going to work, Maria had no way of contacting him. There had been numerous periods of marital discord, but Juan's departure was totally unanticipated by Maria. She had no idea where Juan went, nor did she receive any financial help from him. After a few weeks, Maria ran out of money and was forced to find a job. The only job that she was able to find was as a maid in a small motel three days per week. She and her children moved in with Maria's older sister, Theresa, and her two children in a less costly area of the city.

Theresa has been a widow for 5 years and she works part-time as an office clerk. She rents a well-kept, three-bedroom apartment on the second floor of an apartment building built for low-income families. Maria and Theresa were always very close when they were growing up; thus, this arrangement provided emotional support for both of them. The living arrangement seemed to work fairly well. However, at times they disagreed on how the children should be disciplined and who was responsible for various household duties.

STUDY QUESTIONS

14-1. What are the beliefs and religious teachings of the Roman Catholic church on the following topics: marriage, family, birth, death, illness, family planning?

14-2. What is a sacrament? What is the value of administering a sacrament?

14-3. Which of these beliefs and religious practices are accepted by Maria?

14-4. What are the common, characteristic beliefs of Puerto Rican people on the following topics: diet, family, courtship, status of women, birth, illness?

14-5. Which of these beliefs are held by Maria?

14-6. Is the Sanchez family eligible for Medicaid? For other welfare assistance?

DISCUSSION QUESTIONS

D-1. What support systems are available to Maria in the event of a situational crisis?

D-2. With only limited financial resources, why did Maria see a private physician instead of a clinic?

D-3. What societal groups (government, church, and private) are available to assist Maria financially?

D-4. Does the state welfare system in your area search for an estranged husband? If yes, how is it done?

D-5. How could a nurse mobilize societal groups to assist Maria?

CLIENT ASSESSMENT

After cleaning the apartment one day, Maria Sanchez noticed what she thought might be blood in the toilet after urinating. This had never happened before during her other pregnancies. Since she wasn't having any pain or discomfort, Maria decided to ignore it for the time being. Despite her constant checking that day, there was no further incidence of bleeding. It was still almost six weeks until Maria's anticipated due date of October 25.

The following morning at 7:00 A.M., Maria awoke to find bright red blood on her underwear and nightgown as well as on the sheets. She sat on the edge of the bed, crying out of fear. Diana, who shared the sofa bed with her mother, awoke to the sound of her crying.

"Go get Aunt Theresa, Diana," Maria commanded through her tears. Theresa was there within minutes and could see what the problem was without having to ask.

Theresa asked, "Are you in pain or anything, Maria?"

Maria replied, "No, no pain. I just woke up and there it was."

Theresa surmised, "Maybe you're in labor?"

After a few moments hesitation, Maria replied, "No, there's been no labor pain." She looked downward. "The bleeding must have happened sometime after I got up to go to the bathroom—probably two or three hours ago." She paused. "Oh, Theresa—I'm not going to lose another baby, am I?"

Theresa embraced Maria and said, "We must pray for the best."

Theresa quickly crossed herself as if finishing a prayer. She went immediately to the phone to call Dr. Martinez, Maria's obstetrician. Theresa was advised to bring Maria to St. Ann's Hospital and that he would meet them there in the labor and delivery unit. (St. Ann's Hospital houses the region's high risk perinatal unit including a special care nursery.) He would contact the hospital so that they would be anticipating her arrival. Maria was surprised, since she had planned to deliver at her neighborhood hospital—not at St. Ann's Hospital; but she thought it best to just do what the doctor said.

She'd always believed Dr. Martinez was responsible for José, her youngest child, being born normal, despite complications.

Theresa quickly went next door to get someone to stay with the children while she took Maria to the hospital. In the meantime, Maria cleaned herself up a bit and put on some clothes. When the neighbor arrived, Maria and Theresa hastily left for the hospital. Maria had kissed Diana good-bye and told her not to worry. The other children had slept through the commotion, unaware of what was happening.

LABOR ROOM

The car ride to the hospital seemed to take forever. They reached the hospital at 8 A.M., but Dr. Martinez had not yet arrived. Maria and Theresa went directly to the labor and delivery unit. Ms. Smith, the charge nurse, greeted Ms. Sanchez and informed her that she was expected. Maria was promptly taken to a labor room. Theresa was instructed to have a seat in the waiting room adjacent to the unit. The nurse assured Theresa that she could be with Maria after the admission procedures were finished and the doctor had completed his examination.

Ms. Smith helped Marie put on a patient gown and then gathered the following assessment data:

DATE: September 15, 8 A.M.

GENERAL HEALTH: Alert, Puerto Rican female 29 years of age; no physical abnormalities apparent, distressed facial appearance.

CHIEF COMPLAINT: Bright red vaginal bleeding observed by client upon awakening this A.M. Client denies discomfort, pain, or labor contraction.

PERTINENT PAST HISTORY: Noncontributory health history; no known allergies.

PREVIOUS OBSTETRIC HISTORY: (See table.)

PREVIOUS OBSTETRIC HISTORY

Birth Date	Present Age	Sex	Birth Weight	Type of Delivery	Comments
Spontaneous abortion	—	—	—	—	1st trimester
Feb. 5	7 years	F	7 lb 5 oz	forceps	ABA no complications
Sept. 17	5 years	F	5 lb 2 oz	NSD	premature

PREVIOUS OBSTETRIC HISTORY (*continued*)

Birth Date	Present Age	Sex	Birth Weight	Type of Delivery	Comments
spontaneous abortion					1st trimester
March 23	2 years	M	6 lb 8 oz	forceps	ABA, cord around neck 2x fetal distress

PRESENT OBSTETRIC HISTORY: Gravida 6 Para 3 Ab 2 (spontaneous) LMP: January 20   EDC: October 25
Medications: prenatal vitamins

PHYSICAL ASSESSMENT
General:
   Height: 150 cm   Weight: 61.4 kg (52.4 kg prior to pregnancy)
   BP: 124/86   P: 86 strong, regular   R: 22
   FHT: 144 in RUQ   Fetal palpation deferred.
   No abdominal tenderness noted.
Genitalia: One partially saturated perineal pad removed from client which was applied 30–45 minutes ago. Bright red blood observed coming from vagina at intermittent slow trickle.
External genitalia has no apparent lesions, masses, or evidence of trauma. Further genital assessment deferred at this time.
Cardiovascular: Radial pulses are bilaterally equal, strong and regular; NSR; AP: 86/min.
Neurological: (see diagram)

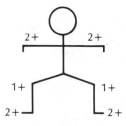

Dr. Martinez arrived at the unit about one-half hour later than expected. Ms. Smith had proceeded with monitoring the mother and fetus every fifteen minutes until his arrival. She recorded Maria's vital signs and had initiated electronic external monitoring of the fetus as per hospital protocol.
   Dr. Martinez spoke with Ms. Sanchez in Spanish for a few moments. He then turned to Ms. Smith and asked about the bleeding that was apparent on

admission, Maria's vital signs, and the location and rate of the fetal heart tones. The following medical orders were written by the physician for Maria Sanchez:

1000 ml of 5% D/W IV c̄ 18 gauge needle to KVO

NPO except ice chips

No vaginal or rectal exams, no enemas

Vistaril 25 mg IM now

Ultrasound scan this A.M.

Type and cross-match 2 units of whole blood

CBC c̄ differential

Urinalysis   stat

Vaginal specimen for fetal hemoglobin

Maria's vital signs and the fetal heart rate remained stable. The vaginal bleeding was beginning to subside by 11:30 A.M. that same day. Theresa stayed with Maria most of the morning. By noon, the ultrasound report and laboratory results had arrived on the unit.

CBC:
  Hgb: 9.5 g
  Hct: 35%
  RBC: $4.0 \times 10^6 mm^3$
  WBC: $6000 \ mm^3$
    Neutrophils: 60%
    Lymphocytes: 30%
    Monocytes: 6%
    Eosinophils: 3.5%
    Basophils: 0.5%

Urinalysis:
  color—straw, cloudy
  Sp. Gr.: 1.021
  pH: 6.0
  Sugar: neg.
  Acetone: tr.
  Protein: 2+
  Fetal hemoglobin in vaginal
    specimen: neg.

Ultrasound report: Placental tissue is visualized in the right lower uterine segment. The fetus appears to be in a transverse lie. Gestational age of the fetus is estimated to be 33–34 weeks.

Later that afternoon, the vaginal bleeding had ceased. Maria was allowed to eat a regular diet at lunch and then slept comfortably. Theresa decided to go home for awhile, since Maria was sleeping and Dr. Martinez had decided that Maria should stay in the hospital for at least another day.

STUDY QUESTIONS

14-7. What are the possible causes of vaginal bleeding during pregnancy?

14-8.   Differentiate placenta previa and abruptio placenta in terms of patho-physiology, symptomatology, treatment modalities, and prognosis.

14-9.   What are the morbidity and mortality rates associated with placenta previa for the mother? the fetus/infant?

14-10. What is an ultrasound scan? fetal hemoglobin test? What is the rationale for having each performed in Maria's case?

14-11. Complete the following laboratory grid on Maria's lab tests:

Test	Normal Range During Pregnancy	Maria's Values	Amount Deviation From Normal	Possible Cause for Alteration

14-12. Complete a drug information card on Vistaril.

14-13. What is the expected effect of Vistaril on the obstetric client?

14-14. What are the nursing care objectives for Maria? What is the rationale for each and how are the objectives achieved? How are they evaluated?

Objectives	Rationale	Nursing Actions	Method and Frequency of Evaluation

14-15. What is the risk of intrauterine infection in clients with placenta previa?

DISCUSSION QUESTIONS

D-6. Why would Dr. Martinez make the decision to have Maria brought to St. Ann's Hospital rather than to the hospital she had anticipated?

D-7. Why would the physician write a specific order for "*no* vaginal exams, etc."?

D-8. Analyze the assessment on Ms. Sanchez. What are her nursing care priorities and what is the rationale for each?

Nursing Care Priority	Rationale

D-9. Identify the conservative management approach and the aggressive management approach for treating the hemorrhage of placenta previa. What factors must be considered prior to determining the management approach?

DELIVERY—CESAREAN SECTION

The physician had hoped to give Maria's baby some more "growing time" by delaying delivery via conservative management. However, Maria had an episode of copious, bright red bleeding from the vagina the next afternoon. Dr. Martinez was notified by the resident, Dr. King. The decision was made to deliver the baby by Cesarean section right away, since Maria's blood pressure had fallen to 106/64 and the fetal heart rate had decreased to 112. In addition, a unit of whole blood was administered to Maria stat in an attempt to replace the apparent loss and reduce the surgical risk.

Maria cried as the resident tried to explain the reason for the Cesarean section. Ms. Simpson, the 3–11 P.M. primary care nurse was rushing to prepare the obstetric OR. However, she did attempt to ease Maria's anxiety as she prepared Maria for surgery.

Theresa was notified by Ms. Simpson and arrived at the hospital within the hour, accompanied by their parish priest. Father Antonio was allowed to visit Maria for a few moments and gave Maria the sacrament for the sick. He conversed briefly with Theresa and encouraged her to call him at the rectory if he could be of any assistance.

Maria's conversation with Theresa was very brief. Maria told her sister that the baby was to be named Juan after her husband if it was a boy, and Theresa if it was a girl. They briefly prayed together as they held each other's hands, fighting back their tears. Soon it was time for Maria to be taken to the obstetric operating room.

Prior to the surgery, Maria's blood pressure was stable at 114/72; pulse rate was 90/minute, the fetal heart rate was 130/minute. The stat hemoglobin and hematocrit results were 10.8 g/100 ml and 39%, respectively.

Even with their masks, Maria recognized Dr. Martinez and Ms. Simpson, but she did not know who all the other masked people were in the operating room. Maria tried to cooperate as the anesthetist inserted a spinal needle into her back. Drs. Martinez and King performed a classical Cesarean section. The surgery was complicated by the transverse fetal position and a blood loss of 750 ml. Twenty units of Pitocin was added to 1000 ml D_5 in Ringer's Lactate promptly following manual removal of the placenta. The IV infused at the rate of 200ml/hr in the delivery room. The surgical procedure took almost 90 minutes. The assessment on Juan, Jr., at one minute was as follows:

Weight: 1.8 kg

Heart rate: 130

Cry: weak, but spontaneous

Respirations: spontaneous but irregular

Mild flexion of extremities

Acrocyanosis, pale

At five minutes after birth, the infant's assessment was as follows:

Heart rate: 134/minute

Respirations: 40/minute

Moderate flexion of extremities

Cry—more vigorous

Generally improved color with mild acrocyanosis still present

His prematurity was evidenced by his size and appearance; however, he did seem to adapt initially to extrauterine life.

Maria was only vaguely aware of the birth, because of the intravenous Valium and spinal anesthesia. But she did realize that it was a boy.

NURSERY

The Sanchez baby was classified as a high-risk infant and taken to the observation nursery. Within the first two hours of life, it became apparent that Juan Jr. was not breathing adequately. As soon as his condition was stabilized, he was transferred to the special care nursery, which was designed to manage ill neonates who needed aggressive therapeutic management. Prior to the transfer, the observation nursery nurse baptized Juan as requested by his mother before the Cesarean delivery.

RECOVERY ROOM

Maria's incision repair was completed and she was taken to the recovery room. A second unit of whole blood was transfused through the IV in her left arm while the 5% dextrose in Ringer's lactate intravenous solution infused through an IV in the right hand. The Foley catheter was draining well, and the patient's condition was reported to be fairly stable. The following medical orders were written by Dr. Martinez:

> Type and cross-match for additional unit of whole blood.
>
> Hgb and Hct 1 hour after present transfusion absorbed.
>
> Slow present IV rate to 150 ml/hr until finished; then start 1000 ml 5% Ringers lactate with 10 units Pitocin q 8 h × 2 liters. Then continue with 1000 ml 5% dextrose in Ringer's lactate q 8 h × 2 liters.
>
> Demerol 75 mg q 3–4 h prn for pain.
>
> Foley catheter to straight drainage
>
> NPO except ice chips
>
> Keep under close observation in the recovery room area for at least 12 hours postoperatively.
>
> CBC and electrolytes in A.M.

The early recovery phase was relatively uneventful. Maria's vital signs remained stable. She was sedated for pain twice during her twelve-hour stay in the recovery room. Following the transfusion, Maria's hemoglobin was 11 g/100 ml and her hematocrit was 39%.

STUDY QUESTIONS

14-16. What is a spinal (epidural) anesthesia? How is the client positioned? How can Maria's cooperation be obtained during the procedure?

14-17. What specific observations would you need to make while the patient is receiving a blood transfusion? Describe the specific techniques that would be carried out when administering blood products and then starting a dextrose solution.

14-18. What items should be explained to Maria before the Cesarean section? What should be explained about each?

Item	Explanation

14-19. What is an Apgar score? How is it determined?

14-20. What was Juan Jr.'s Apgar score at 1 minute? 5 minutes?

14-21. What are the potential allergic reactions to a blood transfusion? What should be observed and how frequently? What should be done for each allergic reaction?

Allergic Effects	Assessment	Frequency	Nursing Action

14-22. Why is an 18-gauge needle used to administer whole blood?

14-23. What precautions should be taken when administering blood? Why? After administering blood? Why?

14-24. Complete a drug information card on the following medications: pitocin, Demerol.

14-25. Compare the hemoglobin and hematocrit results on Maria given to this point. Analyze the effect of the blood transfusion.

14-26. What are the nursing objectives for Maria's postpartal period? What is the rationale and nursing action for each objective? How would Maria's progress be evaluated?

Objectives	Nursing Actions	Rationale	Evaluation of Progress

DISCUSSION QUESTIONS

D-10. What are the possible explanations for the fetus being in a transverse lie this late in pregnancy?

D-11. What is the rationale for choosing to perform a classical Cesarean section? What are the ramifications of this procedure?

D-12. Describe Maria's ability to cope with stress. How effective is her use of her support systems?

D-13. What might be done to facilitate Maria's understanding and cooperation when she was taken to the obstetric operating room?

D-14. Given that you had about five minutes to interact with Maria in her labor room while preparing her for the Cesarean section, what would you say to her that might be therapeutic?

D-15. How might the nurse assist the pregnant client who is receiving a spinal anesthetic?

D-16. How is an infant baptized by a nurse? When should an infant be baptized by a nurse?

POST PARTUM

The following orders accompanied Maria as she was transferred to the post-partum unit from the recovery room:

Ergotrate 0.2 mg qid × 6 doses

Demerol 75 mg q 4 h prn for pain

D/C Foley catheter tomorrow in A.M.

Progress to full liquid diet as tolerated

1000 ml 5% D/W IV for 10 hours, then D/C IV

Blow bottles qid

Iron dextran 100 mgm IM today

Ms. Torres was the primary care nurse assigned to Maria Sanchez. By the second postoperative day, Ms. Sanchez seemed more comfortable and open to conversations with Ms. Torres. Maria admitted to Ms. Torres that although she had planned to breast feed, she no longer had the desire since she couldn't even see her infant. Ms. Torres discussed this issue with Maria at length to clarify the patient's decision and the reason behind it. A phone order for chlorotrianisene (Tace) 64 mg bid was obtained and administered by the nurse.

Maria did not really initiate much discussion about Juan Jr. until the third postpartal day. Up until that time, Maria would ask, "How is my baby now?"; but her interest in any detailed answer was minimal. On the fourth day, however, she was strong enough to tolerate being taken to the special care nursery in a wheelchair to see and touch her infant. Maria expressed a lot of apprehension as she spoke of his small, frail body and all of the equipment to which Juan Jr. was connected.

Maria Sanchez experienced an episode of heavy postpartum bleeding the evening of the fourth day after delivery. Until that time, light to moderate lochia rubra had been noted. Additional IV pitocin therapy was initiated to control the bleeding. Ten units of pitocin in 500 ml of 5% D/W was administered over the next four hours.

The vaginal bleeding was minimized; but Maria experienced subsequent breast engorgement. Breast binders, cold compresses, and Percodan 4.9 mg po q 3–4 h were used to relieve the condition.

Maria was finally discharged after ten days. She was visibly disappointed when she was told that the baby would not be discharged on the same day. However, she accepted the pediatrician's decision and recognized that Juan Jr. was premature and still "sick" despite his improvement.

Since Theresa had to return to her job, Maria's twenty-year-old sister, Bonita, arranged to stay with Maria for a few days. Bonita enjoyed the children and would manage the household while Maria recuperated. While the children were in school, Bonita would drive Maria to the hospital to see Juan Jr.

STUDY QUESTIONS

14-27. Complete a drug information card on the following medications: ergotrate, iron dextran, chlorotrianisene, Percodan.

14-28. Describe the technique that is used when administering an irritating medication such as iron dextran.

14-29. Identify the indications for and implications of intravenous pitocin therapy postdelivery.

14-30. What are some of the factors that contributed to the breast engorgement in Maria?

14-31. Explain the purpose of each of the following treatments of breast engorgement. What is the expected response to each treatment item? What nursing actions are necessary and what is the method and frequency of evaluating Maria's response?

Treatment	Purpose	Nursing Action	Method and Frequency of Evaluating Response
Breast Binder			
Cold Compresses			
Percodan			

14-32. Identify the stages of acceptance of motherhood that Maria is exhibiting during the early postpartum period. How does Maria compare to the normal postpartum mother?

DISCUSSION QUESTIONS

D-17. What might be the cause for Maria's episode of postpartum bleeding on the fourth day following delivery?

D-18. What other treatments of breast engorgement are available?

D-19. Upon discovering a postpartum client bleeding vaginally, what data should be collected? What are the priorities of care and what is the rationale of each?

Assessment	Nursing Priorities	Rationale

CHAPTER DISCUSSION QUESTIONS

1. Due to the condition of the mother and the newborn immediately following delivery, it was not appropriate to focus on the maternal-infant attachment. Describe the nursing intervention that might be implemented to positively influence the attachment and bonding process during the recovery and early postpartal phases. (Assume that the infant cannot be brought to the mother in the recovery room nor to the postpartum unit.)

2. Prior to Ms. Sanchez's discharge, discuss some of the arrangements that should be made for the client. What kind of assistance can be offered to her? Who would be the most appropriate health professional to implement the various components of the discharge plan?

3. What factors support the classification of Maria Sanchez as a high-risk pregnancy?

4. Discuss how you would deal with Maria's concerns for her ill newborn infant.

5. How can a professional nurse assist Maria with the
   a. Loss of a spouse
   b. Loss of a normal pregnancy?

SUGGESTED ACTIVITIES

1. Interview a priest. How can a nurse assist a Roman Catholic client? How can a nurse assist a priest in giving the sacraments?

2. Observe a Cesarean section. What is the role of each of the health professionals in attendance?

3. Interview a client who has had an emergency Cesarean section. What are her feelings about the Cesarean section? the loss of a vaginal delivery? Observe her reaction with her infant.

4. Observe a baptism of an infant by a nurse.

BIBLIOGRAPHY

Babson, S. Gorham et al. *Management of High-Risk Pregnancy and Intensive Care of the Neonate.* 3d ed. St. Louis: C. V. Mosby Co., 1975.

Bergersen, Betty. *Pharmacology in Nursing.* 13th ed. St. Louis: C. V. Mosby Co., 1976.

Brunner, Lillian Sholtis, and Suddarth, Doris Smith. *The Lippincott Manual of Nursing Practice.* 2d ed. Philadelphia: J. B. Lippincott Co., 1978.

Clark, Ann L., and Affonso, Dyanne D. *Childbearing: A Nursing Perspective.* Philadelphia: F. A. Davis Co., 1976.

Garb, Solomon. *Laboratory Tests in Common Use.* 6th ed. New York: Springer Publishing Co., 1976.

Greenhill, J. P., and Friedman, Emanual A. *Biological Perspectives and Modern Practice of Obstetrics.* Philadelphia: W. B. Saunders Co., 1974, pp. 415-425.

Jensen, Margaret D.; Benson, Ralph C.; and Bobak, Irene M. *Maternity Care—The Nurse and the Family.* St. Louis: C. V. Mosby Co. 1977.

Lewis, Oscar. *La Vida.* New York: Vintage Books, 1966.

Little, Dolores E., and Carnevali, Doris L. *Nursing Care Planning.* 2d ed. Philadelphia: J. B. Lippincott Co., 1976.

Malasanos, Lois et al. *Health Assessment*. St. Louis: C. V. Mosby Co., 1978.

Mercer, Ramona Thieme. *Nursing Care for Parents at Risk*. Thorofare, N.J.: Charles B. Slack, Inc., 1977.

Oxorn, Harry, and Foote, William R. *Human Labor and Birth*. 3d ed. New York: Appleton-Century-Crofts, 1975.

Pritchard, Jack A., and MacDonald, Paul C. *William's Obstetrics*. 15th ed. New York: Appleton-Century-Crofts, 1976, pp. 416–421.

Pumphrey, John B. "Recognizing Your Patient's Spiritual Needs." *Nursing '77* 7 (December 1977): 64–70.

Scarlato, Michael. "Blood Transfusions Today—What You Should Know and Should Do." *Nursing '78* 8 (February 1978): 68–72.

Spellacy, William N., ed. *Management of the High-Risk Pregnancy*. Baltimore, Md.: University Park Press, 1976.

Stroot, Violet R.; Lee, Carla A.; and Schaper, C. Ann. *Fluid and Electrolytes: A Practical Approach*. 2d ed. Philadelphia: F. A. Davis Co., 1977.

CHAPTER FIFTEEN

Covert Health Problem: Battered Women

ANDREA B. SAVITZ

SARAH SATTIN

OVERVIEW

Madeline Lang is divorced and is raising two children. Her common-law "husband" has physically abused Madeline for over one year. When she sustained chest injuries and a fractured arm, Madeline finally confided to the nurse that her "husband" frequently "beats her up." A public health nurse is assigned to the family. Between the two professional nurses, Madeline is finally ready to attend the battered woman center in her area.

CONTENT EMPHASIS

- Characteristics of battered women
- Case finding—battered women
- Interpersonal Relations (IPR)—resistent client
- Battered women's centers

SETTINGS

- Emergency room
- Home setting—public health nurse

OBJECTIVES

Upon completing this chapter the student will be able to:

1. Analyze the personality characteristics of battered and abused women.
2. Design intervention techniques to assist battered and abused people.
3. Analyze strategies of interpersonal relationships regarding interviewing and counseling.
4. Comprehend the legal rights of the abused.

DEFINITION OF TERMS

The following terms are used in this case study and should be defined before proceeding:

Abuse   Masochist
Battered woman   Sadist
Battered women's centers   Common-law husband

FAMILY ASSESSMENT

Mike Hoffman and Madeline Lang have been living in common law for two years. Their home is a small, crowded converted beach house in an area that had once been a resort. The house has four rooms. With them live Madeline's two children from her previous marriage. The children are thirteen-year-old Joey and eight-year-old Susan. (See genogram.)

Madeline's father, Fred Moore, had been a physically abusive alcoholic. When Rita, Madeline's mother, died of cancer, Fred became more abusive. If he noticed that something was out of place at home or if the meal Madeline had cooked was not to his liking, Fred would explode. Usually Madeline tried to explain her shortcomings to her father. Fred rarely listened to Madeline. He would just start to beat her.

Madeline stayed at home for about one year after her mother's death. Then she found herself pregnant by Harry Lang. Harry, Madeline thought, was the man of her dreams. Plus, Harry represented a way out of the Moore home for Madeline. She clung to Harry and emotionally broke off all ties with her own family of origin.

Nine years later, Harry left Madeline, saying he simply could not take her absolute dependence on him any longer. He said to Madeline, "You're smothering me. You always must know everything I'm thinking... and if that's not enough, you then insist on my hearing every little thing you're thinking... Enough is enough... I can't be your crutch anymore."

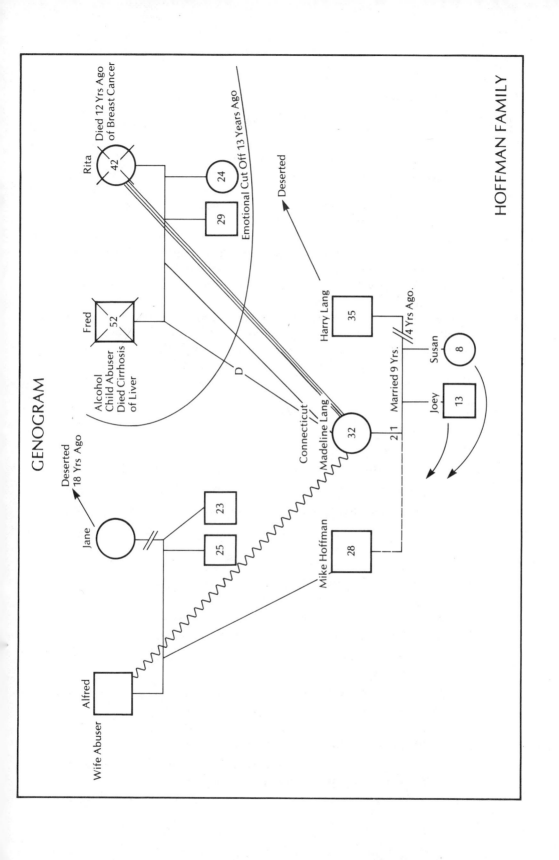

GENOGRAM

HOFFMAN FAMILY

Mike Hoffman had never been married. However, he did have one thing in common with Madeline. His father, Alfred, had been an abuser also. However, in the Hoffman home it was the wife who was beaten, not the children. When Jane Hoffman left her family in fear of her life eighteen years ago, Alfred had started a campaign against her to the boys. Alfred would say, "She wanted a career more than she wanted you." After a while Mike found himself accepting his Dad's story, because "after all she did desert her children." The merciless beatings she had received at the hands of his father began to be remembered as Jane's "just reward."

Mike and Madeline met three years ago. Madeline was waitressing at the truck stop Mike frequented when doing local trucking of appliances. Mike was fascinated with her. Instead of the slick good listener-type waitresses he met all the time, Madeline was somehow helpless and soft. Madeline told him her problems.

Mike and Madeline dated for a year before combining homes. Madeline wanted the children to have time to know Mike before he took on the role of stepfather. At first the combined household of Hoffman and Lang worked very nicely. However, after two years, the relationship was not as satisfying to Madeline and Mike.

STUDY QUESTIONS

15-1. What are the classical characteristics of an abused individual?

15-2. Is there a relationship between child abuse and wife abuse? Explain.

15-3. What is the most common personality type demonstrated in abused women? Explain.

DISCUSSION QUESTIONS

D-1. How would you describe Madeline's personality?

D-2. Does Madeline's personality put her at risk for abuse?

D-3. How much do you believe the abused person contributes to being abused? Explain.

D-4. What behaviors were common to all the adult male-female relationships Madeline had?

D-5. Do the family communication systems from which Mike and Madeline come put them at risk as an abusive couple? Explain.

D-6. Do the family communication systems from which Mike and Madeline come put them at risk as abusive parents? Explain.

CLIENT ASSESSMENT

At about midnight Saturday, Madeline Lang was brought into the emergency room of Barnard Hospital by a female friend. Madeline was crying silently as she held tight to her friend's right arm.

Ms. Reaves, R.N., showed Madeline Lang and her friend into an emergency room cubicle. Madeline did not raise her eyes, but she did follow directions. She walked to the examining table and cautiously sat down. By observing the way Madeline moved, Ms. Reaves assessed that she was in some degree of pain, but in no acute distress. The nurse then filled in the admission fact sheet as fast as Madeline could answer the questions. The biographical data were recorded as follows:

NAME: Madeline Lang
AGE: 32
SEX: Female
ADDRESS: 42 Seaview Way
        Oceanside, Conn.
MARITAL STATUS: Divorced
DEPENDENTS: Son 13 yrs.; daughter 8 yrs.
HEALTH INS.: None
FINANCIAL SUPPORT: Supported by common-law husband (approx. salary
    $16,000/yr.) Children on Aid to Dependent Children.
OCCUPATION: Unemployed waitress
SUPPORT SYSTEMS: Friend—Alice Newton

As Madeline spoke, Ms. Reaves continued to be struck by how familiar the client seemed to her. However, rather than quiz Madeline, Ms. Reaves proceeded with the history. The nurse recorded the following:

CHIEF COMPLAINT(S): Pain rt. lower arm; pain lt. ant. chest aggravated
    inspiration.
HISTORY OF CHIEF COMPLAINT: Fell down stairs at about 11:15 P.M. tonight
MEDICAL HISTORY: nonsignificant

Ms. Reaves's physical assessment yielded the following abnormal findings:

HEENT: Red swollen eyes; lacerations of face.
CHEST: Softball-size hematoma (painful to palpatation) lower lt. ant. chest
    wall.
RT. FOREARM: Multiple hematomas.
GENERAL IMPRESSION: Thin, pale female; disheveled.

Ms. Reaves placed Madeline in a position of good body alignment and excused herself to arrange for a medical assessment.

While Donald Carton, M.D., reviewed the emergency room intake sheet, Ms. Reaves followed up her hunch about having seen Madeline previously in the ER. She consulted the ER file of previous contacts and learned that this client had been treated four times in the last year for bodily injuries reported as accidents. These previous injuries included hematomas around her spine and burns on her abdomen and chest. This was the first time that Madeline's injuries were visible to casual observation. Ms. Reaves immediately notified Dr. Carton of her suspicions of abuse. He did his medical-physical assessment with this in mind.

Then Dr. Carton met privately with Ms. Reaves. He told her that he would support all nursing efforts to get Madeline to accept help against abuse. He left the following orders:

Cleanse facial wounds with 3% peroxide solution and apply dressings.

Apply cold compresses to rt. forearm

X-rays: PA and lat. chest, rt. forearm.

Encourage acceptance of referral to Battered Women's Center

While Madeline was in the Radiology Department, Alice Newton asked to speak to Ms. Reaves. Alice, Madeline's friend, said that she was very worried. She believed that there was a very good possibility that Mike Hoffman had injured Madeline earlier that evening. Ms. Reaves assured her that the staff would do everything possible to help Madeline. Lastly, Ms. Reaves asked that Alice wait in the lounge, so that a private conference could be held with Madeline on her return from X-ray.

NURSING INTERVENTION FOR ABUSE

When Madeline later returned from the radiology department, this interaction took place between Ms. Reaves (Ms. R.) and Madeline (M):

Ms. R: You look terribly upset, Madeline. Tell me what is bothering you.

M: Well, wouldn't you be upset if you fell down the stairs? (*defensively*)

Ms. R: Yes, I would be, but I get the feeling that there is something else going on.

M: No, there isn't (*sharply*). I just want to get these bruises taken care of so I can get home to my kids. (*Silence.*)

Ms. R: Madeline, I see that you've been here before with similar kinds of injuries.

M: (*Looked surprised.*) I guess I'm just accident-prone (*indifferently*).

Ms. R: In the last year you've had many accidents at home. Are you having trouble managing at home?

M: Yeah, sometimes.

Ms. R: Do you have any help at home?

M: Yeah—Mike helps me sometimes (*long pause*).

Ms. R: Tell me more about Mike.

M: Oh, he's good to us—generous with money.

Ms. R: What does he think about your frequent injuries?

M: He thinks I'm stupid and careless. That's all. He doesn't talk much. (*Becomes tearful.*)

Ms. R: Is that a problem, that he's so quiet?

M: Yeah, but no matter what I do he won't tell me what he's thinking or feeling. He just gets angry with me. (*Silence.*) Why are you asking me all these questions? (*Stares at Ms. Reaves.*)

Ms. R: You look very upset, and I'm interested in helping you. (*Pause.*) Do my questions make you feel uncomfortable?

M: Not really (*softly*).

Ms. R: You were telling me about you and Mike.

M: Ya—I guess I shouldn't depend on him so much.

Ms. R: What else do you two fight about?

M: The kids. He's rough with them. I don't want him near my kids.

Ms. R: You seem to have strong feelings about that.

M: Yes, I do. I know how it was with my own father. He gave me nothing but problems. When he got drunk, he beat me. That's not going to happen to my kids (*angrily*).

Ms. R: Do you have any reason to believe that it might happen to your kids?

M: Ah—well, yeah—he pushes them around some. And he's rough with me, too.

Ms. R: What do you mean, rough?

M: He hits me sometimes.

Ms. R: Madeline, did he do all this to you?

M: (*She nodded her head.*) Yes. (*Now sobbing.*) It's terrible. I'm no good anyway. I probably deserve it . . . but it's terrible.

Ms. R: (*Puts her arm around Madeline's shoulder.*)

M: How could I let it go on for so long?

Ms. R: (*While holding Madeline's hand.*) You've just taken the first step toward making things better.

M: I shouldn't have said anything. Mike will get in trouble.

Ms. R: The only way he'd get in trouble is if you call the police and press charges against him.

M: No, No . . . I'd never do that. But I don't know how much longer I can stand being beaten. (*Silence.*) You know it hasn't always been this way—I guess I keep hoping it will get better again.

Ms. R: It might help you to know that you're not the only woman in this situation. There are even agencies set up to help women with just this problem. . . . We can talk more about this after your arm is taken care of.

The X-ray reports read as follows:

PA & lat. chest: Fracture 6th and 7th ribs of left anterior chest

Rt. forearm: Fractured rt. ulna

Dr. Carlton applied a cast to Madeline's right forearm and taped her fractured ribs. He then attempted to convince Madeline to allow herself to be admitted for observation and ventilation exercises. However, Madeline refused, stating that she must get home to her children. Then Madeline became very anxious to leave the hospital.

Ms. Reaves explained cast care, circulatory monitoring of her distal extremities beyond the cast, and ventilation exercises. Then the nurse gave Madeline the ER phone number along with the Battered Women's Center phone number, saying that she should use the ER number if she had any questions.

Lastly, Ms. Reaves mentioned that she would be making a public health nurse referral for Madeline. The nurse would check on Madeline's physical progress at home. However, Ms. Reaves emphasized, the public health nurse would also know all about the Battered Women's Center. So, if Madeline had any questions about the center, she could ask her.

Good-byes were said. Then Alice took Madeline home.

STUDY QUESTIONS

15-4.   To which parent does the abused child publicly cling: the abusive parent or the nonabusive parent? Explain.

15-5.   Does abuse and/or battering happen more frequently in any given socioeconomic level? race? area? age group? relationship categories (that is, common-law marriages)?

15-6.   When does the adult abused person usually call for help? (Early or late in the history of abuse/battering.) Explain.

15-7. State the theories that explain abuse from a psychodynamic approach, from a sociological approach, and from a family systems approach.

15-8. What principles and strategies of interviewing/counseling did Ms. Reaves use while speaking with Madeline?

15-9. What laws exist in your state for the protection of the abused?

15-10. What must the abused/battered person do in your state to legally curtail the activities of the abuser?

15-11. Make a teaching plan for Ms. Reaves to use to educate Madeline about cast care, circulatory monitoring, and ventilatory exercises:

Objective	Content	Method of Teaching	Evaluation of Learning

15-12. Can silences be considered a part of good counseling/interpersonal relationship techniques? Explain.

15-13. What kind of question phraseology should be avoided by the interviewer when interviewing a relatively nonverbal person? Explain.

15-14. What kind of question phraseology is best for the interviewer to use when the information desired is more than a "yes" or "no" answer?

15-15. What methodology of intervention is used by the organizations in your area that help the abused, that is, group, family, or individual therapy?

DISCUSSION QUESTIONS

D-7. Why do you believe Madeline avoided reporting to the ER staff the source of her injuries?

D-8. When a member of a couple is abused, does that necessarily mean that the abuser dislikes the abused? Explain.

D-9. As an emergency room nurse, what patterns would you consider to be indicators of possible abuse?

D-10. What organizations in your state or county are focusing most or part of their programs on the needs of battered persons? Who are the organization's target groups (that is, battered women, battered children, battered men)? What are they doing for them?

D-11. What attitude must the health professional have toward abusive family systems in order to intervene effectively?

D-12. Do you believe Ms. Reaves used good nursing judgment when she arranged to see Madeline alone? Explain.

D-13. Do you believe Ms. Reaves used good nursing judgment when she told Madeline about the public health nurse referral, rather than asking if Madeline wanted a referral? Explain.

PROGRESS

The public health nurse, Ms. Evans, started her visits to Madeline within a couple of days. As a part of her intake assessment, she recorded Madeline's family genogram. Madeline's physical progress was going well, and even though it was terribly painful for Madeline to do the ventilation exercises, she continued as instructed.

On the third visit to Madeline's home, Ms. Evans found her client particularly tired. It had been raining, the kids had been indoors all day, and her cast was itching. Ms. Evans noted tears on the brim of Madeline's eyes. As Madeline started to expand her chest with her ventilation exercises she said, "You know, no one deserves this kind of pain."

Ms. Evans stated, "I agree."

Then there was a long silence.

Madeline collapsed down into one of her kitchen chairs. She gestured to Ms. Evans to take another chair. Madeline said, "I've been thinking a lot about how I ended up in all this pain. And I've decided I just never want to get hit again. Ms. Reaves over at the ER said that there was help for women like me . . . you know . . . women that get hit. Do you know about the Battered Women's Center?"

Ms. Evans said, "Yes, they have a fine program."

"Well," said Madeline, "I just have to ask you something, just like I asked Ms. Reaves. Could Mike get in trouble if I go there? Because, even though he hits me, God knows I love him."

Ms. Evans assured Madeline that no harm, legal or otherwise, would come to Mike from the center. "The center's only purpose is to help you. And, in helping you to learn how to avoid physical fights, Mike might end up happier, too."

Madeline phoned the Battered Women's Center later that day.

During the coming months, Madeline attended group therapy sessions with other battered women. Madeline was beginning to learn about the part she played in arguments with Mike that resulted in violence. Just by listening to other group members' histories and advice, Madeline was gaining more insight into the problem. Also, she was beginning to feel better about herself, because, as she reported to Ms. Evans, "A few times my advice has been helpful to others in the group."

Further, she has been learning to behave differently around Mike. When Mike is upset she attempts not to nag him for that reason. She lets him alone when he wants to be alone. Recently, she reported that she had seen a change in Mike and the children's behavior toward each other. There is a more relaxed feeling in the house.

Finally, Madeline reports that the fights have not completely ended with Mike, but she is less likely to get injured. The group at the Battered Women's Center has pointed out that Madeline is not as self-sacrificing or masochistic as she reported herself to be months earlier. To put it neatly, Madeline has been heard to say, "If you don't like yourself and take care of yourself, no one else will."

STUDY QUESTION

15-16. What is the value of the genogram as a tool for assessment of a client/ family when abuse is a reality? Explain.

DISCUSSION QUESTIONS

D-14. Discuss the effect of Madeline's changed behavior on her relationship with Mike.

D-15. Why do you believe Madeline pursued/nagged men?

D-16. Discuss potential behaviors of persons who are feeling pressured–nagged and/or pursued.

D-17. In the case of abuse, what value, if any, do you believe group therapy has over other clinical approaches?

D-18. Why is it difficult for an emotional pursuer or nagger to give up that behavior?

SUGGESTED ACTIVITIES

1. Critique a group therapy session at a battered women's center or an equivalent setting.

2. Research your local police department's attitude toward the abuser and the abused.

3. Interview a formerly abused person and ask:

   a. What understanding do they have of the relationship in which abuse occurred?

    b. What behavioral changes does the formerly abused person consider to be related to the cessation of the battering?

4. Research how your local area hot line manages abuse phone calls.

5. Interview a mental health professional who works with the abused.

BIBLIOGRAPHY

Bell, Joseph, "Rescuing the Battered Wife." *Human Behaviors* 6 (June, 1977): 21–22.

Benson, Evelyn, and McDevitt, Joan. "Care of the Patient and the Family in the Home." In *Community Health and Nursing Practice.* Englewood Cliffs, N.J.: Prentice-Hall, Inc., 1975.

————. "Mobilizing Community Resources for Family Health." In *Community Health and Nursing Practice.* Englewood Cliffs, N.J.: Prentice-Hall, Inc., 1975.

Burgess, A. W. et al. "Assault: Patterns of Emergency Visits." *Journal of Psychiatric Nursing* 14 (November, 1976): 32–36.

Burgess, Ann W., and Johansen, Pamella M. "Assault Patterns of Emergency Visit." *Journal of Psychiatric Nursing* 14 (November 1976): 32–36.

Burton, Genevieve. "Families in Crisis: Knowing When and How to Help." *Nursing '75* 5 (December 1975): 36–43.

Curtis, Lynn. "Victim Precipitation and Violent Crime." *Social Problems* 21 (April 1974): 594–605.

Elbow, Margaret. "Theoretical Considerations of Violent Marriages." *Social Casework* 58 (November 1977): 515–526.

Flynn, John. "Recent Findings Related to Wife Abuse." *Social Casework* 58 (January 1977): 13–20.

Geller, Richard. "Abused Wives—Why Do They Stay?" *Journal of Marriage and the Family* 38 (November 1976): 659–668.

Hanks, Susan E., and Rosenbaum, Peter. "Battered Women: A Study of Women Who Live with Violent Alcohol-Abusing Men." *American Journal of Orthopsychiatry* 47 (April 1977): 291–306.

Pendagast, Eileen G., and Sherman, Charles O. "A Guide to the Genogram Family Systems Training," *The Family* 5 (1978): 3–14.

Von Hentig, Hans. "Remarks on the Interaction of the Perpetrator and Victim." In *Victimology.* Edited by Israel Drapkin and Emilis Orano. Lexington: Lexington Books, 1974.

CHAPTER SIXTEEN

Maladaptation to a Maturational Crisis: Parenting

LINDA K. HARRISON

SARAH SATTIN

OVERVIEW

Ted and Shirley Clinton are successful career-minded individuals. When Shirley becomes pregnant, the couple attend natural childbirth classes. Since Shirley is in her mid-thirties, an amniocentesis is performed and is followed by genetic counseling. The nurse clinician at a maternity center provides support and counsel throughout the pregnancy and postpartal period. Due to stress factors upon the family system, the couple's ability to adjust to the maturational crisis is impaired. When Shirley develops "postpartal blues" bordering on depression, the clinician successfully treats the maladjustment with the use of family therapy and crisis intervention techniques.

CONTENT EMPHASIS

- Genetic counseling—amniocentesis, sickle cell screening
- Developmental tasks of pregnancy and parenthood
- "Postpartum blues"—assessment and treatment
- Family developmental process

SETTINGS

- Maternity center
- Labor and delivery
- Nurse clinician's office

231

OBJECTIVES

Upon completion of this chapter the student will be able to:

1. Analyze the process of pregnancy and childbirth as a family maturational crisis.
2. Comprehend some of the methods of determining the genetic health of a fetus.
3. Analyze the factors which contribute to the development of depression following the birth of the first-born.
4. Determine specific intervention techniques useful for working with expectant and new parents.
5. Describe the effect of a first pregnancy and childbirth upon a married couple.

DEFINITION OF TERMS

The following terms are used in this case study and should be defined before proceeding:

Amniocentesis	Nuclear family system
Antepartum	Postpartum
Extended family system	Postpartum blues
Family therapy	Postpartal depression
Genetic defects	Prepared childbirth classes
Grief reaction	Role deprivation
Intrapartum	Sickle cell disease
Maturational crisis	Sickle cell trait
Natural childbirth classes	Ultrasound scan

FAMILY ASSESSMENT

Anna Marie Pfeiffer, R.N., nurse clinician, met the Clintons at registration for natural childbirth classes at a maternity center. Anna Marie was their group leader for the eight childbirth classes dealing with La Maze techniques for labor and delivery, in addition to general education about maternal and infant health. She would assist the couple during labor and delivery as well as counsel them, upon request, during the antepartum and postpartum periods. As was her practice, Anna Marie interviewed each of the six couples enrolled in her group in order to gather information that would contribute to her ability to teach and counsel them.

During the initial interview with Ted and Shirley Clinton, the following data was collected:

NAME:	Clinton, Ted and Shirley	STATUS:	Married (1½ years)
ADDRESS:	111 Scenic Drive	RACE:	Black
	Seattle, Washington	RELIGION:	Presbyterian

FAMILY MEMBERS:

Shirley—35 years old; Gravida-1 Para-0 Ab-0; EDC, April 10; employed as assistant professor, history department, Washington University.

Ted—37 years old; employed as engineer consultant/sales representative with Beck Industry, Inc., in Seattle.

MARITAL HISTORY: Shirley and Ted met four years ago at a Washington University social event. At the time, Ted was attending graduate business college and Shirley was on the faculty. After dating for ten months, they were married and moved to an apartment in Seattle. Married 1½ years. They share similar interests in theatre and the arts and have a number of mutual friends. Both consider their marriage to be a rewarding relationship. They describe their life together as "busy, but rewarding."

FAMILY BACKGROUND:

Shirley—Raised in a predominantly white, middle class, suburban neighborhood in the Midwest. Only child in her family; describes her family relationship as "extremely close to my parents, grandparents, and aunts." Both parents are living and in good general health.

Ted—Raised in a lower-class neighborhood in the Chicago southside. One of 4 brothers and 2 sisters, he is the second oldest child and oldest son. "I became the man of the family when my father died fifteen years ago." "My mother died five years ago. That was the last time all us kids were together."

PSYCHOSOCIAL BACKGROUNDS:

Shirley—Recalls her childhood and experiences in school as enjoyable. Considers herself ambitious, motivated, and intelligent. Throughout her life she has always been involved in various academic/professional groups, social events, and organizations. She enjoys the challenge and involvement required by her career.

Ted—Recalls his childhood days and school experiences to be a combination of good times and hard times. States that he "had to be responsible for my brothers and sisters throughout most of my life." Determined to get himself and his siblings "out of the

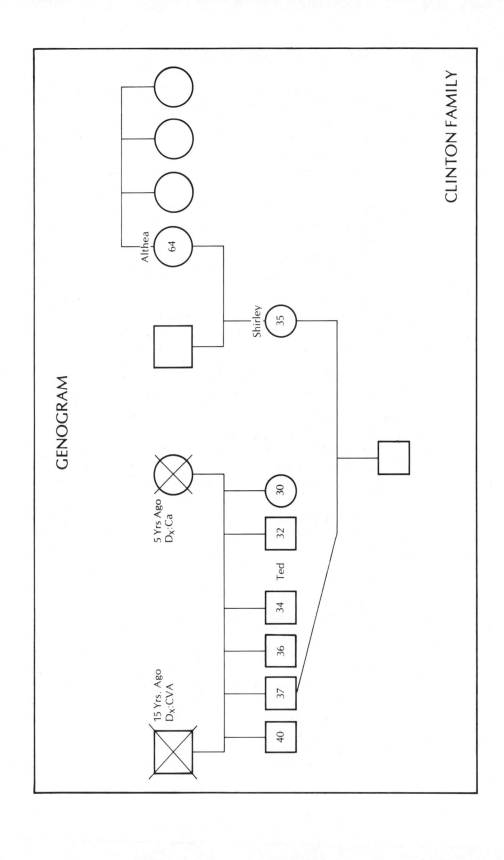

GENOGRAM

CLINTON FAMILY

poor neighborhood" since the age of 16 years. Enjoyed college, which he attended in the evening while working full-time. Was working toward a graduate degree in business when he met Shirley. Moved to Seattle area from Chicago as a result of job transfer and promotion.

During the interview, Shirley and Ted both expressed great delight about the pregnancy. When Anna Maria asked Shirley how she felt about the pregnancy, Shirley responded: "At first I couldn't believe I was pregnant since I felt so well. After a while I started to have mixed feelings about it. I really wanted to share a baby with Ted but I was worried about how a child would affect our marriage and my career. I was also afraid that the baby would be abnormal because I'm kind of old to have a baby." Shirley also said that she had discussed the latter concern with her obstetrician who recommended that an ultrasound scan and amniocentesis in addition to sickle cell screening be done with subsequent genetic counseling as indicated. Shirley said that she found the genetic counseling helpful, but she tried not to think about her pregnancy while she waited for the eighteenth week of gestation when the ultrasound scan and amniocentesis was scheduled.

The nurse-client interaction related to this issue was as follows:

Shirley: The test itself was easy. It was the wait for the results that was hard—especially because I'd begun to feel the baby move. But I wouldn't let myself get excited about it.

Nurse: Why not?

Shirley: Well, you see, Ted and I had decided I would have an abortion if there was a genetic defect. (*Voice lowered and with her eyes downcast.*)

Nurse: You seem uncomfortable telling me that.

Shirley: I guess I am. I feel guilty that we would decide to have an abortion if necessary.

Nurse: Where did those feelings come from?

Shirley: Well, I guess my upbringing. My family thinks abortions are murder.

Nurse: Do you share that opinion?

Shirley: Not really; but I've never told anyone about our plans.

Ted: We were so happy when we heard that the amniocentesis revealed no abnormalities in the genes.

Nurse: I can appreciate that those must have been very uncomfortable days while you waited. (*Pause.*)

The Clintons faithfully attended the childbirth classes and practiced the breathing exercises at home as recommended. The Clintons would often stay after class to ask questions and converse with Anna Marie. Consequently, the rapport between the nurse and this couple was especially good.

One night, Anna Marie noticed that Shirley had a tense facial expression and her usual smile was gone. Ted smoked incessantly during that class. They were not talking to each other as they usually did. After class, Anna Marie took a few extra minutes to talk with them. They told the nurse that they were going through the difficult process of choosing a neighborhood suitable for raising their child. They explained that they had different ideas about how to go about making the decision.

At later classes they looked more relaxed. Shirley said she was really enjoying being pregnant. Fetal growth was reportedly normal, her weight gain was not excessive, and she felt well. She told the nurse about the special treatment she had been receiving from her relatives, friends, and Ted. Shirley seemed very happy about being the center of attention wherever they went. She commented that her colleagues were more cooperative than ever; her family called more often; and Ted had given her a very "chic" maternity dress and taken her out for a special dinner the previous week. She confided to Anna Marie that her own behavior had changed quite a bit too. "I feel like I can ask for and receive help more easily from others now." She generally allowed herself more relaxation; she began spending "time doing absolutely nothing." In fact, she told Anna Marie in a joking voice, "I am going to hate to give this all up when I have the baby." In later conversations with Anna Marie, Shirley expressed fear of labor and delivery as well as anxiety about her mothering abilities.

STUDY QUESTIONS

16-1. What risks related to pregnancy and delivery are involved for a middle-aged primigravida?

16-2. During the interview, Shirley verbalized mixed feelings about her pregnancy. Is this indicative of any major conflict or pathology at this point?

16-3. What are the developmental stages of pregnancy? of parenthood?

16-4. Determine the etiology and pathophysiology of sickle cell disease. What screening method(s) are used to determine the presence of the sickle cell trait?

16-5. What are the chances of having an infant with sickle cell anemia if one parent has the trait? Both parents? What are the chances that the newborn infant will carry the trait?

16-6. What are the indications for an amniocentesis? Why is an ultrasound scan performed prior to an amniocentesis?

16-7. How is an amniocentesis performed? What information about the fetus can be gained from an amniocentesis? What nursing care is indicated for a client who has had an amniocentesis?

16-8. How is genetic counseling useful to a couple who are anticipating a pregnancy? To a couple who are already pregnant?

16-9. When can an abortion be done without danger to the mother?

DISCUSSION QUESTIONS

D-1. How might Ted and Shirley's earlier life experiences affect their choice of a spouse?

D-2. What other information might be obtained during an interview such as the one described here?

D-3. What are some possible effects of the first-born child upon a marriage? Explain.

D-4. What insurance companies will pay for the expense of an abortion in your area?

INTRAPARTUM EVENTS

When Shirley went into labor at 3 A.M., Ted showed some anxiety. He grabbed Shirley's packed suitcase and rushed it to the door. Then he went to the phone to call the hospital. In the middle of dialing the phone, he suddenly stopped and said to himself, "What am I doing?" Ted then walked back to the bedroom and started to coach Shirley. After arriving at the hospital at 7:30 A.M., Ted called Anna Marie, who supported the couple through the remaining eight hours of labor and then the delivery. Jason was born at 3:30 P.M., a healthy 3400 g newborn. There were no complications for either the mother or the infant, much to everyone's satisfaction.

In a telephone conference with Anna Marie, Shirley said she enjoyed her three-day hospital stay. She and Ted had had a good opportunity to become acquainted with their son and they were grateful for Anna Marie's assistance. Either Shirley's mother or aunt was there each day following Shirley's discharge. They insisted on Shirley getting her rest while they did the housework and looked after Jason.

STUDY QUESTIONS

16-10. What are the five phases of fatherhood? Explain each. What phase is Ted experiencing?

16-11. During Shirley's late antepartal and intrapartal phase of pregnancy, how can Anna Marie best support the couple's teamwork? Develop a plan of care that correlates with the nursing diagnoses she would make.

Nursing Diagnosis	Therapeutic/Educational Interventions	Rationale

DISCUSSION QUESTIONS

D-5. What are the policies relating to the involvement of the father in the birth process in a hospital in your area?

D-6. How can the nurse assist in the changing and/or updating of the above policies?

POSTPARTUM—A CRISIS

Around the seventh postpartum day, Shirley began to worry. Her mother and aunts were almost always there taking care of everything in the house in addition to much of Jason's care. There was nothing left for Shirley to do except to breast-feed the baby. Between feedings Shirley was spending long periods of time alone. It was as though Jason had replaced Shirley in the affections and concerns of her family. She felt she was being ignored.

During the third postpartum week, Shirley and Ted requested a conference with Anna Marie. Almost immediately, the nurse noted that Shirley was pale and had dark areas around her eyes, and she talked slowly. The following discussion occurred:

Shirley: I don't know what's wrong with me, (*wringing her hands*). I feel so depressed all the time. I know about postpartum blues; but this is something more. I have trouble sleeping at night and I have no appetite and I'm tired all the time. Sometimes I even have trouble breast-feeding Jason. The worst thing of all is that I don't care about the baby (*tearful*). I wanted him so much and now I feel like this—it's terrible (*crying*).

Ted: She's always crying and saying she does not know how to take care of the baby.

Nurse: How do you respond when she says those things?

Ted: I lose my temper. Here she's getting all this help and she has a beautiful baby. I don't understand it. It scares me to see her like this. She was never like this before.

Shirley: (*Begins to sob.*)

Nurse: Put your tears into words.

Shirley: I have let him down too.

Nurse: Where do you get the idea that you have let Ted down?

Shirley: Well, he gets angry when I tell him how I feel.

Ted: No honey, that's not it. I get angry because I do not know how to help you. I think you are doing a great job!

Nurse: What is your response to what Ted just said, Shirley?

Shirley: It's good to hear it (*a faint smile*).

Nurse: Ted, you can help Shirley at home with that same kind of reassurance.

Nurse: Shirley, tell me how it came about that your family became involved in the baby's care.

Shirley: My mother and aunts wanted to help and I knew they would love to take care of the baby. I did not want to hurt their feelings and besides they are better at it than I am (*pause*). But now it bothers me how they hover over him and they don't care about me.

Shirley later talked about missing teaching, the people at work, and the satisfaction of doing a job well. She felt lonely—especially now that Ted was out of town more frequently.

STUDY QUESTIONS

16-12. What factors should be assessed in order to assist the mother, father, and their first-born infant to adjust to discharge from the hospital?

16-13. What behaviors do mothers and fathers often exhibit that indicate a healthy transition to their roles as parents?

16-14. In this case, Anna Marie uses a family-therapy approach in counseling the Clintons. What advantages does family therapy have as compared to individual therapy? Explain.

DISCUSSION QUESTIONS

D-7.   Discuss how the nurse can offer her services and expertise to clients and families in a nonthreatening manner during the postpartum phase.

D-8.   Analyze the interviewing techniques employed during the family-nurse interaction. Discuss the dynamics of this interaction.

D-9.   What behavioral changes are normal with the progression of a pregnancy? Compare the textbook picture with Shirley's behavior.

D-10. Analyze the discussion presented here and determine the method of verbal communication used by the nurse in this interview.

NURSING DIAGNOSIS

Anna Marie made her nursing diagnosis based upon her past data and the current interview. In order to provide them with the support and counseling, Anna Marie agreed to conduct six, 1-hour weekly sessions with the Clintons. At that time, the need for further sessions would be evaluated. Having determined that Shirley's anorexia and inability to sleep had significantly affected her physical health, Anna Marie made a referral for Shirley to contact her obstetrician for a medical evaluation and possible treatment.

STUDY QUESTIONS

16-15. Based upon the data presented thus far, determine the nursing diagnosis and support each diagnosis with behaviors and dialogue as a part of the data base. Pay special attention to the dynamics of the couple as well as the relatives.

Nursing Diagnosis	Supporting Behaviors/Dialogue

16-16. In light of the diagnosis, formulate a plan of nursing intervention that could feasibly be accomplished during six 1-hour family sessions. What is your rationale for the chosen interventions?

Nursing Intervention	Rationale

DISCUSSION QUESTIONS

D-11. What would be the benefit of giving Shirley a medical referral? Discuss the particular medical treatment regimes (pharmacologic agents) that might be prescribed to manage the physical problems.

D-12. Role play or outline the therapeutic communication (interviewing) techniques (tools) that you would use during a specific session with the Clinton family. Focus on one nursing goal at a time (for example, facilitate more effective verbal communication between Ted and Shirley).

D-13. Why do you suppose that Anna Marie suggested a schedule of multiple weekly sessions with the Clintons (rather than just one long session)?

D-14. In what way(s) did Anna Marie encourage the Clintons to assume responsibility for their health care? Their infant's care?

PROGRESS

Following six 1-hour sessions, Anna Marie had noted the following behavioral changes in the Clinton family system:

- Shirley was assuming nearly all of the responsibility for the household maintenance and infant care with assistance from Ted on the weekends and, sometimes, on weekday evenings.

- Shirley, Ted, and Jason were visiting one or two of Shirley's relatives for not more than three hours weekly.

- Shirley was verbalizing how much fun it was to bathe Jason and how much smoother the breast-feeding was going. "He has been such a good baby lately."

- Whenever Ted was out of town on business in the evening, he would phone Shirley to see how she and Jason were doing at home.

- Ted cared for Jason at least twice a week while Shirley had her "free time."

- Ted and Shirley had set aside one evening each week during which the two of them would share a relaxed candlelight dinner at home, or would go out to dinner.

- Ted and Shirley both commented that their relationship had improved considerably. They responded that they were able to discuss their feelings and resolve their differences more readily.

- Jason weighed 12 lb. He was eating every 4 hours and sometimes sleeping 6 hours through the night without awakening.

• Shirley was seriously considering an offer to return to the university to teach part-time.

Anna Marie and the Clintons jointly decided that they had gained what they wanted from their counseling sessions. She complimented Ted and Shirley on their progress in successfully adjusting to their new family situation. Everyone agreed that they felt comfortable about terminating their sessions at this time. The Clintons were informed that they were free to contact Anna Marie at her office if they felt she could be of further service to them. The nurse requested the couple's permission to make a home visit for a follow-up evaluation, to which they agreed. The final session was then terminated.

STUDY QUESTIONS

16-17. What do the listed behavioral changes indicate to you about the couple's progress in coping with a family crisis? What other behaviors might one observe as a family begins to function more effectively following the birth of a child?

16-18. What information can be gained by the nurse and the Clintons by making a follow-up home visit in three months?

16-19. What is the purpose of terminating a client/family–nurse relationship? Explain.

DISCUSSION QUESTION

D-15. Role play the terminating interview between Anna Marie and the Clintons.

SUGGESTED ACTIVITIES

1. Observe an ultrasound scan and amniocentesis procedure.

2. Attend a natural childbirth class in your area. Become familiar with the various relaxation and breathing techniques that can be used by women in labor and delivery. What is the role of the husband?

3. Interview a couple who are expecting their first child or who have recently had their first baby. Explore with them the changes that have occurred in their life-styles and their perceptions of parenthood.

4. Visit a genetic counseling clinic and/or a genetic laboratory.

5. Explore the agencies and organizations available to expectant parents and new parents in your community.

BIBLIOGRAPHY

Aguilera, Donna C., and Messick, Janice M. *Crisis Intervention—Theory and Methodology.* 3d ed. St. Louis: C. V. Mosby Co., 1978, pp. 21–28, 47–52, 63–72, 79–80, 146–54.

Arieti, Silvano, ed. *American Handbook of Psychiatry.* New York: Basic Books, Inc., 1966, pp. 239–254; 345–352.

Doswell, Willa M. "Sickle Cell Anemia—You Can Do Something to Help." *Nursing '78* 8 (April 1978): 65–70.

Feldman, Larry B. "Depression and Marital Interaction." *Family Process* 15 (December 1976): 389–395.

Ferrer, Thelma L. "Counseling Patients in Genetic Abnormalities." *Nursing Clinics of North America* 10 (June 1975): 293–305.

Hall, Joanne E., and Weaver, Barbara R. *Nursing of Families in Crisis.* Philadelphia: J. B. Lippincott Co., 1974, pp. 33–50; 64–83; 138–157.

Jensen, Margaret Duncan; Benson, Ralph C.; and Bobak, Irene M. *Maternity Care—The Nurse and the Family.* St. Louis: C. V. Mosby Co., 1977, pp. 80–103; 138–167; 429–446; 641–645.

Kalkman, Marion E., and Davis, Anne J., eds., *New Dimensions in Mental Health-Psychiatric Nursing.* 4th ed. New York: McGraw-Hill, 1974, pp. 129–154; 451–478; 520–546; 547–574.

Little, Dolores E., and Carnevali, Doris L. *Nursing Care Planning.* Philadelphia: J. B. Lippincott Co., 1976.

McFarlane, Judith. "Sickle Cell Disorders." *American Journal of Nursing* 77 (December 1977): 1948–1954.

McGowan, Madeline N. "Postpartum Disturbance—A Review of the Literature in Terms of Stress Response." *Journal of Nurse-Midwifery* 22 (Summer 1977): 27–34.

Murray, Ruth, and Zentner, Judith. *Nursing Concepts for Health Promotion.* Englewood Cliffs, N.J.: Prentice-Hall, Inc., 1975, pp. 44–72; 157–184; 206–248; 346–370.

Pendagast, Eileen G., and Sherman, Charles O. "A Guide to the Genogram Family Systems Training." *The Family* 5 (1977): 3–14.

Ritchie, C. Ann. "Depression Following Childbirth." *Nurse Practitioner* 2 (March/April 1977): 14–17.

Ruff, Coralease. "Childbearing in Sickle Cell Anemia: A Nursing Approach." *Journal of Obstetric, Gynecologic and Neonatal Nursing* 6 (May/June 1977): 23–25.

Skolnick, Arlene S., and Skolnick, Jerome H. *Family in Transition.* Boston: Little, Brown, 1971, pp. 331–341; 419–431.

Toman, Walter. *Family Constellation.* New York: Springer, 1969.

CHAPTER SEVENTEEN

Postoperative Management of Complications: Cholecystectomy

MARGARET MERVA

OVERVIEW

Joyce Cowgill is a thirty-seven-year-old recently widowed woman with three children. They live on a farm in the Midwest. After several episodes of abdominal pain, Joyce visits a family health clinic and is immediately admitted to a medical-surgical unit in a nearby hospital. A cholangiogram confirms the diagnosis of gall stones and a cholecystectomy is performed. Several complications are dealt with by the nursing staff before Joyce's condition is stabilized and she is allowed to return home.

CONTENT EMPHASIS

- Assessment and treatment of cholelithiasis
- Management of nausea and vomiting
- Management of fever
- Postoperative control of pain

SETTINGS

- Farm home
- Family health clinic
- Medical-surgical unit

OBJECTIVES

Upon completing this chapter the student will be able to:

1. Describe the pathophysiology and etiology of gall bladder disease.
2. Determine an effective approach to the promotion of respiratory gas exchange in preoperative and postoperative clients.
3. Develop health outcomes specific to the care of acutely ill clients in both the preoperative and postoperative phases.
4. Develop health outcomes specific to the care of clients who experience postoperative complications.
5. Determine the effectiveness of nursing interventions designed to control nausea, vomiting, fever, and pain.

DEFINITION OF TERMS

The following terms are used in this chapter and should be defined before proceeding:

Bacteremia
Cholangiogram
Cholecystectomy
Cholecystitis
Cholelithiasis
Commodities market

Department of Youth and Family Services
Home health aide
Hypothermia
Hypothermia machine
IPPB

FAMILY ASSESSMENT

Joyce Cowgill is a thirty-seven-year-old mother of three children who was widowed eleven months ago and lives on a 150-acre farm. The Cowgill farm, in Millstone Township, produces cabbage and tomatoes. This is the Cowgill's first harvest season since the death of Mr. Harvey Cowgill (age 42) following a farm accident. Joyce's family of origin lives in nearby Freehold borough. Harvey's parents moved back to the farm to be with Joyce and the children after the death of their son. They had retired to Florida three years ago. The farm was formerly owned by Harvey's parents. They signed it over to Harvey and Joyce before they moved to Florida. Mr. Cowgill, age 62, is managing the farm with the help of migrant workers.

When Harvey Cowgill died, sufficient life insurance was collected to protect the farm investment; but the current cost of living far exceeds the income

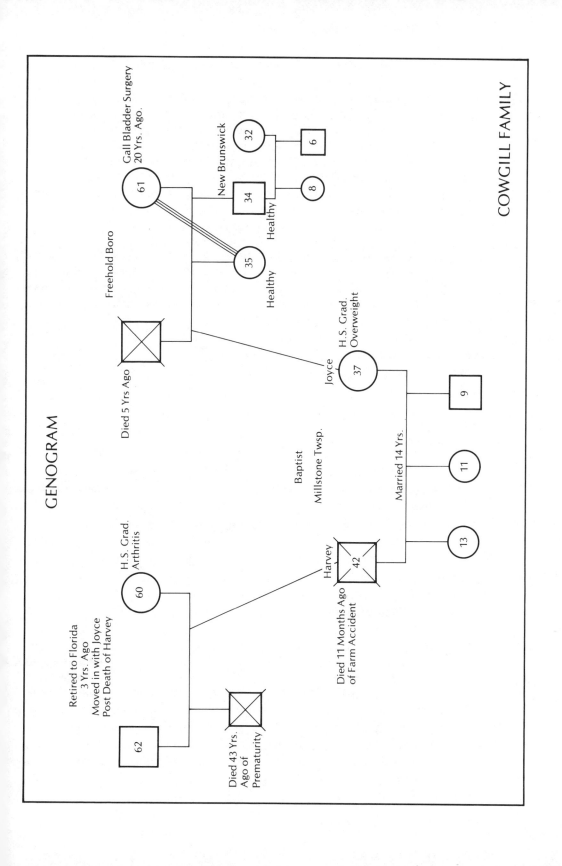

GENOGRAM

COWGILL FAMILY

from the commodities produced. However, the value of the land in this area continues to increase. Therefore, Joyce is attempting to retain the property until a good opportunity to sell at a considerable profit presents itself.

The family lives in a sturdy, ten-room farm house heated by oil. Harvey insulated the attic and installed new storm windows just prior to his death. Each of the children has his own room, as do Mr. and Mrs. Cowgill, Sr.

The Cowgills are practicing Baptists. Joyce met Harvey through their church in Heightstown while Harvey was home on leave from the service. They married soon after his military discharge.

As required by law, the Cowgill farm was visited periodically throughout the migrant season. Mary Dowling, the community health nurse, was assigned to monitor the health care needs of the migrant families for the summer. Joyce Cowgill would greet Ms. Dowling each time she visited, since she was anxious to talk about the migrants as well as her own family. From their conversation, the nurse recognized that Joyce apparently had some health problems that needed attention. Ms. Dowling's strong encouragement to seek care at the Freehold Health Center at the Tuesday evening family clinic seemed to be disregarded by Joyce, despite Joyce's constant complaining.

STUDY QUESTIONS

17-1. What are the stages of grief? What behaviors are typical of these stages?

17-2. According to Erikson's theory, determine the developmental phases that the Cowgill children are presently experiencing. (See genogram.)

17-3. What are the major beliefs and practices of the Baptist religion?

DISCUSSION QUESTIONS

D-1. Would it be advisable for Ms. Dowling to discuss Joyce's health status with her in-laws? Explain.

D-2. There are a number of Baptist congregations that are separate and distinct as defined by their beliefs and practices. What questions might the nurse pose to the client that would more specifically identify her religious beliefs and the religion's impact on her life-style? How would this information be useful in the assessment and future nursing interventions with this client?

D-3. How would you expect the sudden death of Mr. Cowgill to affect the family's functioning? Consider the relationship between (1) Joyce and her in-laws; (2) the in-laws and their grandchildren; (3) Joyce and her children.

D-4. What health and supportive services are available to migrant farm workers in your state?

D-5. Identify the stage of grief that Joyce Cowgill is probably experiencing.

CLIENT ASSESSMENT

Following increasingly painful episodes of gastric discomfort, Joyce Cowgill is seen at the Family Health Clinic by Ms. Clayton, the family nurse practitioner, for complete physical examination. The following health history and physical assessment findings are recorded:

GENERAL APPEARANCE: Well-developed, 37-year-old, widowed female who is alert and oriented.

VITAL SIGNS: T: 37.8°C, P: 94, R: 20, BP: 132/88, Height: 165 cm   Weight: 86.4 g

CHIEF COMPLAINT: Client states that she has an increasing intolerance to fatty foods over the past six months. Also has considerable right upper quadrant abdominal pain radiating to the mid-epigastric area. The pain has increased in severity throughout the past week with pain radiating to the tip of the right scapula and the right chest wall.

PAST HEALTH HISTORY: Seasonal (fall and winter) episodes of "headcolds" that are self-treated with aspirin and cold tablets. No past hospitalizations or surgeries; Gravida 3 Para 3 with uneventful labors and deliveries. No known allergies to foods or drugs. Last medical examination was about three years ago.

FAMILY HEALTH HISTORY: Gallbladder disease with cholecystectomy experienced by mother at age 44 years. Father deceased—unknown cause of death. No history of diabetes, heart or lung disease, cancer, or mental illness in family.

SOCIAL HABITS AND HISTORY: Attends Baptist services with family weekly; a high-school graduate employed as a secretary for six years prior to husband's death. Consumes about 1 glass of alcoholic beverage (wine) weekly; denies smoking tobacco.

DIET HISTORY: Readily admits to overeating until the last few weeks. Drinks coffee with cream and sugar throughout the day. Twenty-four-hour diet recall:

Breakfast: coffee, sweet roll or muffin with butter and jelly.
Lunch: cheeseburger on bun, 4 chocolate chip cookies, apple.
Supper: fried pork chops, hash browns, green beans, coffee.
Snacks: coffee, apple pie.

ELIMINATION HISTORY: Normally has a soft brown stool every one to two days in A.M. Has experienced occasional bouts of constipation in the last month. No urinary frequency or burning, voiding 4–5 times daily.

HEALTH ATTITUDES: Client states, "I try to take care of my health, but sometimes I just don't care that much about myself and other things are more important; besides doctors cost money."

PHYSICAL ASSESSMENT:

Integument	Skin is slightly warm and moist to touch; good turgor; mild cutaneous icterus but denies pruritus.
HEENT	Noncontributory findings
Chest	Clear and symmetrical lung sounds; dullness noted over right lower lobe on percussion.
Heart	NSR; AP: 94, regular; no murmurs or bruits; S-1 and S-2 sounds differentiated; peripheral pulses are equal, but difficult to locate in legs.
Gastrointestinal	Stools are light brown without evidence of blood. Active bowel sounds in RUQ. Presence of rebound tenderness and pain upon palpation of the right hypochondrium and the epigastric area. Gall bladder palpated near the right costal margin at the midclavicular line.
Extremities	Varicosities present in both lower legs. Edema 1+ in lower extremities. No ulcerations nor abrasions evident.
Genitourinary	Pelvic exam deferred. Concentrated, dark amber urine specimen obtained.

Following the completion of the client assessment, Ms. Clayton alerted Dr. Booker, the clinic physician, of her findings. Dr. Booker confirmed the abnormal findings and advised immediate hospitalization. The nurse practitioner counseled Ms. Cowgill, explaining her findings and the urgent need for further tests to determine the cause of her pain, nausea, jaundice, and fever. Although Joyce consented, she was greatly concerned about her family. The children had not stayed alone with their grandparents in over five years and she wondered how they would all manage. She phoned her own parents and her in-laws from the clinic.

The client's hospital admission was arranged by telephone. A referral form was completed by the nurse practitioner and the physician with a copy of the assessment findings attached. While the in-laws stayed at the house with the children, Joyce's mother and younger sister met her at the hospital, which was about five miles from the clinic.

By 9:00 that evening, Joyce had been admitted to a semi-private room on a medical/surgical unit in the 250-bed community hospital. The attending physician, David Jones, M.D., wrote the following admitting orders after reviewing the clinic's referral form, interviewing Joyce, and completing a brief physical examination:

Bedrest with BRP

Vital signs q 4 hrs

Low-fat diet

NPO after midnight for cholecystogram

Demerol 50 mg }
Vistaril 50 mg } IM q 3 h prn for pain

Aqua mephyton 10 mgm IM now

Seconal 100 mg po HS

IVs #1 1000 ml of 5% D/W with 1 ampule Berocca-C at 125 ml/hr
    #2 1000 ml 5% D/W at 125 ml/hr
    #3 1000 ml 5% D/W with 20 mEq KCl at 125 ml/hr

CBC with differential prothrombin time, serum electrolytes, urinalysis, blood chemistry, chest X-rays, abdominal flat plate, and EKG in A.M.

Fleets enema tonight

Once Joyce was settled and her mother had met the physician and nurse who would be responsible for Joyce's care, they returned to their home. Their phone numbers were left at the nurses' station with instructions to call if there was any change or anything they could do.

The next morning, the cholecystogram was completed and the following laboratory results were available:

HgB: 11.5 g/100 ml

Hct: 35%

RBC: $4.0 \times 10^6/mm^3$

WBC: $13,000/mm^3$

Neutrophils: 70%

Lymphocytes: 20%

Platelets: $219,000/mm^3$

Direct bilirubin (post-hepatic): 0.5 mg/100 ml

Icterus index: 15 units

Prothrombin time: 34 seconds (29 sec-control)

Alkaline phosphotase: 6 u/ml

SGOT: 225 u/ml

SGPT: 275 u/ml

Serum amylase: 11 u/ml

Sodium: 130 mEq/L

Potassium: 4.2 mEq/L

Chloride: 97 mEq/L

CO_2 content: 28 mEq/L

Abdominal X-ray findings: Calcified stones seen in upper right quadrant of abdomen.

Chest X-ray: Nonadventitious lung tissue; no evidence of fluid or disease. Heart size is normal.

EKG: R: 92, NSR, normal QRS complex.

Cholecystogram: Multiple calcified stone shadows visualized in the gall bladder and near the bile duct. Outline of the bladder is diffuse.

Joyce continued to experience frequent nausea and occasional vomiting throughout the second day of her hospitalization. Her right upper quadrant abdominal pain persisted despite analgesic medication.

Dr. Jones discussed the diagnostic test results with the client Thursday morning, informing her of the diagnosis—cholecystitis and cholelithiasis. He highly recommended that surgery be done to remove the gall bladder as soon as possible. This did not come as a total surprise to Joyce since she readily recalled her mother's similar illness. Joyce signed the necessary surgical consent forms and was scheduled for a cholecystectomy with a cholangiogram to be performed Friday morning.

Ten minutes later when Ms. Johnson, R.N., entered Joyce's room, she found Joyce sobbing. Offering her some words of consolation as she gently held the client's hand, the nurse listened while Joyce explained that her main worry was for her children and "how long they would be without their mother." Having regained her composure, Joyce followed through with the nurse's suggestions that she phone her children at home after school. She could hear from them about how things were going at home and she could help them understand that she would need to stay in the hospital for a while to have surgery.

The following preoperative orders were written by Dr. Jones Thursday evening:

NPO at midnight

NG tube to low Gomco suction in A.M.

Preoperative on call medications:

  Demerol 75 mg IM

  Vistaril 75 mg IM

  Atropine 0.4 mg IM

Skin prep

Seconal 100 mg po HS

Change IV to 5% D in ½ NS at 100 cc/hr

Type and cross-match for 2 units whole blood

Joyce Cowgill received her on-call medications at 7 A.M. and was taken to the operating room at 7:30 A.M.

STUDY QUESTIONS

17-4. Describe the function and physiology of the gallbladder. Trace the flow of bile from its point of origin to the duodenum.

17-5. Compare the pathophysiology and etiology of cholelithiasis and cholecystitis.

17-6. What foods contribute to the exacerbation of biliary tract disease? Why?

17-7. What causes the changes in the characteristics of Joyce's urine and fecal matter? Explain.

17-8. What complications can result from not treating bilary tract disease? Explain.

17-9. Analyze Joyce's 24-hour diet recall in terms of nutritional needs. What foods consumed by Joyce increase her symptoms described under "chief complaint."?

17-10. Why is Demerol the analgesic of choice for Joyce's right upper quadrant pain? Why is morphine not an alternative drug of choice in this instance?

17-11. The following medications are given at some time prior to Joyce's surgery. Complete a drug information card on each of the following: Demerol, Vistaril, Aquamephyton, Seconal, atropine, intravenous potassium solution.

17-12. What is the purpose of prescribing a low-fat diet, particularly the evening prior to a cholecystogram? Explain.

17-13. State the rationale for the choice of parenteral fluids. Why is $D_5/.45$ NS infused following the insertion of an indwelling nasogastric tube? Explain.

17-14. Complete the following laboratory grid:

Lab Test	Normal Range Adult Female	Joyce's Value	Cause for Alteration (Where Applicable)
Hgb			
Hct			
RBC			
WBC			
Neutrophils			
Lymphocytes			
Platelets			

Lab Test	Normal Range Adult Female	Joyce's Value	Cause for Alteration (Where Applicable)
Prothrombin Sodium Potassium Chloride Carbon dioxide Direct bilirubin Icterus index Alk. phos. SGOT SGPT Serum amylase			

DISCUSSION QUESTIONS

D-6. Based upon the assessment data and the client's condition, determine the nursing diagnosis at admission. What are the nursing care objectives and the rationale for each? What are the nursing actions and the rationale for each? How is the effectiveness evaluated?

Nursing Diagnosis	Objective	Rationale	Nursing Action	Rationale	Method and Frequency of Evaluating Effectiveness

D-7. What revisions should be made preoperatively in the care plan?

D-8. What alternative methods might be employed by the nurse in dealing with Joyce's concern for her children?

D-9. Compare Joyce's disease process with the classical textbook picture of this disease.

POSTOPERATIVE PHASE

Following the surgical procedure, Joyce was transferred to the recovery room. The anesthesiologist remained with her until she was fully awake and responding. The report of surgery read as follows:

Postoperative Diagnosis: Cholelithiasis, cholecystitis

Surgical Procedure: Cholecystectomy; operative cholangiogram

Time: 3 hrs. 15 min.

Estimated Blood Loss: 150 cc

Drains: 6-in. penrose—inserted into subhepatic area

Condition: Good

Specimen: Gallbladder

Findings: Multiple calcified stones; blocked biliary duct

Last Vital Signs: BP: 120/70   P: 76   R: 16

Anesthesia: General

Joyce was transferred from the recovery room to her hospital room. She was in considerable pain, even though she had been medicated three hours ago while in the recovery room. Her vital signs were as follows: T: 37.2°C, P: 88, R: 24; BP: 120/78. Her abdominal dressing was dry and intact. Joyce was transferred to her bed and placed in a semi-Fowler's position. The Levine tube was connected to low intermittent suction.

Joyce's mother and sister were waiting in the hospital lobby to learn of her condition. Joyce's inlaws had called the unit to learn of her return to the floor, and they left word that they would visit her that evening. The following orders were written for Joyce's postoperative care:

Vital signs q 15 min. until stable; then q 2 h for 8 h.; then q 4 h and prn.

N/G tube to low suction; irrigate q 2–4 h prn with normal saline

NPO

Bedrest; OOB in A.M. with assistance

Intake and output

Straight catheterization if unable to void in 8 hr.

Blow bottles, cough and deep breathe q 2 hr.

3000 ml of 5% D in .33 NS with 20 mEq KCl added to each liter—to run 24 hr.

Demerol 75 mg } IM q 4 h prn for pain
Vistaril 50 mg

IPPB therapy with 10 ml Mucomyst 10% qid × 15 min.

Antiembolus hose

Joyce's first postoperative day was uneventful. She dangled in the morning and was OOB in the chair for 15 minutes. Her vital signs were stable and she was cooperative with the IPPB therapy. However, she slept most of the day and required pain medication every 4–5 hours.

On the second postoperative day, Ms. Cowgill's N/G tube was clamped as she ambulated to the bathroom with the assistance of the nurse and voided 300 cc of dark amber urine. The nurse instructed Joyce to support her incision as she walked. Upon her return to bed, Joyce vomited 100 cc of dark bile-colored fluid and the abdominal dressing was stained with serosanguinous drainage. The nurse noticed that Joyce was diaphoretic, flushed, and warm to the touch. Joyce said that she was dizzy and felt cold. The nurse reassured her and returned her to bed. She checked the status of the wound, irrigated and connected the N/G tube and monitored the vital signs. They were as follows: T: 39°C (rectal), P: 110, R: 30, and BP: 124/78. After the surgeon was notified about Joyce's changes, he changed her dressing. The wound area was red, tender, and draining purulent material around the penrose drain. A specimen of the wound drainage was taken. Then the surgeon left the following orders:

NPO

5% D in ½ NS with 20 mEq KCl to run @ 150 ml/hr × 4 hrs; then 125 ml/hr

Change dressing prn; cleanse wound with 1:1 H_2O_2 and NS

Sputum and wound for culture and sensitivity

Clean catch urine for culture and sensitivity

Ampicillin 1 gram IV q 6 h

ASA 600 mg supp. q 3–4 h for temp. over 38.3°C

Cool water sponge bath for temp over 38.8°C (rectal)

The nurse explained to Joyce the need for an aspirin suppository. After giving the ASA suppository, the nurse auscultated Joyce's chest and abdomen. Chest sounds were clear however, no bowel sounds were heard. After bathing Joyce and changing her bed, the nurse gave Joyce an opportunity to rest. She had been medicated for pain prior to ambulation. One hour later Joyce had an IPPB treatment by the inhalation therapist. A sputum specimen was obtained at that time for culture and sensitivity.

On the third postoperative day, Joyce's temperature was 38.6°C (rectally). Her vital signs were: BP: 106/60, P: 88, R: 24. Urinary output was averaging 70 to 100 ml per hour. Blood cultures were drawn during the period of fever and were thus far found negative.

The surgeon visited and ordered the following:

IV 5% D in .45 NS, run at 125 ml/hr

Blood cultures for temp. above 38.8°C

Hypothermia blanket for temp above 39.4°C

Ampicillin 1 g IV q 6 hours to continue

Urine ph and specific gravity qid

Valium 5 mg IM q 4–6 h prn for anxiety

Administration of corticosteroids was deferred at this time in order to evaluate Joyce's response to the Ampicillin therapy.

A summary of the nursing care given to Joyce Cowgill read as follows:

JOYCE COWGILL   surgery date: 7/14
NURSING POSTOPERATIVE FLOW SHEET   surgery: cholecystectomy

Date/Time	Vital Signs	Temp.	Significant Lab Findings	Oral Intake	Intravenous Intake	Urine N/G Others	Medications	Comments
7/14 11 A.M.	120/70, 76-16	37°C		NPO	5% D in ⅓ NS, 125 cc/hr	Blood loss: 150 cc	Demerol, 50 mg IM Vistaril 50 mg IM	Recovery room abdomen soft, afebrile
7/15 P.O. #1	120/78, 88-24	37.2°C (R)	Hgb: 11.7 g Hct: 37% WBC: 13,000 K⁺: 3.2 mEq	NPO	5% D in ⅓ NS, 125 cc/hr	N/G: 800 cc urine: 650 cc	Demerol, 75 mg IM Vistaril, 50 mg IM	Awake and respond Dressing dry and intact
7/16 P.O. #2	124/78, 100-30	39°C (R)	K⁺: 3.9 mEq	NPO	5% D in ½ NS, 125–150 cc/hr	Vomited 100 cc bile N/G: 150 cc urine: 1200 cc	Demerol, 75 mg IM Vistaril, 50 mg IM Ampicillin, 1 g × 4 IV ASA suppository 600 mg	Serosanguinous wound drainage; and wound sputum specimens sent for C and S
7/17 P.O. #3	102/60, 112-30	38.6°C (R)	K⁺: 3.5 mEq		5% D in ½ NS, 125 cc/hr		Ampicillin, 1 g × 4 IV	Blood culture: negative to date

STUDY QUESTIONS

17-15. What is IPPB therapy? What is the rationale for this therapy and what nursing responsibilities are connected with the treatment modality? What adverse reactions can occur with the use of IPPB therapy? What symptoms would you assess?

17-16. Why is IPPB an important adjunct to coughing and deep breathing?

17-17. List the reasons for changing the surgical dressing.

17-18. List the steps in changing a postoperative dressing using the surgical aseptic technique. What precautions must the nurse take to ensure prevention of nosocomial infections?

17-19. Complete a drug information card on the following medications: Vistaril, aspirin, Valium, Ampicillin, Mucomyst.

17-20. Why is Ampicillin the preferred choice in Joyce's case?

17-21. How is Ampicillin prepared for IV administration? What side effects would you watch for while supervising a client on this medication?

17-22. With the onset of Joyce's postop fever the nurse administered ASA 600 mg suppository. What is the expected action of this drug in this situation? What adverse reactions would you look for knowing Joyce's preoperative history?

17-23. If Joyce's fever does not respond to ASA, the nurse will institute hypothermia. Develop a postop nursing care plan for this treatment modality, including appropriate goals, intervention, rationale, and evaluation. List the various methods for inducing hypothermia.

Goal	Objective	Rationale	Nursing Action	Rationale	Method and Frequency of Evaluating Effectiveness

17-24. What postoperative complications might be responsible for Joyce's increased body temperature? As the body temperature increases, so do oxygen requirements increase as cellular metabolism increases. How do body fluid requirements change? Give your rationale.

17-25. Can you explain why Joyce vomited 100 cc of bile-colored fluid? What action might the nurse have taken immediately to correct this fluid loss?

17-26. What electrolytes are being lost through Joyce's N/G tube? Through the penrose drain? How might these fluids and electrolyte losses affect wound healing?

17-27. What effects might Joyce's obesity have on her postoperative care? Explain.

17-28. What does Joyce's concentrated urine indicate in terms of her body's postoperative physiological response? Explain.

17-29. What are the causes of postoperative wound infection? What might be the etiology of Joyce's infectious process?

17-30. After Valium is ordered how should Joyce's pain medication be adjusted? What adverse reactions can Valium precipitate?

17-31. What are the therapeutic effects of short and long GI tubes? What are the characteristics of each? Complete the following chart.

Tube	Therapeutic Effect	Characteristics of Tube	Potential Problems	Client's Responses to Unwanted Effect (Physiologically and Psychologically)	Nursing Objectives and Actions	Method and Frequency of Evaluating Its Effectiveness
Short naso-gastric tubes: Levine Rehfuss Salem Sump						
Long intestinal tubes: Miller-Abbott Cantor Johnston Harris						

17-32. What are the nutritional needs of postoperative patients with infections? Be specific as to nutritional composition, caloric intake, vitamins and minerals.

17-33. Which of the GI tubes listed in the chart is being used for Joyce?

17-34. What are the therapeutic effects of drains and what are their nursing implications?

Type	Principles of Usage	Therapeutic Effect	Unwanted Effect	Client's Responses Physiologically and Psychologically	Nursing Objectives and Actions	Method and Frequency of Evaluating Its Effectiveness
Gauze						
Penrose						
T-tube						

17-35. What are therapeutic effects of using antiembolitic stockings for Joyce Cowgill after the surgery? What are the nursing responsibilities related to the client's use of antiembolitic stockings? What other nursing measures can achieve similar therapeutic effects?

DISCUSSION QUESTIONS

D-10. What was the extended family's response to Joyce's acute illness? What emotional support systems and coping mechanisms are being used? Explain.

D-11. Discuss the nursing implications for clients receiving massive doses of antibiotics.

D-12. Discuss the body's inflammatory response to an acute infectious process. (Consider Selye's local adaptation syndrome and general adaptation syndrome.) How does it apply to Joyce?

D-13. What factors besides medical intervention influenced Joyce's ability to successfully cope with the stress of acute illness? Explain.

EVALUATION AND FOLLOW-UP

Within the following 48-hour period, Joyce's clinical picture improved significantly. Her blood values and her body temperature returned to within the normal limits. Joyce's children were allowed to visit for a short period each day. This seemed to alleviate much of her anxiety about her family.

The utilization review nurse advised Joyce's physician as to the length of hospital stay permitted under her Blue Cross plan for a complicated abdominal surgical procedure. Plans were then made to discharge Joyce by the fourteenth postoperative day. An order was written for a home care referral that was developed by the nurse in conjunction with David Jones, M.D. This included a physician's order for a home health aide.

Since the Cowgill's medical insurance does not reimburse for a home health aide, the Department of Youth and Family Services assisted with this expense until a nursing assessment determined that it was no longer necessary to ensure Ms. Cowgill's safe convalescence and prevention of complications.

DISCUSSION QUESTIONS

D-14. What changes should Joyce expect to see in terms of her elimination status? Explain.

D-15. What is the approximate length of time for recovery from a cholecystectomy? A complicated cholecystectomy? Explain.

D-16. Prior to discharge, what teaching should Joyce receive regarding activity level and diet?

Goal	Objective	Content	Method of Teaching	Evaluation of Learning

D-17. Develop a home health care referral for Joyce Cowgill based on her condition at discharge.

D-18. Develop a nursing care plan based on this referral. What home care benefits are available under Blue Cross in your state?

Objective	Rationale	Nursing Action	Rationale	Client Response	Method and Frequency of Evaluating Effectiveness

D-19. What activities would a home health aide perform in caring for Joyce? Who would be responsible for teaching and supervising the aide? Explain.

SUGGESTED ACTIVITIES

1. Apply the knowledge gained in this case study to care of a client experiencing a cholecystectomy.

2. Investigate the social support services available through your state's Department of Youth and Family Services.

3. Spend some time with a utilization review nurse to learn her role.

4. Interview a client who has been discharged home after having had major surgery. Explore the feelings, expectations, and experiences of the client and his or her family as it relates to hospitalization and homebound recuperation.

5. Have someone administer a 5-minute IPPB treatment to you.

BIBLIOGRAPHY

Baer, Ellen; McGowan, Madeline; and McGivern, Diane. "Taking a Health History." *American Journal of Nursing* 77 (July 1977): 1190–1193.

Beland, Irene. *Clinical Nursing* 3d ed. New York: Macmillan, 1975, pp. 528–535.

Benson, Evelyn, and McDevitt, Joan. "Care of the Patient and Family in the Home." In *Community Health and Nursing Practice.* Englewood Cliffs, N.J.: Prentice-Hall, Inc., 1975.

Bergersen, Betty. *Pharmacology in Nursing.* 13th ed. St. Louis: C. V. Mosby Co., 1976, pp. 394, 196–198, 223–224, 297, 232–236, 464–470.

Carey, Larry C., and Catalano, Philip W. "Acute Cholecystitis." In *Davis-Christopher Textbook of Surgery.* 11th ed. Edited by David C. Sabiston. Philadelphia: W. B. Saunders Co., 1977.

Condon, Robert E. et al. *Manual of Surgical Therapeutics.* 3d ed. Boston: Little, Brown and Co., 1975, pp. 286–287.

Davis, Ann, and Aroskar, Milia. "Rights of Patients in the Health Care System." In *Ethical Dilemmas in Nursing Practice.* New York: Appleton-Century-Crofts, 1978.

deTornyay, Rheba. "Nursing Decisions: A Patient Requiring a Cholecystectomy." *RN* 39 (February 1976): 43–49.

Guyton, Arthur C. *Textbook of Medical Physiology.* 5th ed. Philadelphia: W. B. Saunders Co., 1976, pp. 671–672, 863, 938–944.

Kuhn, Janet S. "Realignment of Emotional Forces Following Loss." *The Family* 5 (1977): 19–24.

LeMaitre, George D., and Finnegan, Janet A. *The Patient in Surgery: A Guide for Nurses.* 3d ed. Philadelphia: W. B. Saunders Co., 1975, pp. 176–180.

Little, Dolores, and Carnevali, Doris L. *Nursing Care Planning.* 2d ed. Philadelphia: J. B. Lippincott Co., 1976.

Luckmann, Joan, and Sorensen, Karen. *Medical-Surgical Nursing.* Philadelphia: W. B. Saunders Co., 1974, pp. 150–162, 317–322, 333–345, 433–435, 545–589, 914–929, 1059–1061, 1116–1138.

McCaffery, Margo, and Hart, Linda. "Undertreatment of Acute Pain with Narcotics." *American Journal of Nursing* 76 (October 1976): 1586–1591.

McConnell, Edwina. "All About Gastrointestinal Intubation." *Nursing '75* 5 (September 1975): 31–37.

Pendagast, Eileen G., and Sherman, Charles O. "A Guide to the Genogram Family Systems Training." *The Family* 5 (1977): 3–14.

Petrillo, Madeline, and Sanger, Sirgay. "A Working Knowledge of Childhood." In *Emotional Care of Hospitalized Children.* Philadelphia: J. B. Lippincott Co., 1972.

Pincus, Lily. *Death and the Family.* New York: Vintage Books, 1974.

Pumphrey, John B. "Recognizing Your Patient's Spiritual Needs." *Nursing '77* 7 (December 1977): 64–70.

Rau, Joseph, and Rau, Mary. "To Breathe or Be Breathed: Understanding IPPB." *American Journal of Nursing* 77 (April 1977): 613–617.

Ryan, Rosemary. "Thrombophlebitis: Assessment and Prevention." *American Journal of Nursing* 76 (October 1976): 1634–1636.

Sommer, Patricia. "Operative Cholangiography: Its Pros and Cons." *RN* 39 (October 1976): 38–39.

Spiro, Howard M. *Clinical Gastroenterology.* 2d ed. New York: Macmillan, 1977, pp. 916–928.

Stahlgren, Leroy H. et al. "Intestinal Obstruction." *American Journal of Nursing* 77 (June 1977): 999–1002.

Stroot, Violet R.; Lee, Carla A.; and Schaper, C. Ann. *Fluid and Electrolytes: A Practical Approach.* 2d ed. Philadelphia: F. A. Davis Co., 1977.

CHAPTER EIGHTEEN

Alteration in Body Image: Radical Mastectomy

ANDREA B. SAVITZ

OVERVIEW

Barbara Livingston is a forty-eight-year-old female who discovers a lump in her left breast while doing a breast self-examination. Barbara and her husband John are Quakers and have three grown children. Her fear of the diagnosis of a tumor is confirmed by Xerography. When the biopsy reveals carcinoma, a radical mastectomy is performed. Barbara needs assistance from the nursing staff when she expresses concern about her body image. She is also encouraged to discuss her sexuality. The nursing staff designs a rehabilitation program for Barbara.

CONTENT EMPHASIS

- Carcinoma of the breast—diagnosis
- Radical Mastectomy—pre- and post-operative nursing management.
- Change in body image—grieving for loss of body part
- Sexual readjustment
- Rehabilitation of mastectomy clients

SETTINGS

- Physician's office
- Surgical hospital unit

OBJECTIVES

Upon completing this chapter the student will be able to:

1. Comprehend the major etiology of and diagnostic methods for cancer of the breast.
2. Support the client's right to completely informed surgical consent.
3. Describe the pre- and post-operative nursing management of a client who has had a mastectomy.
4. Promote the client's adjustment to an altered body image.
5. Facilitate the sexual adjustment of the client who has had a mastectomy.

DEFINITION OF TERMS

The following terms are used in this chapter and should be defined before proceeding:

Body image	Metastatic
Breast lesion	Radiation therapy
Carcinoma	Thermography
Chemotherapy	TNM system
HemoVac	Transillumination
Hormonal therapy	Tumor
Mammography	Xerography
Metastasis	

ASSESSMENT

John and Barbara Livingston have been married twenty-four years. On wedding anniversaries they always laughingly mention the luck of their accidental meeting. The whole family knew that Bernie Grant, Barbara's father, had arranged the meeting. (See genogram.)

Twenty-six years ago, Mr. Grant was the consulting certified public accountant used by the company that employed John as a junior accountant. John spent a lot of time with Bernie, particularly at tax return filing time. Eventually Bernie invited John home to dinner and introduced his daughter Barbara to John.

By the time Barbara and John's courtship had become an engagement, the Livingston and Grant families knew each other quite well. The families had often mentioned that the couple would make a compatible pair. Both Barbara and John came from Quaker homes that dated back to Colonial times. It was

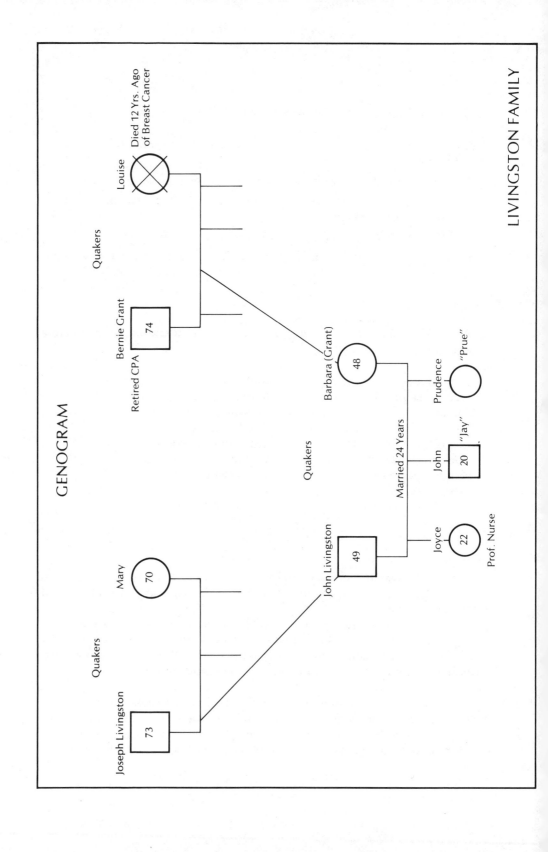

GENOGRAM

LIVINGSTON FAMILY

understood by the couple that child rearing was an essential part of marital life. Over the years the families were delighted when John and Barbara had three healthy infants; who were named Joyce (now 22), John, Jr., or "Jay" (now 20), and Prudence, or "Prue" (now 17).

The only tragedy the John Grants had to face was the death of Louise Grant twelve years ago. Barbara's mother Louise died of metastatic cancer of the breast. Barbara had tirelessly cared for her before her death.

On May 28, Joyce Livingston, age 22, returned home to visit her parents, John and Barbara. She had just graduated from Eagle College of Nursing. Still excited about her education, Joyce started to instruct everyone about health. In a threatening but light tone, she stated, "Mom, I know you must be doing your monthly breast self-examination." Barbara tried to change the subject because she had been lax in doing her self-examination of the breast. As Barbara began to move away from her daughter, Joyce continued, "Look Ma, now I'm serious. . ." Then Barbara became cross and said, "I'm old enough to take care of myself."

Later that night, Barbara did do the examination of her breasts for the first time in five months. John thought he heard Barbara say, "Oh my God." When he asked from the hallway, "Is anything wrong?" Barbara replied, "No, it's nothing."

During the night Barbara was up out of bed several times. She could not sleep. When John found her missing from their bed at 4:00 A.M., he called her name. He knew that she was normally a sound sleeper. Since there was no response, he got up and found Barbara sitting in the den staring out into space. He quietly sat down on the couch next to her and asked, "What's the matter, honey?"

Barbara said, "I was just thinking about how proud my mother would have been of Joyce." John turned to her and said, "That's true but that's no reason to loose sleep. . ." he noticed then that tears were falling down his wife's cheeks. Demandingly he asked, "Honey, what's wrong?"

Barbara winced and blurted out, "I've got a breast lump." Many tears later and with her husband's encouragement, Barbara decided to call Franklin Sands, M.D. for an appointment in the morning. Dr. Sands was the general surgeon in their physician's family practice group.

When Barbara entered Dr. Sand's office, she was greeted by Ms. Sandra Buys, R.N., who ushered her into an adjoining room to obtain Barbara's history. Ms. Buys recorded this updated health history:

NAME: Barbara Livingston

AGE: 48

DATE: 5/29/_____

WEIGHT: 59 Kg

HEIGHT: 140.8 cm.

LMP: 5/14/_____

CHIEF COMPLAINT: Left breast lump discovered yesterday; it was not palpable 5 months ago.

EATING/ELIMINATION: Always maintained good dietary habits, eating foods from the basic four food groups daily; formed stool regularly every 2–3 days.

ILLNESS: Negative history except for chicken pox, measles, German measles, and very occasional URIs.

IMMUNIZATIONS: Immunizations were updated at last physical examination.

EXPOSURE TO DISEASE: None.

ALLERGIES: None.

HABITS: Denies smoking and alcohol consumption. Enjoys golf, needlepoint, and crocheting.

GROWTH/DEVELOPMENT: First menstruation at age 11; Birthed first child at age 26; Gravida three, para three (Children ages 22, 20, and 17); all births unremarkable; breast-fed each child; still menstruating regularly.

FAMILY HISTORY: Mother died at age 58 of metastatic breast cancer.

SOCIOECONOMIC: Lives in five-bedroom house on two wooded acres; has Blue Cross/Blue Shield with Rider J and Major Medical.

During the entire interview, Ms. Buys noted that Barbara continued to manipulate her handkerchief. At one point Barbara's eyes filled with tears, and Ms. Buys attempted to support Barbara emotionally. Having explained what Barbara could expect in the examining room, Ms. Buys led her to examining room B.

After the physical examination, Dr. Sands recorded his impression on Barbara's record as follows:

Nontender tumor of approx. 1 cm diameter with attachment located in upper outer quadrant of left breast.

Then he had the secretary arrange for a Xerographic mammography of Barbara.

When Dr. Sands left the examining room, Ms. Buys remained with Barbara, who just sat quietly in her examining gown. Ms. Buys softly stated, "The documentation of a breast lump is often as upsetting as finding it yourself." After placing her hand lightly on Barbara's arm, Ms. Buys continued with an explanation of the events to date. She also explained the Xerography that would be taken the next morning. Barbara was to return to Dr. Sand's office in the afternoon, with her husband, to receive the results of the Xerography. Then Barbara was given an opportunity to ask questions, which Ms. Buys answered as completely as possible.

Dr. Sands's office received the following Xerography report on Ms. Livingston the afternoon of May 30:

LT. BREAST: Possible cancerous lesion with attachment lt. outer quadrant; approximate size 1.4 cm.

RT. BREAST: Unremarkable.

Consequently, Dr. Sands added the following to his diagnostic impression:

Stage I $T_1N_0M_0$

With Ms. Buys present, Dr. Sands discussed his impression with Barbara and John Livingston. He mentioned that a number of surgical approaches were available. If, on biopsy, the left breast lesion were found to be cancerous, he would perform a radical mastectomy because he had found that treatment to be the best chance for complete recovery. He concluded by saying that if a mastectomy was necessary, he would discuss reconstructive surgery with them at a later date.

Ms. Buys stayed with the Livingstons after Dr. Sands left the room. She noted that John had drawn his wife closer to him. Both Livingstons looked slightly bewildered. Ms. Buys started by saying, "You have just heard distressing news. I will attempt to answer all of your questions now." The discussion lasted thirty minutes.

Hospitalization for Barbara was scheduled for June 3. Barbara needed a pHisoHex scrub of the surgical area twice a day until surgery, and Ms. Buys explained the procedure to her.

STUDY QUESTIONS

18-1. What are the beliefs of the Quakers (Society of Friends) about the following: family life, children, industrialism, death, health? What are the Ten Talents of Quakerism?

18-2. Describe the normal development of the female breast and its lymphatic drainage.

18-3. Design a teaching plan to instruct a 40–50-year-old woman in self-examination of the breasts.

Goal	Objectives	Content	Method of Evaluating Learning

18-4.   What is the procedure for doing a complete examination of a client's breasts? How are abnormalities described?

18-5.   Compare the differences between the following descriptions of breast lesions: mobile, attached, fixated.

18-6.   What are the "high risk" factors for the development of breast cancer? Which of these factors did Ms. Livingston's assessment reveal?

18-7.   Besides cancerous lesions, what benign lesions can occur in the breast?

18-8.   Describe the following breast cancer detection techniques:

Techniques	Indication for Use	Advantage/Disadvantage
Mammography		
Thermography		
Xerography		
Transillumination		

18-9.   Describe the abridged TNM system of classification of carcinoma of the breast. What does "stage I T_1 No Mo" mean? How does metastasis of breast cancer occur?

18-10. Complete a drug information card on pHisoHex.

18-11. Why is Barbara to do a pHisoHex scrub? What area should she scrub? Why?

18-12. Design a teaching plan for instructing Ms. Livingston to perform a pHisoHex scrub of the surgical site.

Goal	Objective(s)	Content	Method of Evaluating Learning

DISCUSSION QUESTIONS

D-1. How might the nursing management of clients who are Quakers be affected by the clients' religious beliefs?

D-2. Why did Ms. Buys request John's presence at the second examination?

D-3. What other support systems are available to Barbara Livingston? How can these support systems be fostered by Ms. Buys?

D-4. Why would the possibility of reconstructive surgery be mentioned prior to the mastectomy?

D-5. How is reconstructive surgery of the breast done? When is reconstructive surgery of the breast possible?

D-6. What items should have been discussed with Barbara and/or John by Ms. Buys? When should each item be discussed? What would you explain about each?

Item	Ideal Time to Explain	Explanation

PREOPERATIVE PHASE

By June 2, the Livingston family and Bernie Grant were extremely upset over Barbara's condition. They were afraid Barbara would die. They all felt helpless. Joyce, particularly, suffered. As the new professional nurse in the family, Joyce had high expectations of herself. She was learning in a very personal way how difficult it is to act in a professional manner when emotionally involved with a client.

Barbara did not mention the word "cancer." Rather, she kept referring to her appearance. When Barbara was alone with John she said, "You know . . . after next week I may not be your 'pretty little package' anymore." John pulled Barbara closer and rocked her in his arms.

By 11:00 A.M. June 3, Barbara was admitted to the hospital. At Barbara's request, John was the only family member who came with her.

Dr. Sands had left the following orders:

OOB

Regular diet

Amputation skin prep of left breast

Skin prep of left anterior thigh

To OR in A.M.

CBC

Urinalysis

Platelet Count

SMA 12   } today

Serology

EKG

Type and crossmatch 2 units whole blood

Ms. Jane Simone, R.N., met the Livingstons on the surgical floor and introduced herself. Ms. Simone explained that she would be Barbara's primary nurse from 7 A.M. to 3 P.M. each day. She then showed them to Barbara's private room.

After Ms. Simone had completed the admission, Barbara was taken to the radiology department for her chest X-rays. John slumped into a chair in Barbara's room. Ms. Simone stayed in Barbara's room to speak to John in private. She said, "You look like the weight of the world is sitting on your shoulders."

John returned, "Is it that obvious?"

Ms. Simone moved closer and asked, "What has Ms. Livingston been able to share with you?"

John remarked, "That's what I can't understand. I'm scared to death about this cancer thing . . . but Barbara seems to be in another world."

"Please give me an example," Ms. Simone quietly demanded.

John said, "Well... for instance, this morning I was trying to tell Barbara that everything would be all right, that if it were cancer, Dr. Sands would get it all...." With his eyes brimming with tears, John continued, "You know what she said? She asked 'What bathrobe do you like best?' I don't know, I feel like I'm speaking another language."

Ms. Simone explained that it sounded like Barbara was upset about her future body image. John listened carefully. When he finally did speak, he asked Ms. Simone for advice on how to help Barbara. Ms. Simone completed her advice just as Barbara was wheeled back into her room. She helped Barbara into the bed and left to give the Livingstons some privacy. John left for work about thirty minutes later.

Barbara was kept busy the rest of the afternoon with her admission work-up. Ms. Simone was careful to explain the purpose of each test.

At 4:00 P.M. Barbara met Ms. Mary Lewis, R.N., her evening primary nurse. John arrived back at 7:00 P.M. Then Dr. Sands came into Barbara's room. After a complete explanation of his surgical plan, which included a biopsy of her breast lesion, Barbara signed a surgical consent. Barbara understood that if the biopsy were cancerous, Dr. Sands would do a left radical mastectomy at that time.

At Barbara's request, her children did not visit. She phoned home after visiting hours had ended and spoke to the children and her father.

The anesthesiologist visited after reviewing Barbara's work-up results. He left these orders:

NPO afer midnight

Nembutal 0.1 g po at HS, repeat 1 hour before surgery

Demerol 75 mg IM
Atropine sulfate 0.4 mg IM } 30 min before surgery

The OR sheet indicated that Ms. Livingston was scheduled for 11 A.M.

When John had left, Ms. Lewis sat down next to Barbara and answered her questions. Then she informed Barbara about the next day's activities. Lastly she explained to Barbara what to expect after surgery. She put particular emphasis on the self-help activities that would speed Barbara's recovery. The possibility of a HemoVac drain and dressings was also mentioned.

STUDY QUESTIONS

18-13. What are the surgical approaches now in use for breast cancer? What tissue is removed with each and what is the rationale for using each approach?

Surgical Approach	Tissues Removed	Rationale for Approach

18-14. Statistically, does one surgical approach to breast cancer have an advantage over another?

18-15. What is a biopsy? What kind(s) of biopsy procedure(s) exist? Is a lumpectomy the same as a biopsy? Explain.

18-16. What is the purpose of a skin prep of the left anterior thigh?

18-17. What is the procedure for doing an amputation skin prep? A left anterior thigh skin prep?

18-18. What is the purpose of the following with regard to Ms. Livingston: crossmatch of 2 units of whole blood, platelet count, SMA-12, EKG.

18-19. Complete a drug information card on the following medications: Nembutal, Demerol, atropine.

18-20. What precautions should be taken when giving preop medications to Ms. Livingston?

DISCUSSION QUESTIONS

D-7.   What understanding of the female body image should the nurse have when emotionally supporting the mastectomy client?

D-8.   Why do you believe Ms. Simone made time to speak with John Livingston?

D-9.   What advice should be given to John while Barbara is in the radiology department?

D-10. What surgical consent should be obtained from Ms. Livingston? What should she know about the surgical procedure before she signs the consent? Who should witness the consent?

D-11. Design a preoperative teaching plan for Ms. Livingston.

Goal	Objectives	Content	Method of Evaluating Learning

POSTOPERATIVE PHASE

At 4:00 P.M. on June 4, John and Joyce Livingston sat anxiously in the surgical waiting room. They had run out of conversation a long time ago. Now they just looked for Dr. Sands to come out of the surgical suite. Finally Dr. Sands arrived.

Dr. Sands told the Livingstons that Barbara was in recovery. She had come through a left radical mastectomy very well. He further explained that the tumor had been cancerous, but there was no evidence of spread. Then before the Livingstons could react, Dr. Sands left, saying, "She's doing fine... I didn't have to do a skin graft. She'll be back in her room soon."

Dr. Sands wrote the following postoperative orders:

1000 ml 5% D/W IV—D/C after present infusion

Demerol 75 mg IM q 4 h prn for pain

Hgb and Hct ⎱
Electrolytes ⎰ in A.M.

Full liquid diet this P.M. as tolerated

Regular diet in A.M.

Elevate left arm in sling over IV pole

I & O

Empty HemoVac q 8 h and prn

Flexion/extension exercises to left hand/wrist/elbow to start in A.M.

Blow bottles q 2 h when awake

Reinforce pressure dressing prn

Dangle in A.M., then OOB as tolerated

Make referral to Reach for Recovery may visit postop day #5

Ms. Lewis prepared for Barbara's return from the recovery room. After transferring Barbara to her bed, she reviewed Ms. Livingston's status and the postoperative orders with the recovery room nurse.

From Barbara's recovery room sheet Ms. Lewis learned the following information:

GENERAL ANESTHETIC USED: Halothane

LENGTH OF SURGERY: 3.5 hours

STABILIZATION OF VITAL SIGNS: 30 min ago, BP: 130/78

LEVEL OF CONSCIOUSNESS: Oriented before leaving RR

Ms. Lewis checked Barbara's vital signs and found that Barbara's blood pressure had dropped to 118/74. She was not alarmed. However, she did monitor Barbara closely until restabilization of her vital signs had occurred. Barbara dozed on and off.

Meanwhile John and Joyce slipped silently into the room. Ms. Lewis reassured the Livingstons about Barbara's condition. They were also given a clear idea of the kind of emotional and physical support Barbara would need.

When Joyce left, John remained by his wife's bedside. During this period Ms. Lewis was in and out of the room frequently. Among other things, she closely observed the couple's behavior. John talked to Barbara, but Barbara did not say a word. However, she remained quietly cooperative during her short wakeful periods.

After visiting hours had ended, Ms. Lewis sat with Barbara. The nurse stated softly, "You know, some people are so traumatized by the suddenness of unexpected surgery that they have difficulty sorting out their thoughts. How is it going for you?"

Barbara responded slowly. Her face tightened, and tears began to flow. Ms. Lewis let her cry for a good five minutes. Then she said softly, "Can you talk now?"

Barbara searchingly asked, "You said that I would have a drain if the surgery was extensive?"

Ms. Lewis stated, "Yes, I did."

"Then my breast is gone, isn't it?" Barbara asked.

Ms. Lewis nodded, "Yes."

Barbara required medication for pain shortly thereafter. Ms. Lewis saw to it that her request was answered quickly. Soon Barbara fell asleep again. In the morning Barbara rediscovered her surgical loss. Ms. Simone was there to emotionally support her.

By the second postoperative day Barbara started working to gain back her strength. Her physical progress was going well. She was introduced to the life-long precautions that she should take to protect her left arm and hand. When Barbara had not brought up the subject of sex by the third postoperative day, the staff believed that intervention was necessary. Since the evening shift allowed for the most privacy with an awake client, the nursing intervention concerning sexuality was assigned to Ms. Lewis on the 3-to-11 shift.

Ms. Lewis started by saying, "When you have sex with your husband, you may feel some pain in your left shoulder." The conversation that followed lasted a full hour. Near the end of the conversation, Ms. Lewis told Barbara about the upcoming visit from the American Cancer Society's Reach for Recovery volunteer.

By the eve of the fifth day postop, Barbara was involved in a full rehabilitative exercise program. She was looking forward to going home and to slowly resuming her daily activities.

STUDY QUESTIONS

18-21. What is the rationale behind each of the postoperative orders?

18-22. What factors should be assessed before giving Barbara Demerol for pain?

18-23. What type(s) of surgical dressing is(are) used for a radical mastectomy? Who changes the first dressing? When is it usually removed?

18-24. If you noted a drainage spot on Barbara's dressing, how would you go about observing the spot over time? What other observations would you make if your client had a drainage spot on her dressing?

18-25. Barbara had a HemoVac. What is the working principle of a HemoVac? What is the expected color of drainage in a HemoVac after a radical mastectomy: postop day 1, 2, 3? Where would the nurse observe to get an accurate impression of the character of the drainage into a HemoVac? After emptying a HemoVac, how would the nurse put it back in working order? On what day post-radical-mastectomy is the HemoVac usually removed?

18-26. What are the therapeutic effects of the dressing? the drains (HemoVac)? What are the undesirable effects of each? What are the nursing objectives used to enhance the therapeutic effects and to prevent and/or diminish the undesirable effects?

Item	Therapeutic Effects	Undesirable Effects	Nursing Objectives (Action)	Method of Evaluating Effectiveness
Mastectomy Dressing				
Drain (HemoVac)				

18-27. Postsurgically Barbara's left arm was wrapped in an elastic bandage. What was the rationale behind this?

18-28. Why was Barbara's left arm elevated in a sling? How is this technique done?

18-29. What are the purposes of exercising the upper extremities following a mastectomy? Which muscles or joints are affected during the exercises? How would these exercises be incorporated into a client's activities of daily living?

Exercise	How is joint or muscle involved?	Precaution during exercise	Incorporating into activities of daily living	Principles of supervising exercise	Method and frequency of evaluating its effectiveness
Elbow elevations					
Elbow pull-in					
Hand pushing on wall					
Pendulum swing					
Rope sliding					
Rope turning					
Wall climbing					
Others					

18-30. Who is the Reach for Recovery volunteer in your area? What is contained in the kit the volunteer will bring for Barbara? What history does the volunteer have that may be extremely helpful to Barbara?

18-31. When does lymphedema stop being a possible complication after radical mastectomy? What action can be taken to lessen the chances of the development of this complication?

18-32. Why wasn't Ms. Lewis alarmed when Barbara's BP dropped slightly after her transfer from the RR stretcher? What caused the drop in BP?

DISCUSSION QUESTIONS

D-12. Who decides on the kind of breast prosthesis Barbara can wear? Who decides when Barbara can first wear a prosthesis? What should the nurse tell Barbara about prostheses? Can Barbara wear the pseudo-prosthesis the Reach for Recovery volunteer brings without a physician's prescription?

D-13. Why did the nursing staff consider a discussion on sexuality with Barbara necessary? What are some of the fears many women have regarding their sexuality after a mastectomy? How can the nurse assist the client to lessen her anxieties related to sex? What other persons might be helpful?

D-14. Why would Barbara need a second documentation of her surgical loss on the first postop day? Explain.

RECOVERY

By the fifteenth postoperative day, Barbara was able to actively take her left arm through the complete range of motion exercises. Therefore Dr. Sands wrote the following order:

Discharge in A.M.
Pt. to be instructed to call for an appt. 3 weeks from now.

John picked up Barbara on the following morning. She wore an appropriate dress of her own that Joyce had picked out of her closet. Barbara was visibly tired, but she met John with a big smile. On the way home John drove them through the local park. He stopped the car long enough to thank God for the safe return of his wife. Barbara started crying tears of joy. She said, "Every wife should have a husband like mine."

Barbara's children and her Dad were at the front door to greet her. After many gentle hugs and kisses, Barbara was overcome by fatigue. She went to take a long nap.

Five days after Barbara returned home the public health nurse (PHN) visited her to check her dressing and progress. Barbara was having difficulty getting her blouses and dresses over her left arm because the arm was enlarged. The PHN made suggestions about Barbara's clothing and answered the rest of Barbara's questions.

STUDY QUESTIONS

18-33. The nurse reinforced Barbara's knowledge about how to protect her left arm from injury. Why does the left arm need protection? What dos and don'ts of left hand and arm care should be given to Barbara?

Dos	Donts

18-34. Barbara's left arm was weak. Explain why.

18-35. What care of the incision should Barbara continue at home? What information should the nurse have given Barbara about the incision area?

18-36. What clothing is appropriate for Barbara in this early postop period?

DISCUSSION QUESTIONS

D-15. What materials can the nurse suggest (without medical clearance) to the postmastectomy client for use as a temporary breast prosthesis?

D-16. Since there is a nurse in the Livingston's household, do you believe that a PHN referral was indicated? Why?

D-17. If Barbara had had metastasis, Dr. Sands might have prescribed additional cancer treatment. Fill in the following grid on other cancer therapies:

Type	Goal	Side Effects	Nursing Implications
Chemotherapy Alkylating agents corticosteroids antimetabolites			
Hormonal Therapy			
Surgical Therapy Hypophysectomy Oophorectomy Adrenalectomy			
Radiation			

D-18. After the postoperative visit to Dr. Sands, what is the most frequently advised schedule for check-ups for the postmastectomy client? What is the rationale behind the frequency of visits? How long should a client continue to have check-ups?

D-19. How does the client's rehabilitation program differ according to the type of surgical procedure?

Type Surgery	Outline of Rehab Program

D-20. What professionals can make client referrals to Reach for Recovery in your area? How is it done?

SUGGESTED ACTIVITIES

1. Contact a self-help group for postmastectomy patients (The American Cancer Society Reach to Recovery, YWCA's Encore, and the like):
   (a) Investigate the education program given to members to become volunteers.
   (b) Investigate the existence or nonexistence of a screening program for judgment of suitability of active volunteer members.
   (c) Critique the group's literature.
   (d) Critique the group's program for the new postmastectomy patient.
2. Interview a postmastectomy patient:
   (a) Evaluate her adjustment to an altered body image, sexuality, and/or resumption of activities of daily living.
   (b) Critique your impression of the person's primary focus of concern (sexuality/body image or cancer phobia).
3. Investigate breast prosthesis(es):
   (a) Predict the product's appearance while in use, comfort, ease of care and durability.
   (b) Critique the preparation of the fitter.
   (c) Report on the availability of the product.
4. Take care of a client who has just had a mastectomy.

BIBLIOGRAPHY

Berry, Gerald D. *Religions of the World.* New York: Barnes and Noble, 1963, 119–20.

Beland, Irene L., and Passos, Joyce Y. "The Patient with Breast Cancer." In *Clinical Nursing.* 3d ed. New York: MacMillan, 1975, 891–895.

Bergersen, Betty. *Pharmacology in Nursing.* 13th ed. St. Louis: C. V. Mosby Co., 1976.

Brunner, Lillian Sholtis, and Suddarth, Doris Smith. *The Lippincott Manual of Nursing Practice.* 2d ed. Philadelphia: J. B. Lippincott Co., 1978.

_____. "Patients with Problems of the Breast." In *Textbook of Medical-Surgical Nursing.* 3d ed. Philadelphia: J. P. Lippincott Co., 1975.

Christopherson, Victor A.; Coulter, Pearl Darvin; and Wolanin, Mary Opal. *Rehabilitation Nursing: Perspectives and Applications.* New York: McGraw-Hill, 1974.

Garb, Solomon. *Laboratory Tests in Common Use.* 6th ed. New York: Springer Publishing Co., 1976.

Giacquinta, Barbara. "Helping Families Face the Crisis of Cancer." *The American Journal of Nursing* 77 (October 1977): 1585–1588.

Guyton, Arthur C. *Textbook of Medical Psychology.* 5th ed. Philadelphia: W. B. Saunders Co., 1976.

Kennerly, Sadie L. "What I Learned About Mastectomy." *The American Journal of Nursing* 77 (September 1977): 1430–1432.

Levene, Martin B. "A New Role for Radiation Therapy." *The American Journal of Nursing* 77 (September 1977): 1443–1444.

Luckmann, Joan, and Sorensen, Karen Creason. "Disease of the Breast." In *Medical-Surgical Nursing.* Philadelphia: W. B. Saunders Co., 1974, 1293–1303.

Malasanos, Lois, et al. *Health Assessment.* St. Louis: The C. V. Mosby Co., 1978.

Mamaril, Aurora P. "Preventing Complications After Radical Mastectomy." *The American Journal of Nursing* 74 (November 1974): 2000–2003.

Martin, Leonide. "Breast Mass." In *Health Care of Woman.* Philadelphia: J. B. Lippincott Co., 1978. 302–329.

Ochsner, Alton. "Diseases of the Breast." *Nursing Digest* 4 (March/April): 5–7.

Pendagast, Eileen G., and Sherman, Charles O. "A Guide to the Genogram Family Systems Training." *The Family* 5 (1977): 3–14.

Perras, Colette, and Camirand, Andre. "Subcutaneous Mastectomy." *The American Journal of Nursing* 73 (September 1973): 1568–1570.

Pumphrey, John B. "Recognizing Your Patients' Spiritual Needs." *Nursing '77* 70 (December 1977): 64–68.

Puhaty, Henrietta Doltz. "Two Rehabilitative Approaches." *The American Journal of Nursing* 77 (September 1977): 1437.

Robinson, Corinne, and Lawler, Marilyn R. *Normal and Therapeutic Nutrition.* 15th ed. New York: MacMillan, 1977.

Schwartz, Morton K. "Hormone Receptor Assay." *The American Journal of Nursing* 77 (September 1977): 1445–1446.

Smith, Dorothy W.; Germain, Carol P. Hanley; and Gips, Claudia D. *Care of the Adult Patient.* Philadelphia: J. B. Lippincott Co., 1971, 929–944.

Strax, Philip. "Cancer Detection Tools." *The American Journal of Nursing* 73 (September 1973): 1570.

Stroot, Violet R.; Lee, Carla A.; and Schaper, C. Ann. *Fluid and Electrolytes: A Practical Approach.* 2d ed. Philadelphia: F. A. Davis Co., 1977.

Thomas, Sally Galbraith, and Yates, Marilyn Mann. "Breast Reconstruction after Mastectomy." *American Journal of Nursing* 77 (September 1977): 1438–1442.

Winkler, W. Ann. "Choosing the Prosthesis and Clothing." *American Journal of Nursing* 77 (September 1977): 1433–1436.

Woods, Nancy Fugate, and Woods, James S. "Concept of Body Image," and "Mastectomy." In *Human Sexuality in Health and Illness.* St. Louis: C. V. Mosby Co., 1975, pp. 141–142 and 148–151.

CHAPTER NINETEEN

Type A Behavior: Myocardial Infarction

SANDRA WARDELL

OVERVIEW

The Shors are a striving upper-class family who encounter numerous stress situations. The family moves from Pennsylvania to Texas when William Shor, who demonstrates Type A behavior, is promoted to the position of acting vice-president of his company. Shortly after the move, William's ailing mother moves in with them. The family's past history reveals dysfunctional coping behaviors when dealing with stress. William suffers an acute myocardial infarction while at work and is taken to the nearby hospital's coronary care unit. He requires intensive nursing management.

CONTENT EMPHASIS

- Situational stress—Type A behavior
- Dysfunctional coping behaviors
- Etiology and management of a client with an acute myocardial infarction

SETTINGS

- Industrial health service
- Coronary care unit (CCU)
- Medical unit

284

OBJECTIVES

Upon completion of this chapter the student will be able to:

1. Analyze the effects of situational stress on a family's health status.
2. Describe the etiological factors that contribute to the development of coronary artery disease.
3. Develop a plan of intervention for a client who experiences an acute myocardial infarction.
4. Design a health teaching plan that will assist a client and his or her family to apply the principles of cardiac rehabilitation.
5. Analyze a client/family's response to situational stress.

DEFINITION OF TERMS

The following terms are used in this case study and should be defined before proceeding:

Anxiety	Premature ventricular contraction
Coping mechanisms	(PVC)
Coronary artery disease	unifocal
Coronary care unit (CCU)	multifocal
Crisis	Pulsus alternans
Myocardial infarction	Pulse pressure
Point of maximum impulse (PMI)	Situational stress
Predisposing factors	Type A behavior
	Type B behavior

FAMILY ASSESSMENT

William Shor is the oldest of five children born to Edith and Chester Shor. The Shors owned a 120-acre grape farm 20 miles outside of Pittsburgh, Pennsylvania. When William was a boy, Edith could frequently be heard remarking to her husband, "that prankish boy of *yours* tears everything apart: he took the kitchen clock apart today just to see how it works." William enjoyed tinkering with mechanical things, but it was not until he was a teenager that he was able to transform the objects back to their original or an improved condition. Chester would often call upon William to repair broken farm equipment. In fact, Chester secretly considered William to be the smartest of his children and he would fondly call him "Tinker."

The Shors had little surplus money after paying the bills each year. But when William expressed a keen desire to enter Drexel Institute's five year work-study program to become a mechanical engineer, Chester consented to pay the tuition of $500 a year. Edith was displeased with her son's desire to become a mechanical engineer, because she expected her eldest son to remain and operate the farm. However, Chester was the head of the house, so William entered college.

William found the competition much stiffer in college than it was in high school, but he just worked that much harder in order to be in the top 10 percent of his class.

On the few occasions that William was able to go home, his mother would always ask him to do certain chores around the farm, particularly when he was just settling down to do some schoolwork. She seldom asked him how college was going because she resented William's refusal of his birth-right, the farm. Chester would sometimes take William into the basement for a drink of "homemade wine," since Edith did not believe in drinking and would not permit it in the house. Chester and William would chat for hours about college and William's dreams of becoming a top executive.

As his parents wished, William regularly attended the Lutheran church located near the college campus. He joined the young people's group, where he met Sarah Logan, a dentist's daughter. Because Sarah was four years younger than William and her family lived in a nearby upper-class neighborhood, William was content to see her at the church. In his senior year, William finally invited her to a college dance. They dated occasionally, but primarily they relied on the church activities to see each other.

Sarah's parents, James and Anna Logan, were not completely satisfied with their second oldest child's relationship with William Shor, but they kept their concerns to themselves. They expected their children to marry individuals from their own social level, not a struggling, bow-tie-wearing country boy. When Sarah expressed her desire to become a grammar-school teacher and attend the University of Pennsylvania, they agreed to support her, assuming that she would meet the "right young man" there and would soon forget her infatuation for the farm boy William. What they did not know was that Sarah and William had discussed the matter at length, and Sarah's intention was made known only after William had accepted a job as a junior mechanical engineer at a large industrial firm just outside of Philadelphia. William intended to marry Sarah, but only after he was earning a salary with which he could support Sarah in the "style to which she was accustomed."

For the next four years, William worked very hard at his job and tried to do even more than was required of him. He even had two processing patents to his credit. William had been promoted to the design division with a sizable increase in salary by the time Sarah graduated from college. He was now making a good salary, but it was not enough to support "a Logan." So the couple decided that Sarah would work for two years and that they would

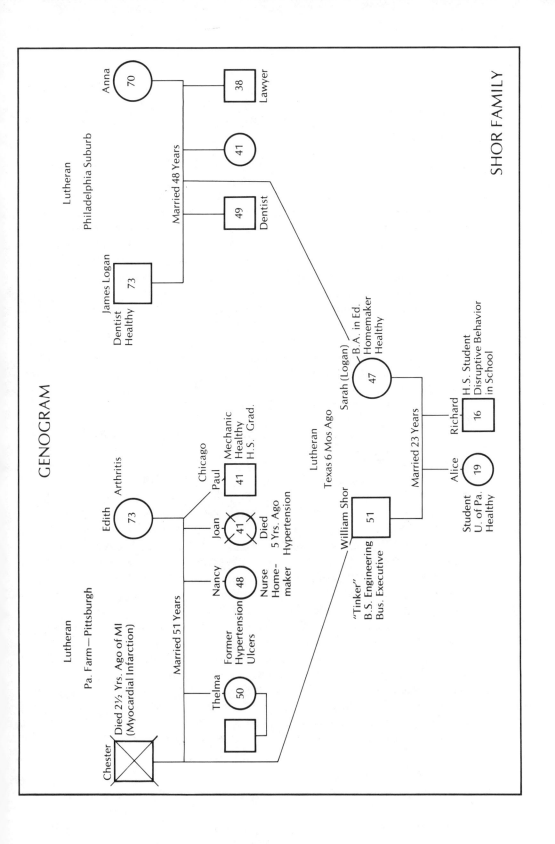

GENOGRAM

SHOR FAMILY

jointly save enough money for a 25 percent down payment on a small, middle-class house. The Logan's were still discontent with their daughter's choice of a mate, but after eight years they had resigned themselves to the intended marriage.

After their marriage, Sarah and William bought a three-bedroom house with a garage near William's company. In order to prove to his in-laws that he could support a wife properly, William insisted that Sarah quit her job and become a housewife. The next few years were a struggle financially, but William continued to receive promotions and corresponding raises in salary. The Shors had two children; Alice was born after two years of marriage and Richard was born three years later. The Shors continued to attend the nearby Lutheran church regularly and William even became a member of the church council. Sarah was an active member of the Ladies' Aid Society and began teaching Sunday school when her children began attending.

The Shors visited the farm at least twice a year, at Thanksgiving and during their summer vacation. William enjoyed the farm visits. However, he always felt uncomfortable when visiting the Logans. William felt that he could never do enough to be successful in James Logan's eyes.

While on their vacation to Myrtle Beach, South Carolina, one summer, the Shors stopped at the farm for the weekend. Chester was as strong as an ox, but Edith was complaining of arthritic pains. Things had changed some on the homestead. Chester was still running the farm. His oldest daughter, Thelma Fields, lived on the farm in an old converted barn with her family. Thelma was gradually taking over the produce-selling at the farmer's market. The Shors had a pleasant weekend and then they proceeded on their vacation.

Tuesday morning of their second vacation week, William was notified of the death of his father. Chester had been found dead in his car in a field. He had died of a heart attack. He apparently died instantly since he had been at a neighbor's house five minutes earlier delivering grapes. William did not cry, he simply told his family to pack immediately. They were leaving. The puzzled family obeyed. Finally Sarah asked William what had happened. William abruptly replied, "Chester is being buried tomorrow. Get packed." The stunned family cried to themselves as they finished packing. Sarah tried to comfort William, but he brushed her aside and continued to pack the car. The family drove all day without stopping. No one said anything. They reached Washington, D.C., and had a flat tire. It was midnight. While the tire was being repaired, Sarah took the children to dinner across the street. She knew that William was determined to make the funeral at 1:00 P.M. that afternoon. Sarah offered to drive, but William simply said "No." He denied being tired. The weary family pulled into the farm at noon. Most of the relatives were already at the funeral home in town. William left without shaving or changing his clothes. His family was to come later with relatives who were still at the house.

Chester had left everything to his wife. Since Thelma expected to inherit the farm, she agreed to take over its operation. Edith refused to leave the farm, so Thelma finally agreed to take care of Edith as well.

STUDY QUESTIONS

19-1. What is meant by "a family in crisis?"

19-2. List and explain at least three types of responses to a crisis situation.

19-3. List and describe the psychological phases of crisis as illustrated by Hymovick and Barnard in *Family Health Care* (see the Bibliography).

19-4. What are the four generalizations about crisis according to Hymovich and Barnard?

19-5. What are the four basic levels of anxiety and how can a nurse assess each level? What can a nurse do to help relieve a client's anxiety?

ANXIETY

Level	Assessment	Client Management
0		
1+		
2+		
3+		
4+		

19-6. List and describe at least five of the primary coping mechanisms used by people who are in a crisis situation.

DISCUSSION QUESTIONS

D-1. How did the William Shor family deal with the crisis of Chester Shor's death? What coping mechanisms were displayed by the family members?

D-2. In the event of a health crisis to William Shor, predict William's behavior. Predict Sarah's behavior.

D-3. What support systems are available to William Shor's family in the event of a future crisis?

PENDING CRISIS

William's income grew steadily over the next two years. The family added a recreation room to their house and they now had the equivalent of one year's salary in savings and investments. William had now become the director of the design department at the Philadelphia branch of his company. Their daughter graduated from high school and was a freshman at the University of Pennsylvania. Their son Richard was now in high school.

William knew that the vice-president of design at the main office in Dallas, Texas, was retiring. He made it known at the office and at the executive parties that he wanted to be considered for the position. He even submitted an outline of changes he would institute, at the request of the present vice-president of design. After six months of vying for the job, he finally received word that he would be given the position on an "acting" basis and that he would be given the permanent position if he could successfully cut the company's expenditures for design by 20 percent within the first year. He accepted the challenge and moved into a hotel near the main headquarters in Dallas. He began reviewing the company's books diligently and in his spare moments he began house hunting.

Meanwhile, back in Philadelphia, Sarah made arrangements to sell their home. Richard would be moving to Texas to finish high school, but it was decided that Alice would become a resident student at the University.

The Shor's purchased a five-bedroom, three-bathroom home on three acres with a swimming pool and tennis court in an upper-class neighborhood of Dallas. Despite the large down payment, the mortgage would initially cost about 40 percent of William's income. The cost for Alice to be a resident student would be an additional 10 percent of his income. However, since William would be expected to entertain and since he had the promise of a sizable salary increase when the vice-president appointment became permanent, the family felt that they should and could manage the considerable change in their budget.

After the move, the family began to settle into their new home. They joined the Lutheran church and attempted to make friends in the neighborhood, but somehow the people back home seemed more sincere. Sarah could not help comparing the two locations. She missed her family and friends in Philadelphia and she frequently made long-distance calls to the old neighborhood. William was seldom home now and he often worked in the den on Saturdays as well. Richard also missed his friends and found it difficult to adjust to the new school. Everyone made fun of his Pennsylvania accent. He didn't even have his father's companionship on outings, as he had had when they lived in Pennsylvania. After two months, Richard began getting into fights at school.

Meanwhile, Edith Shor was doing poorly. Her arthritis was getting worse in the hips and she could not negotiate the stairs at the farm. Thelma was too busy running the farm to help Edith, so Edith's children decided that the best place for her was in the warm climate of Texas. William rushed up and drove Edith to Texas. She was unhappy in these strange surroundings and began to argue with Sarah about the food and the way Sarah kept cleaning up after her. Both women would confide in William, but William did not side with either Sarah or Edith.

The usual diet for William Shor consisted of the following:

7 A.M. Breakfast:	2 eggs or scrapple or pancakes
	bacon
	2 slices of toast with butter and jelly
	coffee
1 P.M. Lunch:	meat sandwhich (usually roast beef or pastrami), with lettuce and mayonnaise
	creamed soup
	potato or macaroni salad
	fruit pie or ice cream
	coffee
7 P.M. Dinner:	meat (usually beef)
	potato, often fried in butter
	vegetable: beans, peas, or beets
	lettuce salad with Russian or blue cheese dressing
	fruit pie or cheesecake
	coffee
10 P.M. Snack:	Cheese and crackers
	2 glasses of wine

STUDY QUESTIONS

19-7. What are the typical characteristics of a client with Type A behavior?

19-8. Does William Shor have Type A or Type B behavior? How do you know?

19-9. Analyze Mr. Shor's diet for the basic nutrients. What does he eat in excess? What is he lacking? What are the potential effects of the inadequacies in his diet?

DIET ANALYSIS

Nutrient	Adequate Diet for Healthy 53-Year-Old Male (Height: 180 cm medium build)	William Shor's Diet Height: 178 cm Weight: 100 kg	Lacks and Excesses in Diet	Potential Effect of Inadequacy
Proteins				
Carbohydrates				
Fats (cholesterol triglycerides)				
Vitamins (A, D, E, K, and B complex)				
Minerals (Na, K, and Ca)				

19-10. What is the effect of coffee (caffeine) on the cardiovascular system?

DISCUSSION QUESTIONS

D-4. What are the stress factors in the Shor family's current situation?

D-5. What coping mechanisms are demonstrated by the Shor family? The paternal extended family?

D-6. Was the use of these coping mechanisms predictable?

D-7. How could a professional nurse assist the family in dealing with stress? What assessments can be made to differentiate between a person with the characteristics of Type A behavior and a client with Type B behavior?

D-8. If requested, how can a professional nurse assist clients with Type A behavior to alter their life-styles?

CLIENT ASSESSMENT

William had had some chest pains in the past, but he always thought it was due to indigestion and ignored the pain. Then, on Thursday morning, while working at his desk, he felt a sharp, sudden chest pain that almost took his breath away. He had some papers that had to be out that afternoon, so he just took a sip of water and relaxed a moment before returning to his work. The pain did not disappear but he kept ignoring it. After 30 minutes his secretary came in and noticed that he was pale and sweating. Upon inquiring whether he was alright, William said abruptly, "yes." Then he added, "Please bring me the Royal papers." After ten minutes, she returned with the papers. By now William was leaning back in his chair grasping his chest. Two of his colleagues came in just then and realized something was wrong. When they started to call the industrial nurse, William said "no," and began to walk toward the door. He said that he would walk over to the health service and get something for his "indigestion." The two men walked with him.

A shortened examination on the 52-year-old Mr. Shor was made by the industrial nurse, Peggy Gray, and it revealed the following findings:

CHIEF COMPLAINT: severe crushing chest pain, sudden onset; no radiation to the left shoulder, arm, or the left side of the neck
BP: 116/62
P: 96 and irregular—5 pauses/min. varying pulse pressures
R: 32 and shallow
T: 37.2°C
HEART: apical impulse (PMI) palpated in the 5th interspace, 8.5 cm from the midsternal line
distant S_1 and S_2 sounds—no murmurs or gallops noted
LUNGS: clear—no rales or ronchi noted
no cough
GI: C/O nausea
last meal was breakfast—3 hours ago

Peggy noted the following items on Mr. Shor's company chart:

Last mandatory company physical—3 mos. ago.
ALLERGIES: Penicillin
HABITS: Smokes 1½ to 2 packs/day
Social drinker
CURRENT MEDICATIONS: none
HEIGHT: 178 cm
WEIGHT: 100 kg

BP: 142/88
P: 78 and regular
R: 18
CHEST X-RAY: negative
EKG: normal sinus rhythm

While Peggy called George Clark, the company physician, Larry Gleason, R.N., instituted the following measures:

Loosened all clothing, semi-Fowlers position

Nasal O_2 at 6 l/min

Vital Signs: q 15 min

Morphine sulfate 15 mg (H)—as per order of George Clark, M.D.

In the 15 minutes it took for the ambulance to arrive, William remained essentially the same. He was transferred to Watson General Hospital. Peggy accompanied him with a copy of the company's health file on William (as per company policy). Dr. Clark was to meet them at the hospital's coronary care unit. A tentative diagnosis of myocardial infarction (MI) was called into the coronary care unit by Dr. Clark.

STUDY QUESTIONS

19-11. What are the most common risk factors associated with a myocardial infarction? Which of these risk factors is demonstrated by William?

19-12. What are the typical signs and symptoms of a myocardial infarction? What is the physiological cause of each?

Sign and Symptom	Physiologic Cause
1.	
2.	
3.	
4.	
5.	
6.	
7.	

19-13. Which of the above signs and symptoms are exhibited by Mr. Shor?

19-14. What are the apparent effects of smoking on the coronary arteries? the lungs?

DISCUSSION QUESTIONS

D-9.   On what findings is the diagnosis of myocardial infarction based?

D-10. What factors in William's diet would predispose him to a myocardial infarction?

D-11. What other factors in William's life style would predispose him to a myocardial infarction?

D-12. What is the reason for each of the actions by the industrial nurses?

Action	Rationale
1. Loosen clothing 2. Semi-Fowlers position 3. Nasal O_2 4. V.S. q 15 m 5. Obtaining a morphine sulfate order from physician 6. Copy of file to hospital	

D-13. Can industrial nurses give IV medications in your area? Explain.

D-14. What is the relationship between IM and/or H injections on a client's blood enzyme levels?

D-15. How can the nurse decrease William's anxiety?

CORONARY CARE UNIT

Peggy Gray gave a report of her findings and the initial treatment to the head nurse of the CCU, while two of the staff nurses transferred William to the bed and began to institute the CCU's standing orders for patients who are admitted with a diagnosis of acute myocardial infarction. The standing orders are as follows:

- Continuous cardiac monitoring—record and mount a tracing q 2 h and prn
- Blood pressure, pulse (apical and radial), and respirations q 30 min × 4, if vital signs are stable, q 4 h. Oral temperature qid
- Bedrest. If there are no complications—may use commode for BM
- Intake and output
- Oxygen at 4–6 liters/min; administer at 2 liters/min if there is a history of chronic obstructive pulmonary disease (COPD).
- Diet: clear liquids on first day, full liquids on second day, no ice or carbonated beverages
- Tranquillizer: Diazepam or Librium
- Hypnotic: Dalmane 15–30 mg po HS
- Stool softner: Colace 100 mg po bid

- EKG now and in A.M. × 3 days
- Portable chest X-ray now
- LDH, CPK, SGOT now and in A.M. × 3 days
- Blood Work now: CBC, electrolytes (Na, K, Cl, CO_2), and BUN. If a diabetic, FBS
- Blood chemistry, erythrocyte sedimentation rate (ESR) and urinalysis in A.M.
- Treatment of premature ventricular contractions (PVCs) if more than 6/min, multifocal or bigeminy: lidocaine of 100 mg IV push; then Lidocaine IV drip at 2–4 mg/min
- Treatment of ventricular fibrillation: Defibrillate at 400 watt sec, Cardiopulmonary resuscitation, sodium bicarbonate 50 cc IV push q 5–10 min, adrenalin IV if indicated

Dr. Clark arrived. Peggy gave the copy of Mr. Shor's chart to him and emphasized that the morphine sulfate had already been given. After examining William, Dr. Clark left the following additions to the standing orders:

NPO until nausea subsides, then clear liquid diet

Morphine sulfate 5 mg IV q 4 h prn for pain

Diazepam 2 mg po qid

1000 ml 5% D/W with minidrip to keep the vein open (KVO)

Dopamine 2 ampules in 500 ml of 5% D/W prn to maintain BP above 100 systolic

Dalmane 15 mg po at HS

William was still having chest pain. He lay quietly and didn't speak unless someone spoke to him. He was very frightened by all the activity and could not understand what was happening. All he knew was that the pain was beginning to subside, so he assumed that whatever was being done was helping. He felt tired and wanted to sleep, but he kept fighting it because he had an awful feeling of impending death.

The nursing staff quietly explained the reason for the wires, tubes, and other medical orders as the treatments were being instituted. He was informed that his family had been notified and would be able to visit shortly. William began to relax, but he still required continued reassurance.

Mr. Shor's initial test reports and laboratory results were as follows:

EKG:
  rate: 88
  occasional unifocal PVC

elevated S-T segment
Impression: Myocardial ischemia, possible acute myocardial infarction
Chest X-ray: negative
Lab results:
  Na: 136 mEq/L
  K: 4.2 mEq/L
  Cl: 100 mEq/L
  CO_2: 25 mM/L
  LDH: 110 U (Wacker)
  CPK: 190 U/L
  SGOT: 35 U (Karmen)
  BUN: 10 mg
  CBC: Hgb: 14.8 g
    Hct: 48%
    RBC: 5.2×10^6
    WBC: 10,500

William wanted to see his family. At 3:30 P.M. Laurie Cohen, R.N., informed William of their arrival and indicated that she would bring his family in for a few moments. Pastor Grey, the Shor's minister, had driven the family to the hospital and was sitting with Sarah and Richard Shor when Ms. Cohen described William's appearance and explained the purpose of the various tubes and wires. Then the family visited William for 15 minutes.

Later that afternoon William's pain had subsided enough for him to fall asleep. His blood pressure ranged between 100 and 110 systolic with the dopamine running. But then at 10:00 P.M. his blood pressure began to show signs of pulsus alternans. He had also developed fine rales in the lower lung base. Dr. Clark was notified and the following orders were obtained:

Lanoxin 0.25 mg IV stat then 0.25 mg IV in A.M.

Lasix 20 mg IV stat

By morning William still had some fine rales. However, his pain was completely gone. His blood pressure was stabilized at 110/70 with the dopamine running at 5 microgtts/min. His pulse was still in the 90s. He had only a few PVCs during the night. His urinary output was 400 cc during the night shift.

STUDY QUESTIONS

19-16. Why is Mr. Shor NPO? Can he receive oral medications? Explain.

19-17. Complete a drug information card on the following medications: diazepam, Librium, Dalmane, Lanoxin, lidocaine, Colace, sodium bicarbonate, Adrenalin, dopamine, regitine, Lasix.

19-18. How is infused Dopamine titrated (regulated) to maintain William's BP? What are the nurse's responsibilities?

19-19. How is infused lidocaine titrated (regulated) to control PVCs? What are the nurse's responsibilities?

19-20. Complete the following laboratory grid:

Test	Normal Male Range	William's Values	Amount of Deviation	Possible Cause of Alteration

19-21. Explain the purpose of each of the following, how they operate, and how they are tested before using them on a client:

Equipment	Purpose	Technique of operation	Testing technique
nasal O_2 (2 prong)			
Cardiac monitor			

19-22. How is a pulsus alternans detected? What is its significance?

19-23. What items should be discussed with the Shor family before they see William? Outline the items in the order in which they should be presented. What would you explain about each?

Item	Explanation

DISCUSSION QUESTIONS

D-16. List each of William's signs and symptoms. What is the nursing management of each?

Sign and Symptom	Basis for Sign and Symptom	Nursing Management

D-17. Determine the nursing care priorities for William. What is the rationale for each?

Nursing Care Priorities	Rationale
1.	
2.	
3.	
4.	
5.	

D-18. Should Pastor Grey have been allowed to visit William? Why?

STABILIZATION

During the second day, William's lungs still had rales in the bases. He had no pain and his BP remained stable at 116/70 with the Dopamine running at only 5 microdrops per minute. He had not had any PVC on the monitor since 9 A.M.

Mr. Shor's A.M. laboratory results and EKG report were as follows:

EKG rate: 88
  elevated S-T segment
  abnormal Q waves in V2-V4
  Impression: acute anterior myocardial infarction
Lab results:
  LDH: 125 U (Wacker)
  SGOT: 98 U (Karmen)
  CPK: 380 U/L
  WBC: 17,000/cm^2
  ESR: 24mm/hr
  Na: 135 mEq/L
  K: 4.0 mEq/L

Cl: 100 mEq/L
CO$_2$: 26 mM/L
BUN: 10 mg
Calcium: 5.0 mEq/L
Creatinine: .8 mg
FBS: 96 mg
Alk. Phos.: 25 U/ml
Cholesterol: 250 mg/dl
Total Protein: 6.4 g/dl
Albumin: 3.1 g/dl
Urinalysis:
Sp. Gr.: 1.012
Sugar: neg.
Acetone: neg.
Protein: neg.
RBC: 0
WBC: 0

Although William's temperature was normal before, at 8 A.M. it was 37.8°C and by 4 P.M. it was 38.5°C. William's intake and output record was as follows:

Day	Time	Intake			Output	
		Oral	IV	Other	Urine	Other
1	12 noon–3 P.M.	30 ml	240 ml	—	200 ml	—
	3 A.M.–11 P.M.	30 ml	850 ml	—	350 ml	—
	11 P.M.–7 A.M.	—	750 ml	—	400 ml	—
2	7 A.M.–3 P.M.	520 ml	210 ml	—	650 ml	—

When George Clark, M.D., visited that afternoon, he left the following orders:

Lanoxin 0.25 mg po OD

Lasix 20 mg IM stat

Dicumarol 250 mg po today

Kaon 5 cc po bid

Full liquid diet

D/C dopamine but KVO c̄ 5% D/W

Prothrombin time (PT) OD

Then Dr. Clark stopped by the waiting room and reported William's progress to the Shor family. Laurie Cohen made a point of reemphasizing the physician's comments.

On the third day William Shor was beginning to wonder whether anything was permanently wrong with him. He felt great. He wanted to get out of bed and indicated that he would like his work brought in to him. His CPK level had dropped to 220 U/L and his BP was stabilized between 120–130 mm Hg systolic. His temperature was ranging between 37.7°C and 38.3°C. His urinary output had increased to 800 ml over the last 8 hours, while his intake was 650 ml during the same time period.

STUDY QUESTIONS

19-24. Complete a drug information card on the following medications: Coumadin, heparin, dicumarol, Kaon.

19-25. What is the difference between an initial dose and a maintenance dose? (i.e., digitalis, dicumarol)

19-26. Why is a PT done daily? What is the desired level at which William should be maintained?

19-27. How does Mr. Shor's output compare to his intake? Explain.

19-28. The nurses should be observant for potential complications of MI. Fill in the following graft:

Complication	Primary Clinical Manifestations	Usual Treatment	Nursing Management

DISCUSSION QUESTIONS

D-19. Compare Mr. Shor's initial laboratory results, EKG reports, and temperature with the present results.

D-20. What is the significance of each of the following and how do the results of each affect the nursing management of Mr. Shor:

	Significance	Nursing Management
Temperature		
Enzymes 　LDH 　CPK 　SGOT		
WBC		
EKG		

D-26. How do the drugs Mr. Shor is taking affect his nursing care?

D-22. Discuss the uses of heparin, Coumadin, and dicumarol for clients with a myocardial infarction. What are the nursing responsibilities when each is administered?

D-23. What should be explained to the Shor family about William's progress?

RECOVERY

After a relatively stable two more days in the CCU, William was transferred to a medical unit. He was now on a 1000 mg sodium diet. He was happy to have bathroom privileges (BRP). (He had been insisting on BRP since the third day because he was unable to have a BM when using the commode.) This was the first BM he had had since before admission.

After an uneventful two more weeks on the medical unit, Mr. Shor was discharged on the following medications:

Dicumarol 25 mg po OD

Lanoxin 0.25 mg po OD

Kaon 5 cc po BID

The rehabilitation program that had been started in the CCU was continued by the staff on the medical unit and other health care workers. The dietition visited him before discharge and explained the 1000 mg low sodium diet that he was to continue on at home. This diet was also explained to Sarah Shor by the nursing staff. Mr. Shor was to rest at home for another month. He was told to visit the industrial health service at work every Thursday to have a blood specimen drawn for a PT and that he was to make an appointment to see Dr. Clark in 4 weeks.

STUDY QUESTIONS

19-29. What are the differences between a 500 mg, 1000 mg, and 2000 mg sodium diet? What is the purpose of each?

19-30. What major foods should be avoided on a 1000 mg sodium diet? What types of food preparation should be avoided?

19-31. Why are Kaon and Lanoxin being administered together?

DISCUSSION QUESTIONS

D-24. What is the probable cause of William's attitude about the commode? What, if anything, should be done about it?

D-25. What are the steps in the cardiac rehabilitation program outlined by the American Heart Association?

D-26. Design a rehabilitation teaching plan for the Shor family. What parts of the plan should be taught before discharge?

Goal	Objective	Content	Method of Teaching	Evaluation of Learning
His condition				
Diet				
Drugs				
PT				
Occupation				
Activities				
Sexual activity				
Life style				

CHAPTER DISCUSSION QUESTIONS

1. Outline the potential roles of the nursing staff at an industrial health service for the following: prevention of coronary artery disease, cardiac rehabilitation.

2. What is the minimal cost of one day's care in a CCU in your area?

3. What insurance plans cover the CCU costs in your area?
4. William Shor had a high risk of having coronary artery disease. Identify these high-risk factors. What could have been done to prevent his MI?

High-Risk Factors	Prevention

5. What are the coronary artery disease screening facilities in your area? Who pays for the screening?

SUGGESTED ACTIVITIES

1. Visit a CCU and observe the nurses' roles. Review the unit's criteria for admitting clients to CCU.
2. Manipulate a cardiac monitor. Attach a fellow student to a monitor and take a tracing.
3. Role play the interaction between the Shor family and the nursing staff before the family's first visit with William on CCU.
4. Visit a health screening facility.
   a. Who does the screening?
   b. What happens to the screening results?
   c. Who attends the facility?
5. Visit an industrial health service.
   a. Who staffs the facility?
   b. What kind of records do they keep?
   c. What "standing orders" do they have in the event an employee has an MI at work? What procedures do they follow?

BIBLIOGRAPHY

Arbeit, Sidney; Fiedler, June; Landau, Thomas; and Rubin, Ira. "Recognizing Digitalis Toxicity." *American Journal of Nursing* 77 12 (December 1977): 1935–1947.

Barnard, Martha Underwood; Clancy, Barbara J.; and Krantz, Kermit E. "Sex for the Cardiac Patient." In *Human Sexuality for Health Professionals.* Philadelphia: W. B. Saunders Co., 1978, 249–257.

Bergersen, Betty. *Pharmacology in Nursing.* 13th ed. St. Louis: C. V. Mosby Co., 1976.

Breu, Christine, and Dracup, Kathleen. "Helping the Spouses of Critically Ill Patients." *American Journal of Nursing* 78 (January 1978): 50–53.

Christopherson, Victor A.; Coulter, Pearl Darvin; and Wolanin, Mary Opal. *Rehabilitation Nursing.* New York: McGraw-Hill, 1974, pp. 363–384.

Friedman, Meyer and Rosenman, Ray H. *Type A Behavior and Your Heart.* New York: Alfred A. Knopf, 1974.

Garb, Solomon. *Laboratory Tests in Common Use.* 6th ed. New York: Springer Publishing Co., 1976.

Gronim, Sara Stidstone. "Helping the Client with Unstable Angina." *American Journal of Nursing* 78 (October 1978): 1677–1680.

Guyton, Arthur C. *Textbook at Medical Physiology.* 5th ed. Philadelphia: W. B. Saunders Co., 1976.

Hymovich, Debra P., and Barnard, Martha Underwood. "Theories of Family Crisis," and "Family Rehabilitation: An Adult with a Myocardial Infarction." In *Family Health Care.* New York: McGraw-Hill, 1973, pp. 271–283 and 390–404.

Little, Dolores E., and Carnevali, Doris L. *Nursing Care Planning.* 2d ed. Philadelphia: J. B. Lippincott, 1976.

Luckmann, Joan, and Sorensen, Karen Creason. "Acute Myocardiac Infarction." In *Medical-Surgical Nursing.* Philadelphia: W. B. Saunders Co., 1974, pp. 669–776.

Malasanos, Lois et al. *Health Assessment.* St. Louis: C. V. Mosby Co., 1978.

Mayer, Gloria Gilbert, and Peterson, Carol Willts. "Theoretical Framework for Coronary Care Nursing Education." *American Journal of Nursing* 78 (July 1978): 1208–1211.

Miller, Margaret Kelly, and Lazure, Linda Armstrong. "Four Steps for Better Cardiac Care in the E.R." *Nursing '78* 8 (August 1978): 40–43.

Mitchell, Pamela Holsclaw. "Responses to Stress." In *Concepts Basic to Nursing.* 2d ed. New York: McGraw-Hill, 1977, 216–233.

Passman, Jerome, and Drummond, Constance D. *The EKG Basic Techniques for Interpretation.* New York: McGraw-Hill, 1976.

Pendagast, Eileen G., and Sherman, Charles O. "A Guide to the Genogram Family Systems Training." *The Family* 5 (1977): 3–14.

Phillips, Raymond E., and Feeney, Mary K. *The Cardiac Rhythms.* Philadelphia: W. B. Saunders Co., 1973.

Proctor, Diane; Fletcher, Ross D.; and Del negro, Albert A. "Temporary Cardiac Pacing." *The Nursing Clinics of North America* 13 (September 1978). Philadelphia: W. B. Saunders Co., 409–422.

Robinson, Corinne, and Lawler, Marilyn R. *Normal and Therapeutic Nutrition.* 15th ed. New York: Macmillan, 1977.

Ross, John, and O'Rourke, Robert. *Understanding the Heart and Its Diseases.* New York: McGraw-Hill, 1976.

Stroot, Violet R.; Lee, Carla A.; and Schaper, C. Ann. *Fluid and Electrolytes: A Practical Approach.* 2d ed. Philadelphia: F. A. Davis Co., 1977.

Widmann, Frances K. *Godale's Clinical Interpretation of Laboratory Tests.* 7th ed. Philadelphia: F. A. Davis Co., 1973.

CHAPTER TWENTY

Urinary Retention: Prostatectomy

FANG-LAN WANG KUO

OVERVIEW

George Martinis is a fifty-six-year-old man of Greek descent who is a member of the Greek Orthodox church. He experiences urinary retention and is taken to the local hospital's emergency room. After admission to the urology unit, several diagnostic tests are performed. When benign prostatic hypertropy is diagnosed, a transurethral resection is performed. Postoperatively, George develops urinary dribbling.

CONTENT EMPHASIS

- Urinary retention—assessment and treatment
- Urologic diagnostic tests—cystoscopy, IVP
- Surgical procedures postoperative management
- Postoperative complication—urinary dribbling
- Sexuality after a prostatectomy

SETTINGS

- Emergency room
- Urology unit
- Operating room

OBJECTIVES

Upon completing this chapter the student will be able to:

1. Analyze the supportive measures for the assessment and testing of a client with acute urinary retention.
2. Compose expected health outcomes for a client with urinary retention who has a prostatectomy.
3. Designate the specific intervention modalities that support the expected health outcomes.
4. Analyze the effect of a prostatectomy on the sexuality of a client and his family.
5. Evaluate the ongoing and rehabilitation health care plan designed for a client who has a prostatectomy and his family.

DEFINITION OF TERMS

The following terms are used in this case study and should be defined before proceeding:

Bladder decompression   Penoscrotal angle
Caliber   Primary nurse
Dysuria   Sedatives
Foley catheter, #16 French   Suppression
Hypnotics   Triage nurse
Nocturia   Urinary retention
Orthostatic hypotension   Urinary urgency

FAMILY ASSESSMENT

Fifty years ago, Lydia and Dimitrios Martinis migrated to the United States from Greece with their six-year-old son George. The Martinis made their residence in Seattle, Washington, in a neighborhood where there were many Greek families, including a few of their relatives. George attended school while his parents worked in a factory.

Other than attending the Greek Orthodox church every Sunday, the Martinis did not attend many other events nor engage in much traveling. They tried to save their money in order to buy a small business. After six years they became naturalized citizens. The following year, Lydia and Dimitrios actualized their dream by buying a small fish market in downtown Seattle.

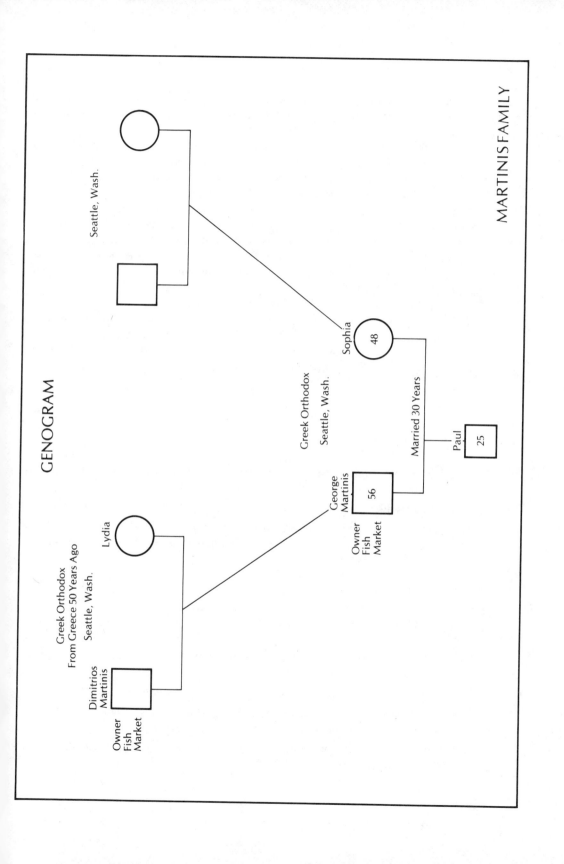

GENOGRAM

Dimitrios Martinis
Owner Fish Market

Greek Orthodox
From Greece 50 Years Ago
Seattle, Wash.

Lydia

Seattle, Wash.

George Martinis
Owner Fish Market
56

Greek Orthodox
Seattle, Wash.

Sophia
48

Married 30 Years

Paul
25

MARTINIS FAMILY

George assisted his parents in the fish market after school and throughout summer vacations. Rarely was it ever necessary for them to employ additional help.

After the first five years the business began to show increasingly large profits. When George graduated from high school, he joined the business full-time. George showed great interest in the management of the market. He was energetic, joked a great deal with his customers, and in general was always willing to please. He was well liked by everyone. Lydia and Dimitrios were able to leave George in charge of the store and take a trip back home.

At twenty-six George married his neighbor's eighteen-year-old daughter Sophia. They then bought a two-family house and gave the downstairs section to George's parents. The next big event for the Martinis was when Sophie gave birth to Paul.

For the next twenty-five years both families remained quite happy. The Senior Martinis' had gradually given over the management of the business to their son and daughter-in-law. The family maintained good health throughout the years. They made infrequent trips to the family physician, Dr. J. Antanakos. They sought his advice only when their home remedies were not successful.

STUDY QUESTIONS

20-1. Complete a growth and development information card on a six-year-old male.

20-2. What is the role of males in the Greek culture? What is the role of females?

20-3. Describe the beliefs and practices of the members of the Greek Orthodox church on the following topics: family, marriage, health and illness, health care providers.

DISCUSSION QUESTIONS

D-1. Discuss the possible reactions of six-year-old George when relocating to a foreign country.

D-2. What are the strengths of the Martinis family? Explain.

D-3. What resources are available to the Martinis family to help them to adjust in Seattle, Washington?

D-4. What are the differences between the Roman Catholic church and the Greek Orthodox church?

CLIENT ASSESSMENT

Until the age of fifty-six, George had enjoyed good health throughout his adult life. Six months ago he experienced hesitation and difficulty in initiating his urinary flow, which gradually progressed to a smaller caliber stream. George denied that there was anything wrong because it was not necessary for him to curtail any of his activities. He neither alerted his wife nor obtained medical attention.

One morning during the winter George had just finished shoveling snow for two hours at the fish market and returned to his apartment to enjoy two cans of beer. He suddenly experienced lower abdominal discomfort that radiated to his lower lumbar and sacral region. George was afraid of catching the flu again, so he took two Tylenol tablets and went to bed under warm blankets. One hour later, he was awakened by chills, headache, nausea, and urinary urgency with inability to void. George had never experienced these symptoms before and did not know what to do. Sophia was frightened and phoned their family doctor, Dr. J. Antanakos. He suggested that George meet him in the emergency room at St. Clare's Hospital as soon as possible. Sophia drove George to the E.R.

STUDY QUESTIONS

20-4.   What are the common causes of urinary retention in an adult male?

20-5.   Review the anatomy and physiology of the male genito-urinary systems. How can enlargement of the prostate effect the urinary system?

20-6.   What are the initial signs and symptoms of prostate disorders?

20-7.   What is the etiology of prostate enlargement?

20-8.   How does the intake of alcohol affect the bladder sphincter control and nerve reflexes?

20-9.   What is the role of the prostate in male sexual functioning?

20-10. What are the potential complications of urinary retention in a male? What is the pathophysiology of each?

Complication	Pathophysiology

DISCUSSION QUESTIONS

D-5. How does the aging process affect urination in males?

D-6. Discuss fears and anxieties of a family when a member is rushed to the emergency room.

D-7. What are the potential emotional effects of urinary retention in a male of Greek descent? Explain.

EMERGENCY ROOM

The triage nurse escorted George to the examining room where she performed a physical assessment.

CHIEF COMPLAINT: Urinary urgency

GENERAL APPEARANCE: apprehensive, pale, in acute distress.

VITAL SIGNS: T: 37.4°C   P: 92   R: 22   BP: 140/80/78

ABDOMEN: rigid, smooth-edged round mass 6 cm above pubic symphysis; tender on palpation.

It was revealed that George had not voided for 13 hours.

The emergency room's resident confirmed the suspicion of acute urinary retention and prescribed the following regimen:

Chest X-ray

EKG

Foley catheter #16 with a 15 cc bag

Bladder decompression, release 100 cc q 1 h

CBC

Blood Chemistry profile

Urinalysis

Culture and sensitivity of urine

Urinalysis

A Foley catheter 16 Fr (French) with 15 cc bag was inserted immediately for straight drainage. The catheter was taped to the lateral thigh to eliminate pressure at the penoscrotal angle. A cloudy, foul-odored, and bloody urine specimen was obtained and sent to the lab. Forty-five minutes later, the reports on Mr. Martinis's tests were returned and read as follows:

COMPLETE BLOOD COUNT

RBC: 4.76 × 10⁶/mm³

Hct: 46%

Hgb: 15 gm/100 ml

WBC: 13,000/mm³

Neutrophils: 50%

Eosinophils: 1%

Basophils: 0.4%

Lymphocytes: 45%

Monocytes: 3%

Platelets: 320,000/mm³

BLOOD CHEMISTRY

K^+: 4.5 mEq/L

Na^+: 140 mEq/L

Cl^-: 109 mEq/L

Ca^{++}: 9 mEq/L

Mg^{++}: 1.9 mEq/L

P^{++}: 4 mg/100 ml

BUN: 21 mg/100 ml

Uric acid: 5 mg/100 ml

Creatine: 6 mg/100 ml

Creatinine: 1.0 mg/100 ml

Acid phosphatase: 4 King
    Armstrong units

Alkaline phosphatase: 6 King
    Armstrong units

Cholesterol: 200 mg/100 ml

Glucose: 115 mg/100 ml

Total protein: 7 g/100 ml

Albumin: 5 g/100 ml

Globulin: 1.5 g/100 ml

URINALYSIS

Color: turbid

Reaction: Alkaline

Sp. gr.: 1.030

Albumin: negative

Sugar: negative

Acetone: negative

Occult blood: large

WBC: 5–7

Bacteria: many

CHEST X-RAY: Unremarkable
EKG: Normal sinus rhythm

Sophia was worried and angry; George had never admitted to a problem until now. On history he said that he had had difficulty urinating for some time. The family physician arrived and reviewed the laboratory test results. He recommended that George be hospitalized for further observations and evaluation. George looked to Sophia to make the decision, but Sophia elected to wait until their twenty-five-year-old son, Paul, had arrived so that it would be a family decision. Paul arrived half an hour later and the family consented to have George hospitalized.

Dr. Antanakos explained to the family that Dr. Henry Young, the urologist would take over the primary responsibility for treating George's urological problem. Following this, George was taken to the urology unit while his wife signed his admission papers in the admitting office.

STUDY QUESTIONS

20-11. Why was the urine cloudy and foul-smelling?

20-12. Complete the following laboratory grid:

Test	Normal Range	George's Values	Amount of Deviation From Normal	Possible Cause for Alteration

20-13. Differentiate urinary suppression from urinary retention.

20-14. What is the French system of grading the size of a catheter?

20-15. What is the rationale for each of the medical orders?

Order	Rationale

20-16. What are the reasons for the hourly decompression of an overdistended bladder?

20-17. What complications might occur from suddenly emptying an overdistended bladder?

20-18. Explain the physiological reason for the pain that is experienced by a client while the Foley catheter bag is being inflated.

20-19. How could this pain be relieved? Explain.

20-20. What is the difference between a Foley catheter and a straight catheter?

20-21. Why is the catheter with a 15 cc bag used instead of a 5 cc bag?

20-22. How does one collect a urine specimen for urinalysis and culture-sensitivity tests from the Foley catheter drainage system using the closed and open method?

20-23. Identify and explain the potential short-term and long-term complications arising from urinary drainage via a Foley catheter. How can these complications be prevented?

20-24. What are the therapeutic effects of the following modalities on a benign prostate hypertrophy (BPH) client? What are the nursing objectives and actions in caring for a client using these modalities?

Modality	Therapeutic Effect	Unwanted Effect	Client's Response to Unwanted Effects	Nursing Objectives and Actions	Method and Frequency of Evaluating Its Effectiveness
Straight urethral catheterization					
Two-way Foley catheterization					
Two-way Foley catheterization with irrigation					

Modality	Therapeutic Effect	Unwanted Effect	Client's Response to Unwanted Effects	Nursing Objectives and Actions	Method and Frequency of Evaluating Its Effectiveness
Three-way Foley catheterization with drip irrigation					
Bladder decompression					

DISCUSSION QUESTIONS

D-8. Why would Sophia elect to wait until Paul had arrived before making the decision?

D-9. What admission papers would Sophia have to sign? Why is it necessary to sign these papers?

PREOPERATIVE WORK-UP

George arrived on the urology ward in a wheel chair with the Foley catheter attached to straight drainage. John Patrick, R.N., the primary care nurse, oriented both George and Sophia to the unit and the hospital routines. He then assessed the functional abilities of the client and the family, and collected the following information while doing the health history and assessment:

RELIGION: Greek Orthodox

EDUCATION: Completed high school

HOUSEHOLD MEMBERS: 2 (wife and son)

ALLERGIES: Erythromycin (manifested by painless skin rashes)
Food—none known
Hay fever every spring (April–June)

T: 37.6°C   P: 92   R: 24   B/P: 140/90

HEIGHT: 160 cm   WEIGHT: 72 kg

PRESENT HEALTH STATUS: Considered health status "very good" prior to admission. Has developed chills, headache, nausea, and urinary urgency for the last 3 hours. Temperature not taken at the time of onset. Denies previous history of similar episodes.

PREVIOUS HOSPITALIZATION AND/OR ILLNESS: "Flu" about a year ago, which lasted seven days; treated with Tylenol and antibiotics (name unknown). Infection of three index fingers on right hand 6 months ago, treated with antibiotics (name unknown). Cholecystectomy 15 years ago, denies having any food intolerance afterwards. Denies history of lung, cardiovascular, liver, blood, or genetic problems.

CHILDHOOD DISEASES: chicken pox. Received all immunizations.

NUTRITIONAL STATUS: always had a good appetite. Prefers seafood and vegetables. Considers himself overweight.

PATTERN OF FOOD INTAKE:
Breakfast: 5:30 A.M. A cup of coffee without sugar. Whole wheat bread, 2 slices of bacon, 2 eggs.
Lunch: meat or fish sandwich, 1 can of beer or glass of wine, dessert.
Midafternoon: 4:30 P.M. A can of beer or cup of tea.
Dinner 7 P.M. Seafood or meat. Vegetable, soup, wine or beer, dessert.

ELIMINATION STATUS: Daily BM without difficulty. Voids 6–7 times daily, experiencing nocturia 1–2 times. Difficulty initiating voiding with decreasing stream of urine within past six months. Denies dysuria prior to the episode.

SLEEP: goes to bed about 10 P.M. and wakes at 5 A.M. Requires no hypnotics or sedatives.

INTEGUMENT: Turgor good; no discoloration; changing hair color from light brown to gray in last 10 years. Nails cut short, well trimmed.

SOCIOECONOMIC: Owner of fish market, Denies any financial difficulties. Has good relationship with wife and son. Enjoys going to church and related functions. Travels occasionally. Drinks 2–3 cans of beer per day. Occasionally drinks with friends. Smokes 1 package of cigarettes per day for 32 years.

PROSTHESIS: Wears glasses for presbyopia for 5 years. Last eye examination 2 years ago. No dentures. Last dental check-up 2 years ago.

MEDICATIONS: Not taking any at present.

FAMILY HISTORY: Parents alive and well. Denies cardiovascular, diabetes, or cancer problems.

George insisted on going to the bathroom to urinate. John Patrick explained the purpose of the catheters, but George kept insisting that he must go and began to pull on the tubes. Finally, Sophia was able to calm George, but he kept on saying, "Why don't you want me to go, when I can go?" John Patrick obtained an order of Demerol 50 mg IM and gave it immediately to George.

Later that afternoon, Dr. Young visited and performed a rectal examination on George. The result was stated as "Rectal examination shows evidence of hypertrophied prostate 2+ with no obvious tenderness or induration." The medical prescription was written as follows:

Regular diet as tolerated

Bed rest with BRP

Forced oral fluid to 3000 ml daily

Record 24 hours intake and output

Vital signs q 4 h

Foley catheter to straight drainage after decompression

Pyridium 220 mg po tid

Mandelamine 1 g po qid

Dalmane 30 mg HS prn

Consent for cystoscopy and needle biopsy in A.M.

For cystoscopy and needle biopsy:

   NPO after midnight except for H_2O

   Fleets enema in A.M.

   Hold breakfast

   Demerol 50 mg IM ⎫ on call to OR
   Vistaril 25 mg IM ⎭

George took an afternoon nap while Sophia and Paul went home to return with his toiletries and pajamas.

Dr. Antanakos, the family physician, visited George in the evening. After reviewing his chest X-ray and EKG, Dr. Antanakos cleared George for cystoscopy and needle biopsy. Sophia's anger was gone; now she just had great concern for her husband's welfare.

The next morning George awoke at 5 A.M. as usual. This time he complained, "How can you sleep alone after you have been married to the same girl for nearly thirty years." Sophia and Paul arrived around 8 A.M.; they had not had a good sleep either. Sophia seemed very nervous.

The routine presurgical procedures were completed. Vital signs were recorded as BP: 140/86, P: 88, R: 20. Temp.: 37°C. An IV of 1000 ml of 5% D/W was started as a KVO before George left for the OR.

At 10:30 A.M. George returned to his room with a three-way Foley catheter with 1000 ml of 0.9% NaCl continuous bladder irrigation. Blood-tinged urine was draining freely from the catheter. His vital signs were: BP: 136/84, P: 88, R: 20. George was awake and did not complain of pain. John Patrick offered him tea and toast.

The C/S report on the urine indicated *Proteus vulgaris,* an organism sensitive to ampicillin. George was then placed on ampicillin 500 mg po q 4 h × 1 day, then 250 mg po q 4 h.

The family was informed about the urine test, but they were anxiously awaiting the pathology report. Paul decided to close the store for the week in order to be with his parents. The members of the family were comforting each other and protecting each other at the same time. John Patrick sensed the strain among the Martinis and he spent some time talking with the whole family.

The next morning Dr. Young discovered from the biopsy report that George had a benign adenoma. He scheduled George for an intravenous pyelography (IVP) the following morning.

George tolerated the procedure well with no signs or symptoms of unwanted reactions. By that evening the family was told by Dr. Young that the IVP indicated that the kidneys and ureters were functioning adequately without any anatomical obstruction or defect. Dr. Young then discussed with the family the various surgical methods of correcting the voiding problem and the urinary obstruction. A transurethral resection of the prostate (TUR) was the treatment of choice in Dr. Young's opinion.

Dr. Young prescribed the following preoperative orders:

Obtain consent for surgery

NPO after midnight

Dalmane 30 mg HS

S.S. enema in A.M.

Demerol 50 mg

Vistaril 25 mg } IM on call to OR

Atropine 0.4 mg

IV at 8 A.M. 1000 ml 5% D/W to KVO

Type and crossmatch 2 units of whole blood

John Patrick reinforced the physician's explanation of the surgery, explained what to expect after surgery, and taught George how to do breathing exercises.

George was transferred to the OR at 8:30 A.M. the following morning. Under low spinal anesthesia, a TURP was performed with an electrode and hemostated by electrocoagulation.

STUDY QUESTIONS

20-26. How would you position George for the rectal digital examination?

20-27. Discuss nursing implementation in carrying out the medical orders.

20-28. What are the components of Foley catheter care? Identify the purpose of each component.

20-29. Is the Foley catheter care an independent nursing function or an interdependent nursing function? Explain.

20-30. What are the complications that might develop from the lithotomy position?

20-31. Discuss the possible complications of cystoscopy and needle biopsy of the prostate.

20-32. What is the reason for having an IVP for a BPH client?

20-33. What is the primary goal of a prostatectomy for a BPH client? Explain.

20-34. What kind of health problems would have developed if irreversible damage to the bladder and kidneys had occurred in George's prostatic hypertrophy?

20-35. If coexisting diseases contraindicates prostatectomy, what would be an alternative treatment for BPH?

20-36. There are five different surgical procedures that can be used to remove adenomatous soft tissue of the prostate gland: transurethral prostatectomy, suprapubic prostatectomy, retropubic prostatectomy, perineal prostatectomy and cryosurgery of the prostate. Compare these five procedures.

Surgical Procedure	Indications	Contraindications	Disadvantages	Post-Op Nursing Implications

20-37. What is the rationale for having a chest X-ray and EKG before cystoscopy and needle biopsy?

20-38. Develop a preoperative nursing care plan for George.

Objective	Rationale	Nursing Action	Rationale	Method and Frequency of Evaluating Effectiveness

20-39. Which muscle(s) and nerve(s) might be traumatized following transurethral resection of the prostate? How will you evaluate the client's functions affected by the above traumatization? What is the nursing responsibility in rehabilitating these functions?

DISCUSSION QUESTIONS

D-10. What is the importance of John Patrick, R.N., taking a health history on George and his family? What areas are identified for health teaching? Develop a preoperative teaching plan for George and his family.

	Objective	Content	Method of Teaching	Evaluation of Learning
George				
Family				

D-11. Discuss the nurse's responsibility in obtaining a surgical consent. What is the liability for the nurse? Explain.

D-12. How is a patient prepared for an IVP? Discuss the nurse's role before and after the IVP.

D-13. Discuss the role of the primary nurse. How does it differ from the team nurse concept?

D-14. What is the chief goal of a primary care nurse in evaluating the functional abilities of a client and family system?

RECOVERY

After staying in the recovery room for two hours, George came back to his room that afternoon with an IV of 5% D in ½ NS running in his left median cubital vein, a three-way Foley catheter (20 Fr. with 30 cc bag) with 1000 ml of NS continuous irrigation to straight drainage. George smiled as he was wheeled into his room and he saw his wife and son waiting for him. The postoperative medical prescription for George was as follows:

Bedrest today

Clear liquid diet to regular diet as tolerated

Discontinue IV after completion

Neosporin G-U irrigation (1:1000)/1000 ml

Peri-Colace 100 mg P.O. tid

Bleeding precaution

V.S. q 4 h, no rectal temperature

Force oral fluids at least 3000 ml daily

I&O

Demerol 50 mg IM q 4 h prn

OOB in chair tid starting in A.M. with Teds stockings

CBC in A.M.

Dalmane 30 mg hs prn

John Patrick, R.N., prescribed the following nursing plan:

- Observe for postspinal anesthesia complications
- Foley catheter care q shift
- Observe for blood clots, bladder spasms
- Force oral fluids, encourage cranberry juice. No ETOH or smoking
- R.O.M. to lower extremities
- Observe for lower abdominal pain

George experienced bladder spasms occasionally, with his reaction changing gradually from one of panic to one of acceptance. Small clots appeared in the urine but never blocked the catheter. George regained total movement and sensation of his lower extremities by the late evening. That night both George and Sophia slept comfortably for the first time since the hospitalization had begun.

First Day Postop. George had no headache, respiratory distress, or lower abdominal pain. Vital signs were stable. George was allowed to be OOB in a chair as tolerated. Precautions were taken against orthostatic hypotension and the condition was prevented. Urine was becoming light pinkish color and fewer bladder spasms were experienced. George continuously made progress.

Second Day Postop. The urine was a light pinkish color without any clots. The bladder irrigation and Foley catheter were discontinued, but the Foley catheter was kept to straight drainage. Urecholine 10 mg p.o. qid was prescribed. The nursing priority at this time was to assist George in maintaining an adequate urinary flow.

Fifth Day Postop. The Foley catheter was discontinued and the tip of the catheter was sent for culture and sensitivity. Urecholine 5 mg p.o. qid was prescribed.

George and Sophia were pleased with his progress. George voided voluntarily and in sufficient amount 3 hours later. Then he realized that he was having dribbling incontinence. He was frightened that his condition might set him back. John Patrick spent some time discussing the problem with George. George understood dribbling and he realized that incontinence would probably improve eventually.

During the afternoon visiting hours, George, Sophia, and John arranged for an informal conference that would provide an opportunity to clear up some misbeliefs. John taught George exercises to strengthen the perineal muscles. John explained to George and Sophia the impact of this operation upon George's sexual activity. John was careful to point out that the prostatectomy should not cause a reduction in George's sexual ability; however, George would be unable to father any more children. Sophia commented to the nurse, "I am glad you explained it to us, because I was a little worried and did not know anyone to ask about it."

On the seventh postoperative day, Dr. Young discharged George. The report from the culture on the Foley catheter tip had been returned negative. John Patrick reviewed with George and Sophia the written instructions that they were going to take home with them.

1. May be up and around at home, but rest when fatigued.

2. No strenuous exercise. Avoid climbing stairs, lifting objects, and riding in a car (except to visit the doctor's office). No sexual intercourse.

3. Drink at least three quarts of oral fluid daily. No alcohol, or caffeinated coffee or tea.

4. Continue Peri-Colace 100 mg three times a day, and Urecholine 5 mg four times a day. Do not strain for BM.

5. Continue perineal muscle exercises 5 or 6 times before arising in the morning and also during each voiding of urine.

6. Expect dribbling, and/or a little bloody urine for the next 4 to 5 weeks at the beginning or end of the urinary stream (this is normal).

7. Empty the bladder at least every 4 hours around the clock. (Including at night.)

8. Please call Dr. Young's office at this number _____, if at any time a problem exists.

9. Your office appointment is _____.

DISCUSSION QUESTIONS

D-15. Discuss the rationale of using the larger size Foley catheter and bag after TURP.

D-16. Discuss the nursing implications of the postoperative medical orders.

D-17. Why is normal saline used for bladder irrigation?

D-18. Discuss how to accurately record intake and output while the Foley catheter irrigation is being used.

D-19. Discuss ways a urine specimen might be collected for sugar and acetone tests from a three-way Foley catheter.

D-20. Identify the possible complications of spinal anesthesia and the nursing intervention relative to complications.

Complication	Nursing Intervention	Rationale

D-21. Discuss the possible signs and symptoms of urinary dysfunction after the Foley catheter is removed.

D-22. Discuss the nursing implications for the prevention and early detection of these urinary dysfunctions.

D-23. Complete a drug card for the following drugs: Peri-Colace, Urecholine, Demerol, Vistaril, atropine, Dalmane, Pyridium, Mandelamine, ampicillin.

D-24. Discuss the desired action of Urecholine for George.

D-25. Explain the rationale for the use of Urecholine. How would you educate George and Sophia about Urecholine?

D-26. Discuss the anatomical bases for George's dribbling incontinence.

D-27. Discuss the perineal muscle strengthening exercises.

D-28. What are the other possible postoperative complications of a TUR prostatectomy? Explain.

D-29. Explain the rationale for the nursing plan prescribed by John Patrick on page 322.

CHAPTER DISCUSSION QUESTIONS

1. Discuss ways Sophia may assist George through his recovery phase at home.
2. Discuss the sexuality of a male client of George's age.
3. What kinds of adjustment problems do you think George may develop?
4. Is it possible for George to develop further prostatic problems? Give the rationale for your answer.

SUGGESTED ACTIVITIES

1. Obtain and read a consent sheet for an operative procedure.
2. Interview a patient and family post-prostatectomy.
3. Observe the role of a primary nurse in a hospital setting.

BIBLIOGRAPHY

Aguilera, Donna C., and Messick, Janice M. *Crisis Intervention.* St. Louis: C. V. Mosby Co., 1978.

Avery, Graeme S. "Geriatric Clinical Pharmacology and Therapeutics." In *Drug Treatment-Principles and Practice of Clinical Pharmacology and Therapeutics.* Acton, Mass.: Publishing Sciences Group, Inc., 1976.

Avery, Graeme S. "Principles and Practice of Antibacterial Chemotherapy." In *Drug Treatment-Principles and Practice of Clinical Pharmacology and Therapeutics.* Acton, Mass.: Publishing Sciences Group, Inc., 1976.

Barnard, Martha Underwood; Clancy, Barbara J.; and Krantz, Kermit E. "The Male Reproductive System and Sexual Response." In *Human Sexuality for Health Professionals.* Philadelphia: W. B. Saunders Co., 1978.

Bergersen, Betty. *Pharmacology in Nursing.* 13th ed. St. Louis: C. V. Mosby Co., 1976.

Bowers, Joan E. "Caring for the Elderly." *Nursing '78* (January 1978): 42–47.

Breu, Christine; Dracup, Kathleen. "Helping the Spouses of Critically Ill Patients." *American Journal of Nursing* 78 (January 1978): 50–53.

Conn, Howard F. "Benign Prostatic Hyperplasia." *Current Therapy.* Philadelphia: W. B. Saunders Co., 1975, pp. 486–491.

Delehanty, Lorraine; Stravino, Vincent. "Achieving Bladder Control." *American Journal of Nursing* (February 1970): 312–316.

Garb, Solomon. *Laboratory Tests in Common Use.* 6th ed. New York: Springer Publishing Co., 1976.

Guyton, Arthur C. *Textbook of Medical Physiology.* 5th ed. Philadelphia: W. B. Saunders Co., 1976.

Garrod, I. P. "Principles and Practice of Antibacterial Chemotherapy." In *Drug Treatment.* Edited by Graeme S. Avery. Massachusetts: Publishing Sciences Group, Inc., 1976, pp. 845–858.

Kettel, Louis J.; Perfetto, Jane; Welty, Mary Jane; Crosby, Alan F.; and Cundiff, Richard J. "Admissions Nurse Practitioners Make a Difference." *American Journal of Nursing* 78 (April 1978): 648–649.

Kratzer, Joan B. "What Does Your Patient Need to Know?" *Nursing '77* 7 (December 1977): 82–84.

Little, Dolores E., and Carnevali, Doris L. *Nursing Care Planning.* 2d ed. Philadelphia: J. B. Lippincott Co., 1976.

Luckmann, Joan, and Sorensen, Karen Creason. "The Nurse's Role in Assessing and Maintaining Adequate Kidney and Urinary Tract Function." In *Medical-Surgical Nursing.* Philadelphia: W. B. Saunders Co., 1974, pp. 716–719.

Malasanos, Lois et al. *Health Assessment.* St. Louis: C. V. Mosby Co., 1978.

Malloy, Jan L. "Taking Exception to Problem-Oriented Nursing Care." *American Journal of Nursing* 76 (April 1976): 582–583.

Marcinek, Margaret Boyle. "Stress in the Surgical Patient." *American Journal of Nursing* 77 (November 1977): 1809–1811.

O'Malley, K.; Judge, T. G.; and Crooks, J. "Geriatic Clinical Pharmacology and Therapeutics." In *Drug Treatment.* Edited by Graeme S. Avery. Massachusetts: Publishing Sciences Group, Inc., 1976, pp. 124–143.

Pendagast, Eileen G., and Sherman, Charles O. "A Guide to the Genogram Family Systems Training." *The Family* 5 (1977): 3–14.

Robinson, Corinne, and Lawler, Marilyn R. *Normal and Therapeutic Nutrition.* 15th ed. New York: MacMillian, 1977.

Roen, Philip R. *Male Sexual Health.* New York: William Morrow & Co., 1973.

Smart, William S. "Benign Prostatic Hyperplasia." In *Current Therapy.* Edited by Howard F. Conn. Philadelphia: W. B. Saunders Co., 1975, pp. 486–491.

Stephenson, Carol A. "Stress in Critically Ill Patients." *American Journal of Nursing* 77 (November 1977): 1806–1808.

Stephens, Gwen. "The Creative Contraries, A Theory of Sexuality." *American Journal of Nursing* 78 (January 1978): 70–75.

Stroot, Violet R.; Lee, Carla A.; and Schaper, C. Ann. *Fluid and Electrolytes: A Practical Approach*. 2d ed. Philadelphia: F. A. Davis Co., 1977.

White, Cheryl L. "Nurse Counseling with a Depressed Patient." *American Journal of Nursing* 78 (March 1978): 436–439.

Woods, Nancy Fugate, and Woods, James S. *Human Sexuality in Health and Illness*. St. Louis: C. V. Mosby Co., 1975.

Zalar, Marianne. "Human Sexuality—A Component of Total Patient Care." *Nursing Digest* 3 (November/December 1975): 40–43.

CHAPTER TWENTY-ONE

Grieving Family: Automobile Accident

ANDREA BRETZ SAVITZ

SANDRA C. WARDELL

OVERVIEW

Harold Arnold is the seventy-two-year-old father of Joan Grayson. When Harold's wife dies, Harold moves in with the Graysons and becomes very attached to Peter, his grandson. Harold and Peter have an auto accident in which Peter is killed and Harold sustains a pneumothorax. Besides the nursing management of an elderly client with a pneumothorax, the nursing staff must complete a family assessment and help Harold and the Graysons to work through the grieving process.

CONTENT EMPHASIS

- Mourning—short-term and long-term reactions
- Death of a family member—child
- Assessment and management of pneumothorax
- Family assessment

SETTINGS

- Site of accident
- Emergency room
- Medical ICU
- Staff conference

328

OBJECTIVES

Upon completing this chapter, the student will be able to:

1. Analyze a client/family's mourning for family members.
2. Evaluate the assessment and management of an elderly client with a pneumothorax.
3. Categorize mourning behaviors according to the various stages of grief.
4. Compose expected health outcomes for an elderly client who is in an acute care setting.
5. Evaluate the ongoing health care plan designed for an elderly client and his family who are mourning.

DEFINITION OF TERMS

The following terms are used in this case study and should be defined before proceeding:

Ecchymotic areas	Mourning
Emotional monitor	Naso-pharyngeal suctioning
Extended family	Nuclear family
Grieving	Pneumothorax
Korotkoff Sounds	closed
Lacerations	open

FAMILY ASSESSMENT

John and Joan Grayson are white, middle class, Protestant adults. They live in a four-bedroom suburban home on two acres. Their female children share a bedroom. Peter, their son, has his own bedroom, as does Harold Arnold, Joan's father. The family lived in their home for two years before Mary Arnold, Joan's mother, died of cancer. Peter was only twelve months old at the time. Later, Harold Arnold joined Joan's nuclear family. Each member of the family is content with the living arrangement.

The John Graysons have been free of known major health problems. Joan seeks medical care for family members only when they are obviously ill. Joan's attitude about health care can be traced back to her family background. Joan's mother, Mary, was of Austrian farm stock. They sought medical help only as a last resort. Mary went to a physician after her cancer had already metastisized. Harold Arnold, Joan's father, is of Ukrainian descent. His parents were bakers who immigrated at the turn of the century and later established a small restaurant. Medical care was a low priority. Harold has disregarded the medical advice he was given three years ago for his bilateral cataracts. John Grayson's family of origin can be traced back to the early 1800s in this country. The male members of the family have, in most cases, been lawyers. Health care was not a high priority, and its maintenance was not sought.

Both John and Joan Grayson's family were and are close to their church. The families of origin were pleased with the marriage of John and Joan. The families had love of family and church in common and they wanted the same orientation of family life for John and Joan.

As years passed, the John Graysons were pleased with and encouraged the relationship between Harold and Peter. Peter had been born at a time of acute personal crisis for Harold, whose wife was dying of cancer. Since then, Harold and the rest of the family still cannot talk about Mary. Mourning has never been worked through.

The anxiety surrounding the death of Harold's wife has been channeled by Harold into energy he uses as "Man Friday" for the John Grayson family. Although his sight has been visibly failing for about a year, John and Joan had not seen fit to curtail his chauffeur duties because he and the children appear to gain so much pleasure from the time spent together. Joan frequently states to John, "His driving only involves going from here to school or church and back."

Harold's presence in the family adds to the family's leisure time. Harold is always willing to pet sit. He enjoys his moments of solitude when "baby sitting the homestead." He presents no economic burden because he receives a handsome share of restaurant revenues from the business he built over the years. Harold also is enrolled in Medicare. In fact, Harold has done so well that he always has money left over to "spoil the grandchildren."

Peter had been the sensitive child in the family. Soon after his birth, he could be recognized as the emotional monitor for the family. Although physical assessments always revealed negative findings in his infant and preschool developmental period of life, Joan has consistently been overprotective in her attitude toward him. She has been uncharacteristically ready to provide (with the assistance of the family's Blue Cross plan) the most extensive of physical work-ups for Peter whenever it seemed to be indicated. The school system had wanted to retain him an additional year in kindergarten, but at the family's insistence he was admitted to first grade. The child study team's findings in second grade were also essentially negative. However, the report did indicate that Peter tests higher than his actual classroom achievement.

Peter's behavior was consistent with a child of low self-esteem. He was shy with his peers and preferred to play within his family. Peter related to his grandfather Harold more than any other family member. The parents were pleased that Harold occupied so much of Peter's time.

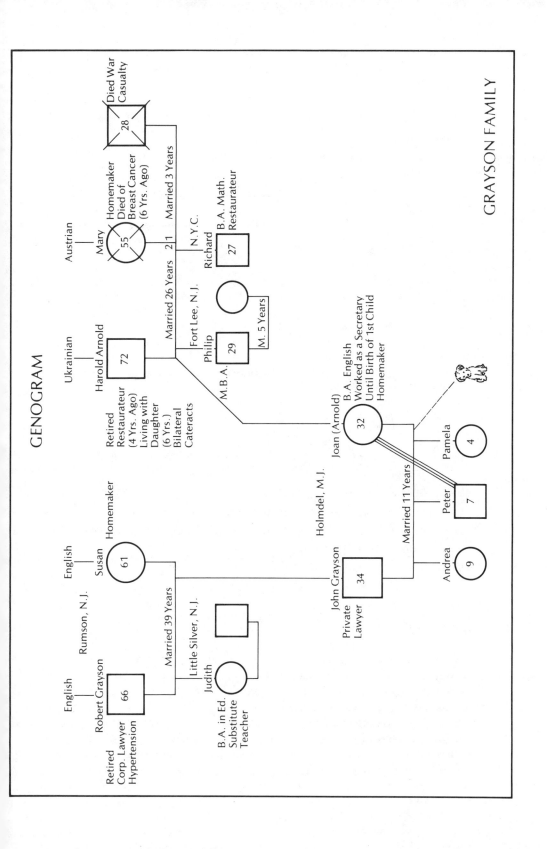

GENOGRAM

GRAYSON FAMILY

STUDY QUESTIONS

22-1. What type of family unit was created when Harold Arnold joined the Grayson's family? Explain.

22-2. Summarize the health status and the attitude about health of each family member:

Member	Health Status	Attitude About Health
Harold Arnold		
Joan Grayson		
John Grayson		

22-3. Complete a growth and development card on a seven-year-old male.

22-4. What are the normal peer relationships for a seven-year-old boy?

DISCUSSION QUESTIONS

D-1. After reading the genogram, what preventive health measures are required for John and Joan Grayson? Harold Arnold? Explain.

D-2. Has Harold Arnold resolved the loss of his wife Mary? How do you know?

D-3. Have the Grayson family members accepted the death of Mary? Explain.

D-4. How does a health professional assist a family to resolve the loss of a significant family member?

D-5. Is Peter Grayson's peer behavior normal? Explain.

THE ACCIDENT

Harold Arnold was driving along a tree-lined road at a quarter to three in the afternoon. His sole passenger was his grandson, Peter Grayson, who was in the right front seat of the automobile. The pair were on their way to a local church where Peter was to attend a scout meeting. It had just begun to snow.

Peter was trying to catch his grandfather's attention by reporting on his day at school. Harold Arnold was uncharacteristically silent with his grandson. He was intent on driving. Visibility had dropped due to the snow. The wind velocity was increasing, and the roads were slick.

Suddenly, as the car crested a hill, a garbage can blew onto the road from the left. Harold Arnold mistook the can for a child. He pulled the steering wheel to the right. The vehicle responded by going into a skid. Arnold was aware that the automobile was out of control. He extended his right arm to brace his grandson against the inevitable impact. However, he could not reach Peter.

Harold's next recollection was of incredible pain in his chest. The automobile had crashed into a tree before halting. The impact had thrown Harold's left thorax against the steering wheel with a resulting chest injury. Harold could see that the windshield was broken, but he could not see Peter. Peter lay huddled in a pool of blood at the base of a tree some feet away.

EMERGENCY ROOM

After a ten-minute ride in the ambulance, while Harold was maintained on 6 liters of oxygen, he was delivered to a local community hospital emergency room. The ambulance team member reported that Harold had exhibited the following:

C/O chest pain

Dyspnea

Dry hacking cough

Cyanosis

Pulse: 110

Blood Pressure: 168/92

While receiving the report, Mark Corry, R.N., the emergency room nurse, wheeled Harold into examining room #3. He was transferred to the examining table, which had been placed in semi-Fowlers position, and Mark started the hospital oxygen at 6 liters via nasal cannula. While carefully loosening Harold's clothing, Mark noted the following:

Left thorax was fiery red and had numerous ecchymotic areas

No paradoxical chest movements noted

Minor facial and hand lacerations

No fractures of extremities or head noted

Restlessness

Temperature: 36.7°C (axillary)

Pulse: 102, regular but thready

Respiration: 32, shallow

Blood Pressure 170/96/78

A more extensive examination revealed the following findings:

- Trachea: slight displacement to right
- Lungs: Lack of breath sounds in the area of the left lower lobe of lung; hyperresonancy in the left upper lobe of the lung and in part of the lower left lobe
- Heart: Apical impulse 9 cm from midsternal line at fifth intercostal space; rate: 104 and regular; no murmurs or gallop noted
- Abdomen: Normal bowel sounds over the entire abdomen; soft, no distention

Dr. Anne Young, the medical resident, arrived and Mark reported his findings to her. After an abbreviated chest exam, Anne Young ordered the following:

Portable A/P Chest X-ray

EKG

1000 ml of 5% D/W to KVO

Oxygen at 6 L/min

Chest tube (#20) to underwater drainage at 20 cm (H_2O) suction

Urinalysis

Arterial blood gases

Blood chemistry

CBC

Transfer to ICU

Based on the medical and nursing assessment, Anne Young listed Harold's tentative diagnosis as a "left pneumothorax."

Meanwhile, Peter was found without detectable vital signs by the ambulance team. The team efforts to re-establish Peter's heart beat and respirations had failed. His head appeared to be crushed like an egg shell. While awaiting Harold's chest films, Dr. Young pronounced Peter Grayson dead on arrival (D.O.A.) and had life-support efforts discontinued.

The John Graysons were notified and arrived at the emergency room asking for their son and Harold. The ER was extremely busy because of the unusually large number of minor accidents due to the snow storm.

When Mark Corry, R.N., heard that John and Joan had entered the waiting area, he notified Anne Young, M.D. He sought relief from Harold's room, and ushered the Graysons to the only available cubicle left in the emergency room area. The task of telling the Graysons about their son was left to him. Although feeling extremely pressed for time, Mark Corry sat down with them. The Graysons waited. Joan was wringing her hands, and John was staring at Mark. Mark reported on Harold and stated he would be transferred to the intensive care unit. Then after a silence, John asked ". . . and our son?" Mark Corry replied softly that Peter was already dead when he reached the hospital.

Tears began to run down John and Joan's faces, but they did not speak or move. Finally, Joan slipped her hand into John's. Mark noted that their hand grasp paled their knuckles. After resting his hands on their shoulders, he excused himself, promising to return.

Mark Corry then checked to see if Peter's body was presentable enough for the family to view. Mark rinsed Peter's face and placed two chairs adjacent to the stretcher holding his body. Then Mark left to find out how Harold was doing.

Harold had been medicated with phenobarbital and Demerol. The medical orders read as follows:

Phenobarbital sodium injection 60 mg IM stat

Demerol 25 mg IV stat

A chest tube to underwater drainage had been inserted without difficulty. Harold was less dyspneic and his acute pain had subsided. He was pleading for information about Peter. The nurse caring for him was trying to calm him. Mark Corry asked his nurse colleague if Harold was stable enough to see his family. To this, the nurse replied, "Yes, someone's got to tell him about Peter, and it might be easier if it were his family."

Mark found the Graysons as they were moments earlier. He told them that they could see their son and Harold now if they so desired. John and Joan slowly stood up. Mark stood close by Joan's side and directed them to Peter's body in the rear hall. When they reached the stretcher, Joan began sobbing and cried, "I can't believe it, I can't believe it." John bit hard on his lip. Neither of them sat down. Mark Corry stood off to one side, remaining silent. Only when Joan began stroking Peter's face did Mark intervene by saying gently, "Mr. Arnold is in a room just off the front hall." Joan was slightly startled by Mark's interruption. John responded by physically coaxing Joan away from Peter.

By the time John and Joan reached Arnold's room, they were quiet again. As they entered the room, Arnold's respirations quickened. For some time nothing was said. Arnold tried to motion Joan to come closer, but was stopped by a resurgence of chest pain. He searched their faces. Then suddenly a pained expression swept over his face and he cried, "Peter's dead, isn't he?" Joan looked up to the ceiling and then closed her eyes hard while nodding her head, "yes." John said nothing.

That was the last time anyone on the staff heard Peter's name mentioned by Harold Arnold or the Graysons; that is, until the nurses intervened.

STUDY QUESTIONS

22-5. Explain the pathophysiology of an open and a closed pneumothorax.

22-6. List some of the most common causes of each type. Explain.

22-7. What are the nursing care priorities for Harold Arnold? Outline them in the order of their importance. Explain your rationale for each.

Priorities	Rationale

22-8. What is the usual medical management of a client with a pneumothorax? Explain.

22-9. Complete a drug information card on each of the following medications: Demerol, phenobarbital.

22-10. What is the effect of the above drugs on the respiratory system? What are the nursing responsibilities?

22-11. What precautions should be taken when administering the above drugs together? Why?

22-12. Explain the rationale for each of Harold Arnold's medical orders:

Order	Rationale

22-13. Why did Mark Corry choose the word "dead," rather than other possible words used for the loss of life?

22-14. What are the stages of grieving? Explain each. How can a client be facilitated through each stage?

Stage	Explanation	Method(s) to Facilitate Each Stage

DISCUSSION QUESTIONS

D-6. What are the nursing diagnoses for Harold Arnold? Joan and John Grayson? Explain each.

D-7. Prepare a nursing care plan for Harold.

Objective	Rationale	Nursing Action	Rationale	Method and Frequency of Evaluating Effectiveness

D-8. In what stage of grieving are the Graysons?

D-9. What family pattern of grieving is unfolding?

MEDICAL INTENSIVE CARE

When Harold Arnold reached the medical intensive care unit, his medical work-up was being called to the floor.

CBC
Hgb: 15.9 g/100 ml
Hct: 48%
RBC: $5.2 \times 10^6/mm^3$
WBC: $6,200/mm^3$

URINALYSIS
color: clear, straw
Sp. gr.: 1.015
pH: 5.8

Glucose: neg.
Acetone: neg.
Protein: neg.
RBC: none
WBC: none

BLOOD GASES (ARTERIAL)
pO$_2$: 84 mmHg
pCO$_2$: 46 mmHg
pH: 7.38

BLOOD CHEMISTRY
Glucose: 100 mg/100 ml
BUN: 28 mg/100 ml
Sodium: 141 mEq/L
Potassium: 3.9 mEq/L
Chloride: 100 mEq/L
CO$_2$: 28 mm/L
Calcium: 5.2 mEq/L
Magnesium: 1.8 mEq/L
Cholesterol: 228 mg/dl
SGPT: 35 U/ml
CPK: 166 mU/ml
LDH: 120 (Wacker units)

EKG
NSR with occasional unifocal PVCs
essentially normal

CHEST X-RAY
Fracture of ribs 5 and 6 at
midclavicular line on left side
No bone fragments noted
Pneumothorax—partial collapse
of left lung

Philip McDuff, M.D. arrived, examined Harold, and added the following
medical orders:

Phenobarbital gr. ½ po tid

Codeine phosphate gr. ¼ po q 4 h prn

Discontinue present IV and start 1000 ml Normosol-M in 5% D/W IV to run
q 8 h

Naso-pharyngeal suctioning prn

Cough and deep breath q 2 h while awake

Cardiac monitoring

Repeat A/P portable chest X-ray in A.M.

Repeat blood chemistry in A.M.

Repeat blood gases in A.M.

Repeat EKG in A.M.

Bedrest

Full liquid diet

Antiemboli stockings

Harold slept that evening. His chest tube container was still bubbling but there was no appreciable drainage. He requested and received two doses of codeine during the night.

The next morning, Jill Maxwell, R.N., noted that Harold's vital signs were essentially stable: Temp. 37.7°C (rectal), Pulse 92, Respiration 24 (shallow), and BP 158/92/74.

Harold cooperated in his care. He coughed, deep breathed, turned, allowed his legs to be sent through range of motion, tolerated his antiemboli stockings, and took fluids upon suggestion. He even learned to do isometric leg exercises.

The repeat laboratory results and examinations were as follows:

EKG: NSR with occasional unifocal PVCs

CHEST X-RAY: essentially the same as previous X-ray, but now there is some reexpansion of the left lung; fracture of ribs 5 and 6 on left side

BLOOD CHEMISTRY
  Glucose: 96 mg/100 ml
  BUN: 30 mg/100 ml
  Sodium: 140 mEq/L
  Potassium: 3.7 mEq/L
  Chloride: 98 mEq/L
  CO_2: 28 mM/L
  Calcium: 5.1 mEq/L
  Magnesium: 1.9 mEq/L
  Cholesterol: 220 mg/dl
  SGPT: 38 U/ml
  CPK: 182 mU/ml
  LDH: 125 (Wacker Units)

BLOOD GASES (ARTERIAL)
  pO_2: 97 mmHg

pCO$_2$: 34 mmHg
pH: 7.46

Over the next two days, Harold Arnold's progress was essentially uneventful. He required less and less codeine. Nonetheless, a certain apathy encompassed him. Harold's mental set was sensed by Jill Maxwell, R.N. She wanted to discuss it with Joan and John, but backed off. The Graysons' almost non-verbal ritualistic visits to Harold unnerved Jill. Jill rationalized, "I never really liked that psychosocial material in college, . . . but I really need it now . . . what shall I do?"

Jill then read over her nursing diagnoses, partly to reaffirm that Harold was receiving "quality nursing," and partly to determine what could be done.

STUDY QUESTIONS

22-15. Complete the following laboratory grid on Harold Arnold:

Test	Normal Range	Harold's Values	Amount of Deviation	Possible Cause(s) for Alteration

22-16. In what physiological condition was Harold's body with respect to acid base balance? Explain.

22-17. What symptom of Harold's was probably responsible for the alterations in his blood pH?

22-18. Complete a drug information card on the following medications: phenobarbital, codeine.

22-19. How does the nurse arrive at the correct drops per minute to set Harold's intravenous drip?

22-20. When checking the intravenous, what should the nurse observe?

22-21. How is a glass intravenous bottle marked to facilitate frequent checks of the rate of flow?

22-22. What is the reason for the change in Harold's IV prescription from 5% D/W to Normosol-M in 5% D/W?

22-23. What cardinal tools of physical assessment would the nurse use to collect data on Harold's fluid balance, and how?

22-24. What is the rationale for the institution of naso-pharangeal suctioning as needed? coughing and deep breathing? Explain.

22-25. How would the nurse determine what size catheter to use for naso-pharyngeal suctioning?

22-26. What are the appropriate positions that the client may be placed in for best results from suctioning of the nasopharynx? trachea?

22-27. For what reason is a Y-tube used in suctioning? Explain.

22-28. What are the steps involved when the nurse institutes the suctioning procedure? Explain each.

22-29. What kind of a seal is maintained in closed chest drainage?

22-30. How does the nurse maintain the seal in closed chest drainage?

22-31. How is the amount of suction regulated in a single-bottle closed-chest drainage system? two-bottle system? three-bottle system?

22-32. What emergency equipment is always maintained at the bedside when chest tubes are being used? Explain.

22-33. How is closed chest drainage equipment secured?

22-34. Under what scientific principle(s) do(es) the chest drainage system(s) operate?

22-35. What is the expected type and amount of drainage from a partial pneumothorax?

22-36. How far below the water level does the glass tube from the client have to be in the closed-chest drainage system, and why?

22-37. When is a malfunction in closed chest drainage system a medical emergency?

22-38. If necessary, by what procedure is the drainage bottle emptied?

DISCUSSION QUESTIONS

D-10. How would you attempt to clear a clogged drainage tube in closed-chest drainage?

D-11. Why is Harold's progress so slow? Explain.

D-12. What revisions should be made in Harold's nursing care plan?

PROGRESS

Jill Maxwell was uneasy about Mr. Arnold's progress. She questioned herself, "Could I have helped in any other way?" She discussed Mr. Arnold in a conference with Philip McDuff, M.D., and a nurse colleague on the unit. Jill learned that she lacked a data base on the man, Harold. She needed more data on his family and his lifestyle. She did not know how he had handled stress in the past, or whether he felt responsible for Peter's death.

When Jill left the conference, she phoned Mark Corry, R.N., and arranged for a luncheon conference. Mark gave Jill his assessment of Harold Arnold and the Graysons. He commented that he was surprised that Jill was asking now for his assessment. He had attempted to give the same report to Jill at the time of Harold's transfer to ICU. Jill had rejected the information. She recalled having said, "I'm busy . . . just read off the medical orders." They ate silently. Then Mark suggested that Jill ask for a client consultation from the hospital's psychiatric nurse clinician. Jill acted on Mark's suggestion.

Jill made a nurse referral to Christine Swift, R.N., psychiatric nurse clinician. It was decided that Jill would introduce Chris as a staff member who helped families through stress, and Chris would take it from there with the Graysons.

Chris's introduction went well. The Graysons showed willingness to speak to her on Harold's behalf. Chris explained that during times of grieving, family members often have difficulty sorting out their feelings. The inability to express themselves to each other often adds to the tension level within a family. She told them that Jill had noted little communication in their family during visits to Harold since the accident. Lastly, she stated that she would like to help the family back to some sense of peace. At this point, Joan started to cry, saying, "Our little boy is gone, I just can't get used to it." Then she looked extremely embarrassed. Chris placed her hand gently on Joan's. John's eyes also filled with tears. Chris went on to explain that the emotional energy that occurs when communications get "stuck" can leave people with little or no energy to meet physical needs. After this, there was a long silence.

John was the first to relate what Chris was saying to Harold's condition. He asked, "Are you saying that Harold might do better if we talk to him about Peter?"

"Eventually, yes," Chris said "But first I want to help you two to talk about Peter."

Although skeptical, the Graysons did enter therapy with Chris the next day. Chris recorded a family genogram. From the genogram, these further diagnoses on Harold were made and acted upon:

- Anxiety (due to the death of his grandson)
- Grieving (due to death of grandson and his wife)
- Sensory disturbance (due to known bilateral cataracts)

An ophthalmological referral was made. For Harold's other nursing diagnoses, Chris coached Joan and John to assist Harold, after she had helped them to grieve for Peter in family therapy. Harold improved as Joan and John's acceptance of Mary Arnold's and Peter's death was worked through.

Chris first coached Joan and John to talk to Harold about missing him. Further, she told them to speak of how empty the house seemed with both Harold and Peter gone, as a way of expressing their need for Harold to be well and home. They always emphasized the positive aspects of Harold's coming home.

After the first silence was broken between Harold and the Graysons, Harold started to recover. He showed steady improvement. In ten days his lung was fully expanded and there was no bubbling in his chest drainage bottle. The next day his chest tubes were clamped on the even hours and opened on the odd hours without consequence. On the twelfth day his chest tube was kept clamped all day. On the fourteenth day his chest tube was removed, and he was ready for discharge on the sixteenth day.

STUDY QUESTIONS

22-39. Why was the chest tube clamped periodically and then continually clamped before removal?

22-40. What assessments should be made when the chest tube is clamped?

DISCUSSION QUESTIONS

D-13. Why did Chris choose to help the Graysons work through the grieving of Mary Arnold as well as Peter?

D-14. What evidence did Chris have that the Graysons had not completed grieving for Mary Arnold?

D-15. Why is it important to work through grieving?

D-16. How does a child Pamela's age assimilate the grieving process and death? What about a child Andrea's age?

D-17. How did Harold gain from family therapy, although he was not an active participant? (Think systems.)

D-18. What are the benefits of Plan A Medicare with respect to hospitalization? home care?

D-19. What is meant by medical authorization, and reauthorization for Medicare?

D-20. Can all Medicare clients be transferred to a nursing home for convalescence?

D-21. Does an extended care facility constitute a new period of hospitalization under Medicare?

D-22. What is considered skilled nursing care?

D-23. What are the benefits under Plan B Medicare?

D-24. Does Medicare pay for medically prescribed pharmaceuticals?

BIBLIOGRAPHY

Aguilera, Donna C., and Messick, Janice M. *Crisis Intervention: Theory and Methodology.* 3d ed. St. Louis: C. V. Mosby Co., 1978.

Benson, Evelyn and McDevitt, Joan. *Community Health and Nursing Practice.* Englewood Cliffs, N.J.: Prentice-Hall, Inc., 1975.

Bergersen, Betty. *Pharmacology in Nursing.* 13th ed. St. Louis: C. V. Mosby Co., 1976.

Brunner, Lillian, and Suddarth, Doris. *Lippincott Manual of Nursing Practice.* 2d ed. Philadelphia: J. B. Lippincott Co., 1978.

Campbell, Claire. *Nursing Diagnosis and Intervention.* New York: John Wiley Sons, 1978.

Garb, Solomon. *Laboratory Tests in Common Use.* 6th ed. New York: Springer Publishing Co., 1976.

Guerin, Philip J., Jr., ed. *Family Therapy.* New York: Gardner Press, Inc., 1976.

Guyton, Arthur C. *Textbook of Medical Physiology.* 5th ed. Philadelphia: W. B. Saunders Co., 1976.

Kübler-Ross, Elizabeth. *On Death and Dying.* New York: Macmillan, 1969.

———. *Death: The Final Stage of Growth.* Englewood Cliffs, N.J.: Prentice-Hall, Inc., 1975.

Kuhn, Janet S. "Realignment of Emotional Forces Following Loss." *The Family* (1977): 19-24.

Lance, Edward. "Chest Trauma," *Nursing '78* 8 (January 1978): 28–33.

Little, Dolores, and Carnevali, Doris L. *Nursing Care Planning.* 2d ed. Philadelphia: J. B. Lippincott Co., 1976.

Luckmann, Joan, and Sorensen, Karen. *Medical-Surgical Nursing.* Philadelphia: W. B. Saunders Co., 1974.

Malasanos, Lois et al. *Health Assessment.* St. Louis: C. V. Mosby Co., 1978.

Mitchell, Pamela H. *Concepts Basic to Nursing.* 2d ed. New York: McGraw-Hill, 1977.

Murray, B. et al. "The Family—Basic Unit for the Developing Person." In *Nursing Concepts for Health Promotion.* Englewood Cliffs, N.J.: Prentice-Hall, Inc., 1975.

Paul, Norman L., and Grosser, George H. "Operational Mourning and Its Role in Conjoint Family Therapy." *Community Mental Health Journal* 1 (Winter 1965): 339–345.

Pendagast, Eileen G., and Sherman, Charles O. "A Guide to the Genogram Family Systems Training." *The Family* 5 (1977): 3–14.

Pincus, Lily. *Death and the Family.* New York: Vintage Books, 1974.

Sandhan, Gayle, and Reid, Barbara. "Some Q's and A's About Suctioning with an Illustrated Guide to Better Techniques." *Nursing '77* 7 (October 1977): 60–65.

Scipien, Gladys M. et al. *Comprehensive Pediatric Nursing.* New York: McGraw-Hill, 1975.

Smart, Mollie S., and Smart, Russell C. *Children.* 3d ed. New York: Macmillan, 1977.

U.S. Department of Health, Education, and Welfare. *Your Medicare Handbook.* Social Security Administration: HEW Pub. no. (SSA) 78-10050 (February 1978).

Wolf, A. W. *Helping Your Child to Understand Death.* New York: Child Study Association of America, 1958.

CHAPTER TWENTY-TWO

Alteration in Mobility: Fractured Hip and Glaucoma

FANG-LAN WANG KUO

OVERVIEW

Mary Papp is an eighty-year-old retired school teacher with osteoarthritis and glaucoma. She fractures her right hip and is treated at the local hospital. An open-reduction of the fracture is done and a Smith-Peterson nail is inserted. Her nursing management is complicated by her age and her failing vision.

CONTENT EMPHASIS

- The aging process
- Glaucoma—assessment and management
- Fractured hip—assessment and management
- Preoperative work-up for an elderly client
- Potential postoperative complications in an elderly client

SETTINGS

- Emergency room
- Orthopedic unit
- Extended care unit
- Home—public health visit

OBJECTIVES

Upon completing this chapter the student will be able to:

1. Recognize the health problems related to the process of aging.
2. Assess the extent of injury when an elderly client sustains a fractured hip.
3. Comprehend the assessment and management of chronic glaucoma.
4. Design a nursing care plan for the aged client with a fractured hip who has an open reduction.
5. Develop a teaching plan for an aged client who has an alteration in his/her ambulation and vision.

DEFINITION OF TERMS

The following terms are used in the case study and should be defined before proceeding:

Activities of daily living (ADL)
Aged
Blanching sign
Extended care unit
Fracture frame
Heberden's nodes
Incentive spirometry
Maturational crisis

Medical clearance
Orthopedic skin prep.
Senior citizen
Situational crisis
Stressful situation
Systems theory
Triage nurse

CLIENT ASSESSMENT

Mary Papp is an eighty-year-old unmarried retired grade school teacher of Irish ancestry. She recently moved from Rochester, New York to a retirement community near Daytona, Florida. She retired from her teaching position fifteen years ago, after forty years of service. She was having some difficulty ambulating due to osteoarthritis. Most of her close relatives are either dead or living at a great distance from her. She moved to a warmer climate in the hope of alleviating some of her arthritic pain. She adopted a stray cat named Pauline from a local animal shelter before she moved to Florida. She is Roman Catholic and does not attend church regularly.

Social Security payments, a small retirement pension, and her bank savings are Mary's only sources of income. She continues to carry Blue Cross and Blue Shield to supplement Medicare.

Mary knew it would be difficult to adjust to her new environment, particularly at her age. But several of her friends moved to Daytona. She socializes with them as well as with the new friends she made in her community.

Even though she had intermittent stiffness in her fingers and knees, Mary was able to maintain her three-room apartment. Except for breakfast, she ate most of her meals with her many friends.

The morning of her accident, Mary Papp was rushing to answer the phone when she bumped into the coffee table and fell. The phone went unanswered. When she attempted to stand, pain surged through her right hip and leg. She lay there for a moment trying to think of some way to get help. Since she couldn't stand and the phone was wall mounted, she dragged herself on her left side the remaining 6 feet to the front door and managed to open it. After what seemed to be many agonizing minutes, her neighbor heard her cries, and came right over.

The ambulance arrived at Mary's ground floor apartment 10 minutes later. Her externally rotated right leg was lying listless in a position of adduction and shorter than the left leg. Mary was not sure whether she had momentarily lost consciousness. The ambulance attendant's observations were as follows:

P: 104

R: 26 shallow

BP: 100/58 (client states normal is 140/92)

C/O: Severe pain in right hip and leg

Right leg: pale and cold to touch, externally rotated in a position of abduction, and shorter than left leg

The ambulance attendants assumed that her right hip was fractured and slipped a fracture frame under Mary. They transferred her to the stretcher.

Mary spotted Pauline huddled in the corner under the table looking at her with frightened eyes. Mary asked, "How can I leave her alone?" The neighbor responded by saying that she would take care of Pauline for her.

During the fifteen-minute ride to the hospital, one of the ambulance attendants notified the emergency room. When Mary arrived, she was conscious and alert but in extreme pain. The fracture frame was carefully transferred to the emergency room stretcher.

The triage nurse collected the following data on Mary Papp:

T: 36°C

P: 106

R: 28

BP: 98/58

Right leg: Shorter than left leg in position of adduction with external rotation; greater trochanter displaced backward into the buttock

Right lower leg: Cold, pale, listless; negative blanching sign; anesthetic to light touch and pinpricks

John Wong, M.D., the orthopedic resident, arrived, and the triage nurse reported her findings. After a brief examination of Mary, Dr. Wong wrote the following orders:

Portable X-ray of both hips and legs, chest X-ray

Demerol 30 mg IM stat

1000 ml 5% D/W IV at 15 gtts./min

Ice bag to right hip

CBC

Urinalysis

EKG

Chemistry profile

Transfer to orthopedic unit

The X-rays revealed the following findings:

- Right intertrochanteric fracture of femur
- Minor osteoarthritic changes in left and right hip joints
- Slight cardiac hypertrophy
- No other remarkable findings in chest or legs

Dr. Wong indicated to Mary that surgery would be necessary but that a medical examination would be required first.

Joan West, a primary care nurse on orthopedics, prepared Mary's bed. She supervised the placement of a fracture board under the mattress. The application of a fracture frame and apparatus for Buck's extension traction with 8 pounds of weight to the traction and an overhead trapeze were ordered by Dr. Wong. When Mary arrived, Joan assisted with the transfer of Ms. Papp from the fracture board on the stretcher to the bed. Mary was surprised that the pain was not as severe now. Joan briefly explained the purpose of the traction and then collected the following data:

80-year-old white single female

Wt.: 65 kg

Ht.: 158 cm

T: 35.8°C

P: 108

R: 28

BP: 94/56

CHIEF COMPLAINT: Severe pain in right hip.

PRESENT HEALTH HISTORY: Fell over coffee table 2 hours ago; unable to move right leg.

PRESENT HEALTH PROBLEMS: *Hypertension*—Diagnosed during an annual health check-up at age 58, with BP ranging from 140/92 to 160/98. Denies any related signs and symptoms. Controlled by a low-sodium diet. Denies requiring any medication.

Glaucoma—Open angle glaucoma; aching eyes and foggy vision in the morning since age 60; Pilocarpine 1.0% gtt T ou bid; denies worsening vision; check-up q 3 months.

Osteoarthritis—Exact time of onset not clear; experienced thoracic spinal curvature, stiff fingers and knees at age 60; Heberden's nodes 2 years later, treated with aspirin, 2 tabs tid and heating pad; put on Motrin 300 mg tid for the last 10 months.

PAST HISTORY: *Surgery and Injuries*—Appendectomy at age 6. D&C for postmenopausal vaginal bleeding at age 47, requiring no further treatment. Sprained left ankle at age 62, immobilized with ace bandage × 3 months, denies sequelae.

Childhood Diseases—Measles, chicken pox, mumps.

Immunizations—unable to remember; smallpox and typhoid fever prior to trip to Orient at age 63.

SPECIAL SENSES
- Auditory ⎫
- Speech   ⎬ Denies alteration in function
- Olfactory ⎭
- Vision—Denies family history of glaucoma; bifocal glasses for reading and shopping only; pupils equally dilated and reacted to flashlight (see PRESENT HEALTH PROBLEMS).
- Tactile—Denies history of impairment; anesthesia to light touch and hypoesthesia by pinprick on right leg distal to the fractured site.

MOTOR STATUS: Symmetrically some limitation on range of joint movement of all fingers, knees, and all toes. Denies requiring any assistance or supportive aid, independent on ADL prior to the accident.

BODY TEMPERATURE STATUS: Normal range unknown, rarely has temperature 39°C with illness.

RESPIRATORY STATUS: Denies having alteration of respiratory function or upper respiratory infection; normal breath sounds, no adventitious sounds; tachypnea—28/min.

CARDIOVASCULAR STATUS: Denies history of edema, chest pain, dyspnea, palpitation, or night sweats. BP range from 140/92 to 160/98 for the last 22 years, controlled only by diet and rest; denies history of headache. Varicose veins in popliteal and ankle areas, bilaterally. Wearing tight corset about 10–12 hours daily. Negative blanching signs on right toes. Diminished pulses distal to fractured site on right leg.

NUTRITIONAL STATUS: Lost 2 kg since moving to Florida. Upper and lower dentures seem to be loosely fitted to gum; difficulty in chewing chunk beef or pork. Prefers chicken and dairy products. Denies history of dysphagia. No known food restrictions except on low-sodium diet. Knowledgeable about diet. Usual diet:

> Breakfast at 7:30 A.M.: Cup black coffee, piece of whole wheat bread, boiled egg, canned fruit.
> Lunch at 12:30 P.M.: Fruit salad or dairy products, tea.
> Supper at 6:00 P.M.: Chicken or meat loaf, frozen vegetable, no dessert.

Morning or afternoon coffee break with friends. Denies having sweet goods. Cup of lukewarm prune juice at 10:00 P.M. for "irregularity."

ELIMINATION STATUS: Denies history of alteration in bowel or bladder. Has BM daily without difficulty. Denies using any cathartics except night-time prune juice. Urinates 4–5 times daily with "good amount." Nocturia once or twice nightly for about 17 years.

REPRODUCTIVE STATUS: Menarche at age 12. Had 28 to 30-day menstural cycle with moderate 3–4 day flow and slight lower abdominal cramping on 2d day of period. Menopause at age 47 (see *Surgery and Injuries* for D&C history). Monthly breast self-examination with negative findings. Last gynecological examination with Pap smear 10 months ago. Pap smear negative.

STATE OF SKIN AND APPENDAGES: Clammy pale skin with poor skin turgor; small brown pigmentations on four extremities and back above the waistline. Ecchymosis around the right hip. Hair color changing from light brown to mixed gray 12 years ago. To beauty salon for hair shampoo weekly. All nails are well-trimmed without clubbing. Showers every other day.

STATE OF PHYSICAL REST AND COMFORT: Right hip area painful to touch. Resting quietly; not interested in her surroundings; sleeps from 10 P.M. to 5 A.M., denies insomnia or drug-dependent sleep, awakes once or twice for urination.

Denies: Allergies to food, drugs, and contact materials.

Denies: Diabetes, heart disease, G.I. bleeding, lung disease, and depression

Denies: Insomnia or use of hypnotics.

EMOTIONAL AND MENTAL STATUS: Oriented to time, day, place, and person. Memory intact.

COMMENT: Enjoys shopping, but tires easily. Enjoys reading, but eyes tire easily. Intends to return to her apartment. Wants to be able to care for cat, "Pauline."

Robert Gilbert, M.D., the attending orthopedist, arrived and discussed the nursing assessment with Joan West. Together they manually reduced the position of the right hip and applied Buck's traction to Mary's right leg. Mary tolerated the procedure without significant pain.

Then the laboratory test results were reviewed:

COMPLETE BLOOD COUNT:
  RBC: 3.2×10^6 mm^3
  Hct: 33%
  Hgb: 10 g/100 ml
  WBC: 12,000 mm^3
  Neutrophils: 62%
  Eosinophils: 3%
  Basophils: 1%
  Lymphocytes: 30%
  Monocytes: 4%
  Platelet count: 200,000/mm^3

BLOOD TYPE: 0 Rh (−)

BLOOD SEDIMENTATION RATE: 40 mm/hr

BLEEDING TIME: 56 sec

CLOTTING TIME: 7 min

PROTHROMBIN TIME: Patient: 12.6 sec   Control: 12 sec

BLOOD CHEMISTRY (VENOUS BLOOD):
pH: 7.40
K$^+$: 3.6 mEq/L
Na$^+$: 144 mEq/L
Uric acid: 2 mg/100 ml
Creatine: 4 mg/100 ml
Creatinine: 1.2 mg/100 ml
Acid phosphatase: 1 unit/ml

Alkaline phosphatase: 10 units/ml
Cholesterol: 250 mg/100 ml
Ca^{++}: 12 mg/100 ml
Mg^{++}: 1.8 mEq/L
P^{++}: 3.2 mg/100 ml
Glucose: 105 mg/100 ml
Total protein: 6 g/100 ml
Albumin: 3.5 g/100 ml
Globulin: 1.5 g/100 ml
VDRL: negative

URINALYSIS:
Color: turbid
Reaction: acid
Sp. gr.: 1.028
Albumin: negative
Sugar: negative
Acetone: negative
Occult blood: negative
WBC: negative
Bacteria: few

EKG: normal sinus rhythm, rate,
    108 beats/min

STUDY QUESTIONS

22-1. Complete a pathophysiology information card (etiology, pathological changing of organ, alternation of normal functions) on the following: chronic glaucoma, osteoarthritis.

22-2. How is glaucoma diagnosed? Explain each method.

Testing Method	Explanation

22-3.   Complete a drug information card on the following: pilocarpine, Phospholine Iodide, Demerol, aspirin, Motrin.

22-4.   What are the signs and symptoms of a suspected fractured hip?

22-5.   What nerves, blood vessels, tendons, or muscles could have been injured by fracture fragments when Mary fell? What would be the resulting injury to each?

Tissue	Resulting Signs and Symptoms

22-6.   Complete a laboratory test grid on Mary's test results:

Test	Normal Range (Aged)	Mary's Values	Amount of Deviation From Normal	Possible Causes for Deviation

22-7.   List the nursing diagnoses on Mary Papp.

22-8.   Prepare a nursing care plan for Mary's initial care.

Objective	Rationale	Nursing Action	Rationale	Method and Frequency of Evaluating Effectiveness

22-9.   What is the purpose of Buck's traction in Mary's situation? How is it applied? What precautions are necessary to maintain this type of traction? List some other situations in which Buck's traction may be used.

22-10. What is the purpose of the trapeze apparatus? What precautions should be taken when a trapeze is used?

22-11. How is an ice bag applied so that the maximum effect is achieved? What precautions must be taken when applying an ice bag to an aged client?

DISCUSSION QUESTIONS

D-1. Does Mary Papp and her cat make up a family? Explain.

D-2. What activities can aggravate the signs and symptoms of glaucoma?

D-3. What are the common causes of accidents in the aged population? How can the nurse assist in the prevention of these accidents?

D-4. Compare Mary Papp's vital signs before and after the accident. What is the probable cause for the alterations? Explain.

D-5. What are the principles of immobilization of the right leg and/or hip so that the client can be transferred to a stretcher? What is the rationale for each?

Principle	Rationale

PREOPERATIVE PHASE

Dr. Gilbert explained to Mary the necessity of surgery. In lay terms he told Mary about the open reduction and the internal fixation of her right hip with a Smith-Peterson nail. He obtained an informed surgical consent.

Joan West spent time with Mary answering questions, orienting her to the setting, and reinforcing the information given by Dr. Gilbert. Ms. West put the side rails up before she left the room. However, Mary was not satisfied by the explanation given for the side rails, and mumbled to herself, "I don't need these."

Dr. Gilbert left the following preoperative orders:

One unit of whole blood this P.M. then KVO with D5W

Obtain a medical clearance from Dr. Lee

1000 mg sodium diet

NPO after midnight

Orthopedic skin preparation this P.M. and repeat in A.M.

Foley catheter to straight drainage in A.M. prior to OR

Fleets enema in A.M. (before skin preparation)

ASA 300 mg with Codeine 15 mg po q 4 h PRN

Obtain premedication from anesthesiology Dept.

After reviewing Mary's laboratory work-up and tests, Dr. Lee briefly examined her. He granted her conditional medical clearance for the surgery in the morning. He wanted her observed throughout the evening and night for any signs or symptoms of brain concussion or contusion. Such symptomatology would be cause for surgical cancellation. Dr. Lee left the following order: Phospholine iodide 0.03% gtt T ou q 12 h.

Later the anesthesiologist visited Mary and left the following preoperative prescription:

Dalmane 30 mg po HS

Demerol 25 mg

Vistaril 15 mg   } 9:00 A.M.

Scopolamine 0.2 mg H

The surgical resident was paged to start Mary's blood transfusion. Her vital signs were as follows:

BP: 96/58

T: 36°C

P: 104

R: 28

The intravenous administration set was flushed with 50 ml of normal saline just before blood transfusion. During the transfusion Mary's vital signs were carefully monitored every 15 minutes. The blood was transfused at 1.5 ml per minute for the first 30 ml. When no unwanted reactions were observed, the transfusion was speeded up to 3.0 ml per minute. After the blood transfusion, Mary's vital signs were as follows:

BP: 102/60

T: 36.2°C

P: 98

R: 24

Further, Mary's complete blood count had changed as follows:

RBC: $3.8 \times 10^6/mm^3$
Hct: 39%
Hgb: 11 g/100 ml
WBC: 13,000 mm^3

Mary was more alert after receiving the blood. She asked many questions before falling asleep for the night.

At 6:00 A.M. Mary was awakened by the nurse. She was given her presurgical preparations. Her vital signs were as follows:

BP: 110/78
T: 36.2°C
P: 90
R: 24

Mary phoned her neighbor to ask about her cat, Pauline, who was reported to be doing fine. Then Mary was taken to the surgical suite in her hospital bed.

STUDY QUESTIONS

22-12. What is the rationale for each of the preoperative medical orders:

Order	Rationale

22-13. Complete a drug information card on the following medications: codeine, Dalmane, Vistaril, scopolamine.

22-14. What is the procedure for an orthopedic skin prep in your hospital? What is the rationale for each step?

Step	Rationale

22-15. What is the purpose of the low-sodium diet for Mary? Explain.

22-16. Why is scopolamine ordered instead of atropine as a preoperative medication? Explain.

22-17. What are the physical changes that occur as a client ages? How could these changes affect Mary Papp's surgery and convalescence? See Appendix I.

System	Change	Possible Effect
Cardiovascular		
Digestive		
Integument		
Musculoskeletal		
Neurological		
Special senses		
Reproductive		
Respiratory		

22-18. How long can refrigerated blood remain at room temperature? Why?

22-19. Compare the advantages and disadvantages of transfusing fresh blood or refrigerated blood, and whole blood or packed cells.

22-20. Identify the potential blood transfusion reactions. What is the cause of each? How are they assessed? What can the nurse do for each?

Reaction	Cause	Signs and Symptoms	Nursing Action	Rationale

22-21. What are the nursing responsibilities in caring for the client who is receiving a blood transfusion?

DISCUSSION QUESTIONS

D-6. What are the disadvantages of inserting a Foley catheter in an aged client? How can these disadvantages be overcome?

Disadvantages	Actions to Overcome Disadvantages

D-7. What preoperative teaching should be done with Mary?

Objective	Content	Method of Teaching	Evaluating Learning

D-8. Compare Mary's laboratory work and vital signs before and after the blood transfusion. What is the rationale for the changes? For the lack of change?

SURGICAL AND POSTOPERATIVE PHASE

Sodium Pentothal, U.S.P., was administered intravenously to facilitate the anesthetic induction prior to nitrous oxide by mask. After a posterior incision to the fractured site, a Smith-Peterson nail was inserted for immobilization. A Snyder HemoVac was connected to the operative site to prevent edema.

By 11:00 A.M. Mary Papp was wheeled to the recovery room, where she received one unit of whole blood. Her vital signs were as follows:

BP: 114/80

T: 36°C

P: 88

R: 24

She was able to move voluntarily and make audible sounds. No respiratory distress was observed. She was responding to her name and simple commands.

At 1:30 P.M. Mary was back in her patient room with an infusion of 1000 ml of 5% D in 0.33% NS with 15 mEq KCl and Berocca-C 2 ml added. The surgical dressing was clean and dry. Her vital signs were as follows:

BP: 120/86

T: 36.5°C

P: 86

R: 22

Dr. Gilbert left the following postsurgical orders:

NPO tonight

Low-sodium clear liquid diet in A.M.; then progress to low-sodium (1000 mg) soft diet as tolerated

1000 ml of 5% D in 0.33 NS with 10 mEq KCl and 2 ml Berocca-C at 100 ml/hr

Colace 100 mg PO tid in A.M.

Demerol 35 mg IM q 4 h PRN

Resume Phospholine Iodide eye drops

Bedrest tonight

OOB in chair 15 minutes × 3 in A.M., no weight-bearing on the right leg

Right hip and chest X-Ray in A.M.

Incentive Spirometry, and cough and deep breathe q 2–3 h

Abduction pillow

Antiembolic stockings to midthighs

CBC this P.M.

The laboratory results were as follows:

RBC: $3.9 \times 10^6/mm^3$

Hct: 39.6%

Hgb: 11.5 g/100 ml

WBC: 12,000 mm^3

The following flow sheet contains Mary's postsurgical progress for the first 5 days after surgery:

		BP	TPR	Intake		Output		BM	Other
				Oral	IV	Urine	Hemovac		
DAY OF SURGERY	1:30 P.M. 3 P.M.	124/80 128/80	36.6 84 20 36.6 84 20	—	250	200	15 ml (bright red)		Rt. leg—positive blanching sign, hypoesthesia on light touch, weak pedal pulses, skin warm
	3 P.M. 11 P.M.	130/82 130/80	36.8 86 22 36.8 86 22	—	800	750	10 ml		Dressing—dry and intact C/O gas pains—expelling flatus, no confusion or disorientation
	11 P.M. 7 A.M.	128/78 130/80	36.4 84 18 36.5 84 18	—	800	800	8 ml		Demerol @ 2 P.M., 9:30 P.M., 2 A.M. Breathing exercises q 2–3 h
P.O. 1		132/80 130/80 128/78	36.4 84 18 36.8 86 20 36.8 86 20	645	2400	2850	7–8 ml		Clear fluids—tolerated Foley D/C @ 11 A.M.—voiding @ 2 P.M. Dressing changed—watching TV OOB in chair 15 min × 2—tolerated well.
2		140/86 138/84	36.8 86 16 37.0 86 18	1330	450	1850	7 ml		Breathing exercises q 2–3 h soft low-sodium diet IV at KVO OOB in wheelchair × 3
3		142/90 138/88	36.4 80 16 36.8 86 18	1165	450	qs		ṫ (enema)	Breathing exercises q 2–3 h Added high-protein foods to diet Fleets enema @ 11 A.M.—good results Hemovac D/C @ 11 A.M. PT at 10 A.M.—friend brought eye-glasses and oxford walking shoes
4		140/84	36.2 80 14	1330		qs		ṫ	Breathing exercises q 2–3 h Rt. leg—pedal pulse strong as left leg IV D/C at 11 A.M. Dressing changed—small amt. of serosanguineous fluid D/C 1PPB PT @ 10 A.M. OT @ 1 P.M.
5		136/78	36 76 14	D/C		qs			Hair shampooed—to solarium in W/C for 1 hour.

STUDY QUESTIONS

22-22. List the nursing diagnosis on the first postoperative day.

22-23. What is an open reduction with an internal fixation of the femur? What are the advantages and disadvantages of this procedure for a fracture?

22-24. What are the advantages and disadvantages of a close reduction with an external fixation?

22-25. Complete a drug information card on the following medications: Sodium Pentothal, nitrous oxide—as an anesthetic, Berocca-C, Colace.

22-26. What are the principles that should be used to turn and position Mary?

22-27. What positions, movements, and activities are contraindicated for Mary? What is the rationale for each?

Contraindicated Position, Movement and Activity	Rationale

22-28. Describe the physiologic process of bone healing. How is this process altered in the aging client?

22-29. What are some of the means by which bone healing can be promoted in Mary? Explain.

22-30. What are the potential postoperative complications of an open reduction with an internal fixation of the femur for Mary Papp? What is the cause of them? How can they be assessed and what nursing care should be instituted to prevent them?

Potential Complication	Cause	Assessment	Preventive Nursing Actions	Rationale

DISCUSSION QUESTIONS

D-9. List the nursing diagnosis for the first postoperative day and design a nursing care plan for Mary Papp.

Objective	Rationale	Nursing Action	Rationale	Method and Frequency of Evaluating Effectiveness

D-10. What revisions should be made in Mary's nursing care plan for the rest of her postoperative phase?

D-11. What are the techniques that can be used by the nurse to maintain function in preparation for Mary's walking? Explain the rationale for each.

Technique	Rationale

D-12. Compare Mary's intake and output for the first 5 postoperative days. How well is her fluid balance being maintained? Explain.

D-13. Compare Mary's preoperative and postoperative blood work. What is the cause for any changes that occurred?

Test	Pre-Op	Value	Post-Op Value	Possible Causes

RECOVERY PHASE

Ten days after surgery, Mary Papp was transferred to the hospital's extended care unit where Ann Smith was her primary care nurse. She learned how to manipulate her walker while being completely independent about activities of daily living. Sutures were removed on the twelfth postoperative day.

A client evaluation conference was scheduled two weeks after surgery. It was attended by the client, Joan West, Ann Smith, Dr. Gilbert, the social worker, the occupational therapist, and the physical therapist. Jointly the decision was made to discharge the client to her home. Prior to the discharge, a home visit was scheduled to evaluate the home environment and make any needed modifications.

Three weeks after surgery, Ann Smith, the physical therapist, and the occupational therapist accompanied Mary Papp to her home for the predischarge home visit. Mary's daily routines were discussed in detail. Some furnishings were arranged in order to allow more room for the walker. A shower chair was ordered for the bath tub. Modifications in the kitchen included removing throw rugs from the floor, positioning a special high chair near the counter, repositioning cupboard items, and the like. The wall phone was replaced by a desk model and two additional phones were ordered. Mary's greatest delight was being able to see Pauline again. They exchanged affection as Mary held Pauline in her lap.

Following discharge, Mary was helped daily by a home health aide. She was visited twice weekly by a public health nurse. Within the first two weeks following the discharge, Mary was maneuvering using her walker with great ease and bearing partial weight on her right leg. She had completed her scheduled visits to the dental and ophthalmology clinics. A prescription for new eyeglasses was filled, and her dentures were adjusted.

DISCUSSION QUESTIONS

D-14. Prepare a discharge plan for the public health nurse:

Objective	Rationale	Nursing Action	Rationale	Method and Frequency of Evaluating Effectiveness

D-15. Prepare a teaching plan for Mary's recovery phase at home.

Objective	Content	Method of Teaching	Evaluation of Learning

D-16. Prepare a teaching plan about glaucoma for Mary Papp.

Objective	Content	Method of Teaching	Evaluation of Learning

D-17. What are the surgical methods of treating glaucoma? Explain each of the surgical methods. Would Mary Papp benefit from the surgery?

Surgical Procedure	Explanation

D-18. Aged clients are particularly susceptible to adverse drug reactions. Explain the factors that may contribute to this phenomenon.

D-19. Why are there an increasing number of hip fractures among the aged population, especially the females?

SUGGESTED ACTIVITIES

1. Take care of an elderly person with a hip fracture.
2. Take care of an elderly person with poor eyesight.

3. Tour a retirement center or home for the elderly. What activities are provided for the elderly client?

4. Visit a rehabilitation department of a hospital. What schedule of therapy would be instituted for a client similar to that presented in this chapter?

5. Contact a local organization for the prevention of blindness. What services are offered for persons with glaucoma or persons suspected of having glaucoma?

BIBLIOGRAPHY

Abel, R., and Leopold, I. H. "Ocular Disease." In *Drug Treatment.* Edited by Graeme S. Avery. Massachusetts: Publishing Sciences Group, Inc., 1976, pp. 275–304.

Beland, Irene L., and Passos, Joyce Y. "Blood Products and Uses." In *Clinical Nursing.* 3d ed. New York: Macmillan, 1975, pp. 957–959.

Bergersen, Betty. *Pharmacology in Nursing.* 13th ed. St. Louis: C. V. Mosby Co., 1976.

Bowers, Joan E. "Caring for the Elderly." *Nursing '78* 8 (January 1978): 42–47.

Combs, Karen L. "Preventive Health Care." *American Journal of Nursing* 78 (August 1978): 1339–1341.

Deyerle, William M. "Broken Legs Are to Be Walked on." *American Journal of Nursing* 77 (December 1977): 1927–1930.

Diekelmann, Nancy. "Pre-Retirement Counseling." *American Journal of Nursing* 78 (August 1978): 1337–1338.

Dresen, Sheila E. "Autonomy: A Continuing Developmental Task." *American Journal of Nursing* 78 (August 1978): 1344–1346.

Garb, Solomon. *Laboratory Tests in Common Use.* 6th ed. New York: Springer Publishing Company, Inc., 1976.

Gotz, Bridget E., and Gotz, Vincent P. "Drugs and the Elderly." *American Journal of Nursing* 78 (August 1978): 1347–1351.

Griggs, Winona. "Sex and the Elderly." *American Journal of Nursing* 78 (August 1978): 1352–1354.

Guyton, Arthur C. *Textbook of Medical Physiology.* 5th ed. Philadelphia: W. B. Saunders Co., 1976.

Hogstel, Mildred O. "How do the Elderly View Their World?" *American Journal of Nursing* 78 (August 1978): 1335–1336.

Kettel, Louis J.; Perfetto, Jane; Welty, Mary Jane; Crosby, Alan F.; and Cundiff, Richard J. "Admissions Nurse Practitioners Make a Difference." *American Journal of Nursing* 78 (April 1978): 648–649.

Kratzer, Joan B. "What Does Your Patient Need to Know?" *Nursing '77* 7 (December 1977): 82–88.

Little, Dolores E., and Carnevali, Doris L. *Nursing Care Planning.* 2d ed. Philadelphia: J. B. Lippincott Co., 1976.

Luckmann, Joan, and Sorensen, Karen Creason. *Medical-Surgical Nursing.* Philadelphia: W. B. Saunders Co., 1974, pp. 324–332, 747–749, 1143–1239, and 1455–1510.

McFarland, Mary B. "Fat Embolism Syndrome." *American Journal of Nursing* 76 (December 1976): 1942–1944.

Malasanos, Lois, et al. *Health Assessment.* St. Louis: C. V. Mosby Co., 1978.

Marcinek, Margaret Boyle. "Stress in the Surgical Patient." *American Journal of Nursing* 77 (November 1977): 1809–1811.

Murray, Ruth and Zentner, Judith. *Nursing Concepts for Health Promotion.* Englewood Cliffs, N.J.: Prentice-Hall, Inc., 1975.

O'Malley, K.; Judge, T. G.; and Crooks, J. "Geriatric Clinical Pharmacology and Therapeutics." In *Drug Treatment.* Edited by Graeme S. Avery. Massachusetts: Publishing Sciences Group, Inc., 1976, pp. 124–142.

Pendagast, Eileen G., and Sherman, Charles O. "A Guide to the Genogram Family Systems Training." *The Family* 5 (January 1977): 3–14.

Robinson, Corinne, and Lawler, Marilyn R. *Normal and Therapeutic Nutrition.* 15th ed. New York: Macmillan, 1977.

Schwaid, Madeline C. "Advice to Arthritics: Keep Moving." *American Journal of Nursing* 78 (October 1978): 1708–1709.

Sculco, Cynthia D., and Sculco, Thomas P. "Management of the Patient with an Infected Total Hip Arthroplasty." *American Journal of Nursing* 76 (April 1976): 584–587.

Sibille, Michael. "Geriatric Care." *Nursing '75* 5(July 1975): 54–55.

Snyder, Joyce C. "Elements of a Psychological Assessment." *American Journal of Nursing* 77 (February 1977): 235–239.

Stephenson, Carol A. "Stress in Critically Ill Patients." *American Journal of Nursing* 77 (November 1977): 1806–1808.

Stroot, Violet R.; Lee, Carol A.; and Schaper, C. Ann. *Fluid and Electrolytes: A Practical Approach.* 2d ed. Philadelphia: F. A. Davis Co., 1977.

Truesdell, Sandra, and Wood, Tom. "Communication—Key to Efficient Patient Care." *Nursing '77* 7 (August 1977): 52–53.

Uhler, Diana M. "Common Skin Changes in the Elderly." *American Journal of Nursing* 78 (August 1978): 1342–1344.

Watson, Jeannette E. "Age—Implications for Nursing," and "Nursing in Disorders of the Eye." In *Medical–Surgical Nursing and Related Physiology.* Philadelphia: W. B. Saunders Co. 1972, pp. 126–143 and 729–744.

Classification of Newborn Infants and Mortality by Birthweight and Gestational Age

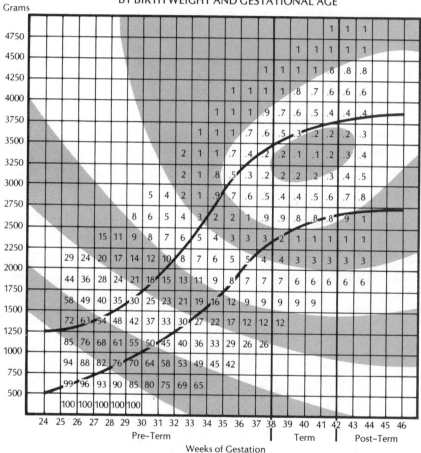

NEWBORN CLASSIFICATION AND NEONATAL MORTALITY RISK
BY BIRTH WEIGHT AND GESTATIONAL AGE

Grams

Weeks of Gestation	24	25	26	27	28	29	30	31	32	33	34	35	36	37	38	39	40	41	42	43	44	45	46
4750																			1	1	1		
4500																1	1	1	1	1			
4250														1	1	1	1	.8	.8	.8			
4000												1	1	1	1	.8	.7	.6	.6	.6			
3750											1	1	1	.9	.7	.6	.5	.4	.4	.4			
3500										1	1	1	.7	.6	.5	.3	.2	.2	.2	.3			
3250									2	1	1	.7	.4	.2	.2	.1	.1	.2	.3	.4			
3000									2	1	.8	.5	.3	.2	.2	.2	.2	.3	.4	.5			
2750							5	4	2	1	.9	.7	.6	.5	.4	.4	.5	.6	.7	.8			
2500						8	6	5	4	3	2	2	1	.9	.9	.8	.8	.8	.9	1			
2250				15	11	9	8	7	6	5	4	3	3	3	2	1	1	1	1	1			
2000		29	24	20	17	14	12	10	8	7	6	5	5	4	4	3	3	3	3	3			
1750		44	36	28	24	21	18	15	13	11	9	8	7	7	7	6	6	6	6	6			
1500		58	49	40	35	30	25	23	21	19	16	12	9	9	9	9	9						
1250		72	63	54	48	42	37	33	30	27	22	17	12	12	12								
1000		85	76	68	61	55	50	45	40	36	33	29	26	26									
750		94	88	82	76	70	64	58	53	49	45	42											
500		99	96	93	90	85	80	75	69	65													
		100	100	100	100	100																	

Pre-Term   Term   Post-Term

Weeks of Gestation

Interpolated data based on mathematical fit from original data University
of Colorado Medical Center newborns. 7/1/58–7/1/69

Silverman Scoring System

Clinical Findings	0	1	2
Expiratory Grunt	Absent	Audible with Stethoscope	Audible without Stethoscope

Retractions
  Intercostal
  Sternal
	Absent
	Absent
		Mild
		Mild
			Severe
			Severe

See-Saw Respirations	Absent	Mild	Severe
Nasal Flaring	Absent	Mild	Severe

Score = or < 4 = clinical RDS; monitor arterial blood gases.
Score = or < 8 = impending respiratory failure.

SOURCE: Courtesy of William A. Silverman. *Pediatrics* 17 (January 1956). Copyright by American Academy of Pediatrics.

Downes or RDS Scoring System

Clinical Findings	0	1	2
Cyanosis	None	In Room air	In 40% F_iO_2
Retractions	None	Mild	Severe
Grunting	None	Audible with Stethoscope	Audible without Stethoscope
Air Entry (crying)	Clear	Decreased or delayed	Barely audible
Respiratory Rate	Under 60	60–80	Over 80 or apneic episodes

SOURCE: Courtesy of Downes, J. J.; Vidyashgar, D.; Morrow, G. N.; and Boggs, T. R., Jr. "Respiratory Distress Syndrome of Newborn Infants: New Clinical Scoring System (RDS Score) with Acid-Base and Blood Gas Correlations." *Clinical Pediatrics* 9 (June 1970).

Key to Genogram Symbols

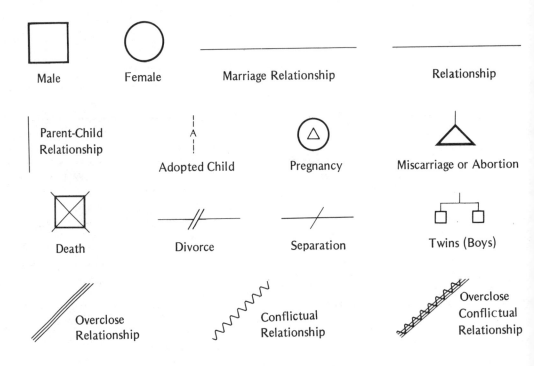

Male	Female	Marriage Relationship	Relationship

Parent-Child Relationship

Adopted Child

Pregnancy

Miscarriage or Abortion

Death

Divorce

Separation

Twins (Boys)

Overclose Relationship

Conflictual Relationship

Overclose Conflictual Relationship

ADDITIONAL AND ALTERNATE GENOGRAM SYMBOLS

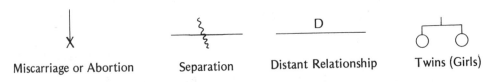

Miscarriage or Abortion

Separation

Distant Relationship

Twins (Girls)

Adapted from Pendagast, E. G., and C. O. Sherman. "A Guide to the Genogram Family Systems Training." *The Family* 5 (1977): 3-14.

Anthropometric Charts

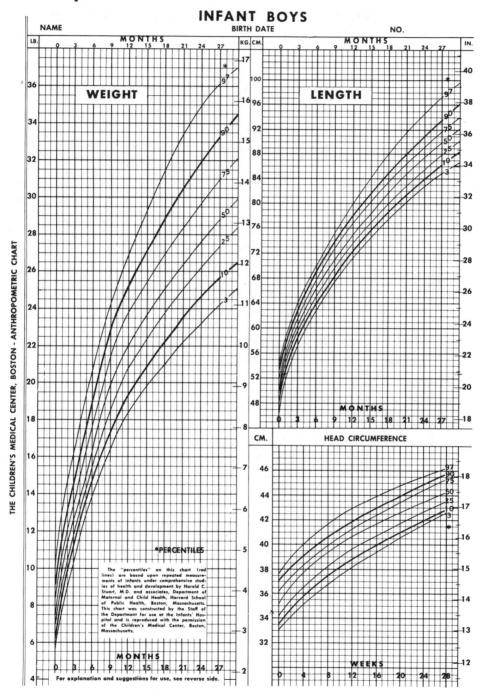

INFANT BOYS

NAME   BIRTH DATE   NO.

THE CHILDREN'S MEDICAL CENTER, BOSTON - ANTHROPOMETRIC CHART

WEIGHT

LENGTH

HEAD CIRCUMFERENCE

MONTHS

WEEKS

*PERCENTILES

The "percentiles" on this chart (red lines) are based upon repeated measurements of infants under comprehensive studies of health and development by Harold C. Stuart, M.D. and associates, Department of Maternal and Child Health, Harvard School of Public Health, Boston, Massachusetts. This chart was constructed by the Staff of the Department for use at the Infants' Hospital and is reproduced with the permission of the Children's Medical Center, Boston, Massachusetts.

For explanation and suggestions for use, see reverse side.

PERCENTILE CHART FOR MEASUREMENTS OF INFANT BOYS

THIS CHART provides for infant boys standards of reference for body weight and recumbent length by month from birth to 28 months and for head circumference by week from birth to 28 weeks. It is based upon repeated measurements at selected ages of a group of more than 100 white infants of North European ancestry living under normal conditions of health and home life in Boston, Mass. The distribution of the measurements obtained from the infants at each age is expressed in percentiles, each percentile giving a value which represents a particular position in the normal range of occurrences. The number of the percentile refers to the position which a measurement of the given value would hold in any typical series of 100 infants. Thus, the 10th percentile gives the value for the tenth in any hundred; that is, 9 infants of the same sex and age would be expected to be smaller in the measurement under consideration while 90 would be expected to be larger than the figure given. Similarly the 90th percentile would indicate that 89 infants might be expected to be smaller than the figure given while 10 would be larger. The 50th percentile represents the median or midposition in the customary range. Here, the 10th and 90th percentiles are presented in heavy lines to show the limits within which most infants remain. The lighter lines in the graphs divide the distributions into segments for ready recognition and description of individual differences as well as of the "regularity" of progress. The 3rd and 97th percentiles represent unusual though not necessarily abnormal findings.

In line with common usage in the United States, the charts are ruled on a scale in pounds to represent weight. They are ruled, however, in centimeters to represent length and head circumference, because this scale facilitates accuracy in measuring and recording and centimeter rules and tapes are readily available. For the convenience of those preferring them, scales for kilograms and inches are placed outside of the principal scales and paralleling them. Therefore, if weights are taken in kilograms and lengths and head circumferences in inches, they may be plotted directly without conversion by placing a ruler at the appropriate points on the outer scales of the charts.

To determine the percentile position of any measurement at a given age, the vertical age line is located and a dot is placed where this intersects the horizontal line representing the value obtained from the measurement. Vertical lines give age by one-month intervals for weight and length and one-week intervals for head circumference; horizontal lines give ½-pound, 1-cm. and 0.5-cm. intervals respectively. This permits by interpolation accurate placement for age to weeks, for weights to 2 ounces and for centimeters to 0.5 cm. Recognition of the position within or outside of the range held by an infant in respect to each measurement recorded calls attention to the relative size and build of the individual at the time. More importantly, comparisons of percentile positions held by these measurements at repeated periodic examinations indicate adherence to or possibly significant deviation from previous percentile positions. Under normal circumstances, one expects an infant to maintain a similar position from age to age — that is, on or near one percentile line or between the same two lines. Occasional sharp deviations or gradual but continuing shifts from one percentile position to another call for further investigation as to their causes. In all cases, readings of measurements should be checked and care should be taken to secure the same position of the infant at all examinations. The following procedures were used in obtaining these norms and therefore are recommended:

Body Weight — The infant is weighed without clothing, preferably on special infant scales.

Recumbent Length — The infant lies relaxed on a firm surface parallel to a centimeter rule or on a special infant measuring board which permits the following procedure. The soles of the feet are held firmly against a fixed upright at the zero mark on the rule, and a movable square is brought firmly against the vertex. Care must be taken to secure extension at the knees, and the head should be held so that the eyes face the ceiling.

Head Circumference — This measurement is more satisfactory if taken with the infant lying on his back. The tape is passed around the head from above and placed anteriorly over the lower forehead just above the supraorbital ridges. With the position of the tape thus fixed anteriorly, the largest circumference is obtained by passing it posteriorly over the most prominent part of the occiput.

Furnished by Mead Johnson Laboratories as a Service in Medicine   Printed in U.S.A.   Lit. 84-B

INFANT GIRLS

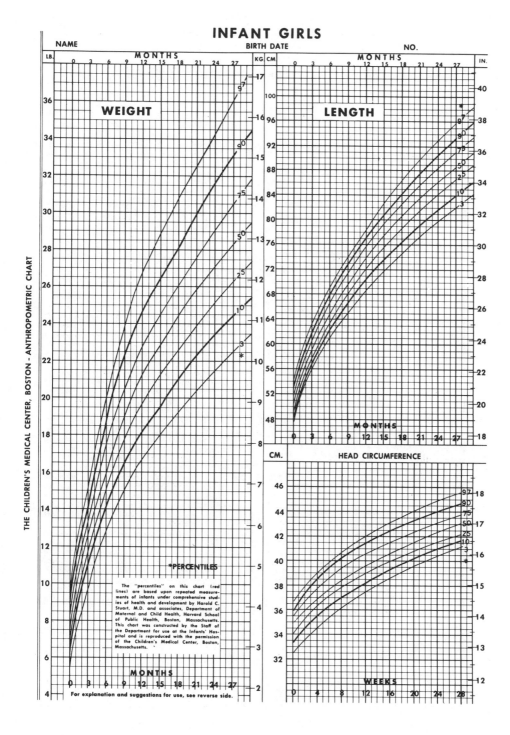

NAME   BIRTH DATE   NO.

THE CHILDREN'S MEDICAL CENTER, BOSTON - ANTHROPOMETRIC CHART

WEIGHT

LENGTH

HEAD CIRCUMFERENCE

*PERCENTILES

The "percentiles" on this chart (red lines) are based upon repeated measurements of infants under comprehensive studies of health and development by Harold C. Stuart, M.D. and associates, Department of Maternal and Child Health, Harvard School of Public Health, Boston, Massachusetts. This chart was constructed by the Staff of the Department for use at the Infants' Hospital and is reproduced with the permission of the Children's Medical Center, Boston, Massachusetts.

For explanation and suggestions for use, see reverse side.

375

PERCENTILE CHART FOR MEASUREMENTS OF INFANT GIRLS

THIS CHART provides for infant girls standards of reference for body weight and recumbent length by month from birth to 28 months and for head circumference by week from birth to 28 weeks. It is based upon repeated measurements at selected ages of a group of more than 100 white infants of North European ancestry living under normal conditions of health and home life in Boston, Mass. The distribution of the measurements obtained from the infants at each age is expressed in percentiles, each percentile giving a value which represents a particular position in the normal range of occurrences. The number of the percentile refers to the position which a measurement of the given value would hold in any typical series of 100 infants. Thus, the 10th percentile gives the value for the tenth in any hundred; that is, 9 infants of the same sex and age would be expected to be smaller in the measurement under consideration while 90 would be expected to be larger than the figure given. Similarly the 90th percentile would indicate that 89 infants might be expected to be smaller than the figure given while 10 would be larger. The 50th percentile represents the median or midposition in the customary range. Here, the 10th and 90th percentiles are presented in heavy lines to show the limits within which most infants remain. The lighter lines in the graphs divide the distributions into segments for ready recognition and description of individual differences as well as of the "regularity" of progress. The 3rd and 97th percentiles represent unusual though not necessarily abnormal findings.

In line with common usage in the United States, the charts are ruled on a scale in pounds to represent weight. They are ruled, however, in centimeters to represent length and head circumference, because this scale facilitates accuracy in measuring and recording and centimeter rules and tapes are readily available. For the convenience of those preferring them, scales for kilograms and inches are placed outside of the principal scales and paralleling them. Therefore, if weights are taken in kilograms and lengths and head circumferences in inches, they may be plotted directly without conversion by placing a ruler at the appropriate points on the outer scales of the charts.

To determine the percentile position of any measurement at a given age, the vertical age line is located and a dot is placed where this intersects the horizontal line representing the value obtained from the measurement. Vertical lines give age by one-month intervals for weight and length and one-week intervals for head circumference; horizontal lines give ½-pound, 1-cm. and 0.5-cm. intervals respectively. This permits by interpolation accurate placement for age to weeks, for weights to 2 ounces and for centimeters to 0.5 cm. Recognition of the position within or outside of the range held by an infant in respect to each measurement recorded calls attention to the relative size and build of the individual at the time. More importantly, comparisons of percentile positions held by these measurements at repeated periodic examinations indicate adherence to or possibly significant deviation from previous percentile positions. Under normal circumstances, one expects an infant to maintain a similar position from age to age — that is, on or near one percentile line or between the same two lines. Occasional sharp deviations or gradual but continuing shifts from one percentile position to another call for further investigation as to their causes. In all cases, readings of measurements should be checked and care should be taken to secure the same position of the infant at all examinations. The following procedures were used in obtaining these norms and therefore are recommended:

Body Weight — The infant is weighed without clothing, preferably on special infant scales.

Recumbent Length — The infant lies relaxed on a firm surface parallel to a centimeter rule or on a special infant measuring board which permits the following procedure. The soles of the feet are held firmly against a fixed upright at the zero mark on the rule, and a movable square is brought firmly against the vertex. Care must be taken to secure extension at the knees, and the head should be held so that the eyes face the ceiling.

Head Circumference — This measurement is more satisfactory if taken with the infant lying on his back. The tape is passed around the head from above and placed anteriorly over the lower forehead just above the supraorbital ridges. With the position of the tape thus fixed anteriorly, the largest circumference is obtained by passing it posteriorly over the most prominent part of the occiput.

Furnished by Mead Johnson Laboratories as a Service in Medicine   Printed in U.S.A.   Lit. 84-G

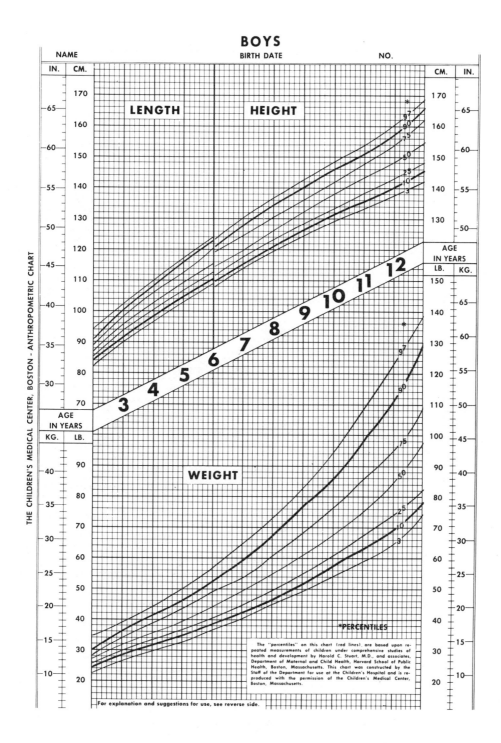

BOYS

PERCENTILE CHART FOR MEASUREMENTS OF BOYS

THIS CHART provides for boys standards of reference for body weight and recumbent length at ages between 2 and 6 years and for weight and standing height from 6 to 13 years. It is based upon repeated measurements at selected ages of a group of more than 100 white boys of North European ancestry living under normal conditions of health and home life in Boston, Mass. The distribution of the measurements obtained from these children at each age is expressed in percentiles, each percentile giving a value which represents a particular position in the normal range of occurrences. The number of the percentile refers to the position which a measurement of the given value would hold in any typical series of 100 children. Thus, the 10th percentile gives the value for the tenth in any hundred; that is, 9 children of the same sex and age would be expected to be smaller in the measurement under consideration while 90 would be expected to be larger than the figure given. Similarly the 90th percentile would indicate that 89 children might be expected to be smaller than the figure given while 10 would be larger. The 50th percentile represents the median or midposition in the customary range. Here, the 10th and 90th percentiles are represented in heavy lines to show the limits within which most children remain. The lighter lines in the graphs divide the distribution into segments for ready recognition and description of individual differences as well as of the "regularity" of progress. The 3rd and 97th percentiles represent unusual though not necessarily abnormal findings.

In line with common usage in the United States, the charts are ruled on a scale in pounds to represent weight. They are ruled, however, in centimeters to represent length under 6 years and height thereafter, because this scale facilitates accuracy in measuring and recording and centimeter rules and tapes are readily available. For the convenience of those preferring them, scales for kilograms and inches are placed outside of the principal scales and paralleling them. Therefore, if weights are taken in kilograms and lengths and heights in inches, they may be plotted directly without conversion by placing a ruler at the appropriate points on the outer scales of the chart.

To determine the percentile position of any measurement at a given age, the vertical age line is located and a dot is placed where this intersects the horizontal line representing the value obtained from the measurement. Vertical lines give age by 2-month intervals and horizontal lines by 2-pound and 2-cm. intervals. This permits by interpolation accurate placement for age to ½ month and for measurements to ½ pound or 0.5 cm. Recognition of the position held by a child within or outside of the range in respect to each measurement recorded calls attention to the relative size and build of the individual at the time. More importantly, comparisons of percentile positions held by these measurements at repeated periodic examinations indicate adherence to or possibly significant deviation from previous percentile positions. Under normal circumstances, one expects a child to maintain a similar position from age to age — that is, on or near one percentile line or between the same two lines. Occasionally encountered sharp deviations or more gradual but continuing shifts from one percentile position to another call for further investigation as to their causes. In all cases, readings of measurements should be checked and care should be taken to secure the same position of the child accurately at all examinations. The following procedures were used in obtaining these norms and therefore are recommended:

Body Weight — The child is weighed without clothing except light undergarments.

Recumbent Length — The child lies relaxed on a firm surface parallel to a centimeter rule. The soles of the feet are held firmly against a fixed upright at the zero mark on the rule, and a movable square is brought firmly against the vertex. The head is held so that the eyes face the ceiling.

Height — The child's heels should be near together, and heels, buttocks and occiput should be against a firm vertical upright mounting the measuring stick. The eyes should be horizontal and approximately in the same plane as the external auditory canals. A right angle triangle or other movable device should be placed firmly on the head at right angles to the measuring stick and the measurement read after a satisfactory position has been adopted.

Furnished by Mead Johnson Laboratories as a Service in Medicine   Printed in U.S.A.   Lit. 85-B

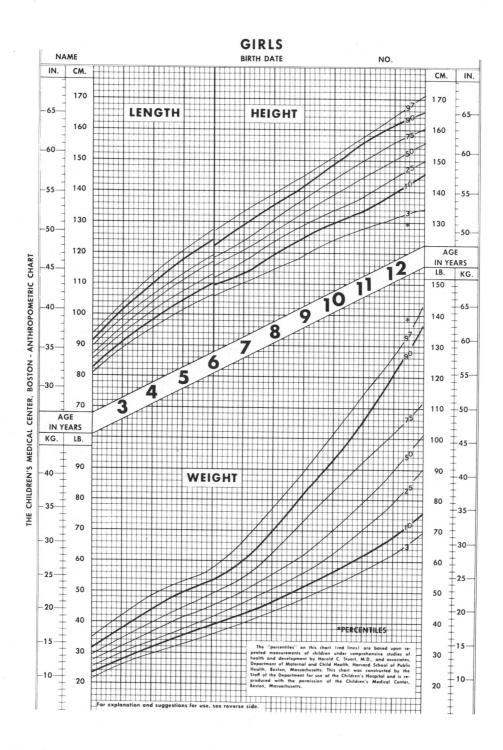

GIRLS

NAME   BIRTH DATE   NO.

LENGTH   HEIGHT

THE CHILDREN'S MEDICAL CENTER, BOSTON - ANTHROPOMETRIC CHART

AGE IN YEARS

WEIGHT

*PERCENTILES

The "percentiles" on this chart (red lines) are based upon repeated measurements of children under comprehensive studies of health and development by Harold C. Stuart, M.D., and associates, Department of Maternal and Child Health, Harvard School of Public Health, Boston, Massachusetts. This chart was constructed by the Staff of the Department for use at the Children's Hospital and is reproduced with the permission of the Children's Medical Center, Boston, Massachusetts.

For explanation and suggestions for use, see reverse side.

PERCENTILE CHART FOR MEASUREMENTS OF GIRLS

THIS CHART provides for girls standards of reference for body weight and recumbent length at ages between 2 and 6 years and for weight and standing height from 6 to 13 years. It is based upon repeated measurements at selected ages of a group of more than 100 white girls of North European ancestry living under normal conditions of health and home life in Boston, Mass. The distribution of the measurements obtained from these children at each age is expressed in percentiles, each percentile giving a value which represents a particular position in the normal range of occurrences. The number of the percentile refers to the position which a measurement of the given value would hold in any typical series of 100 children. Thus, the 10th percentile gives the value for the tenth in any hundred; that is, 9 children of the same sex and age would be expected to be smaller in the measurement under consideration while 90 would be expected to be larger than the figure given. Similarly the 90th percentile would indicate that 89 children might be expected to be smaller than the figure given while 10 would be larger. The 50th percentile represents the median or midposition in the customary range. Here, the 10th and 90th percentiles are represented in heavy lines to show the limits within which most children remain. The lighter lines in the graphs divide the distribution into segments for ready recognition and description of individual differences as well as of the "regularity" of progress. The 3rd and 97th percentiles represent unusual though not necessarily abnormal findings.

In line with common usage in the United States, the charts are ruled on a scale in pounds to represent weight. They are ruled, however, in centimeters to represent length under 6 years and height thereafter, because this scale facilitates accuracy in measuring and recording and centimeter rules and tapes are readily available. For the convenience of those preferring them, scales for kilograms and inches are placed outside of the principal scales and paralleling them. Therefore, if weights are taken in kilograms and lengths and heights in inches, they may be plotted directly without conversion by placing a ruler at the appropriate points on the outer scales of the chart.

To determine the percentile position of any measurement at a given age, the vertical age line is located and a dot is placed where this intersects the horizontal line representing the value obtained from the measurement. Vertical lines give age by 2-month intervals and horizontal lines by 2-pound and 2-cm. intervals. This permits by interpolation accurate placement for age to ½ month and for measurements to ½ pound or 0.5 cm. Recognition of the position held by a child within or outside of the range in respect to each measurement recorded calls attention to the relative size and build of the individual at the time. More importantly, comparisons of percentile positions held by these measurements at repeated periodic examinations indicate adherence to or possibly significant deviation from previous percentile positions. Under normal circumstances, one expects a child to maintain a similar position from age to age — that is, on or near one percentile line or between the same two lines. Occasionally encountered sharp deviations or more gradual but continuing shifts from one percentile position to another call for further investigation as to their causes. In all cases, readings of measurements should be checked and care should be taken to secure the same position of the child accurately at all examinations. The following procedures were used in obtaining these norms and therefore are recommended:

Body Weight — The child is weighed without clothing except light undergarments.

Recumbent Length — The child lies relaxed on a firm surface parallel to a centimeter rule. The soles of the feet are held firmly against a fixed upright at the zero mark on the rule, and a movable square is brought firmly against the vertex. The head is held so that the eyes face the ceiling.

Height — The child's heels should be near together, and heels, buttocks and occiput should be against a firm vertical upright mounting the measuring stick. The eyes should be horizontal and approximately in the same plane as the external auditory canals. A right angle triangle or other movable device should be placed firmly on the head at right angles to the measuring stick and the measurement read after a satisfactory position has been adopted.

Furnished by Mead Johnson Laboratories as a Service in Medicine   Printed in U.S.A.   Lit. 85-G

Pulmonary/Kidney Functions in Acid-Base Balance

MARGARET MERVA

Ratio of acid to base in venous blood
pH = 7.35 to 7.45 is H_2CO_3 = 1:20

Normal	Metabolic Acidosis	Respiratory Acidosis	Metabolic Alkalosis	Respiratory Alkalosis
Acid-Base Imbalance	Blood pH <7.35; ↓ HCO_3^- Urine pH <6.0	Blood pH <7.35; ↑ pCO_2 Urine pH <6.0	Blood pH >7.45; ↑ HCO_3^- Urine pH >7.0	Blood pH >7.45; ↓ pCO_2 Urine pH >7.0
Possible Etiology	Uremia; Diabetic Ketoacidosis; Prolonged or severe diarrhea; Intoxications: salicylates; methanol; and paraldehyde. Lactic acidosis; Starvation.	Hypoventilation; Respiratory obstruction: hyaline membrane disease in infants; emphysema; cardiovascular disease. Retained CO_2 causes ↑ H_2CO_3	Loss of H^+ by vomiting; Nasal gastric suction; Cushing's disease; prolonged administration of corticosteriod/diuretics; Hypokalemia from vomiting and drug-induced diuresis.	Psychogenic hyperventilation; hypermetabolic state: Fever; thyrotoxicosis Gram - negative bacteremia; Excessive - ventilation by mechanical ventilators; Early stage of Salicylate intoxication; Central Nervous System lesions.
Kidney Compensation	Regenerates biocarbonate Na^+ and H^+ exchange is decreased results in the excretion of H^+ as NH_3^+	Retains HCO_3^- and Na^+; Excretes H^- ion as NH_4^+ and carry Cl^- out in the urine.	Excretes: H^+ reabsorbs: Na^+ and K^+ Na^+ carrying HCO_3^- back to blood.	Increase HCO_3^- excretion
Respiratory Compensation	Hyperventilation	Hyperventilation	Hypoventilation	Hypoventilation
Clinical Manifestations	Kussmaul respirations apathy; disorientation; delirium; weakness; stupor; coma; cardia arrhythmias; cardiac arrest.	Wheezing; tachycardia; disorientation.	Irritability; disorientation; lethargy; tetany; convulsion, cyanosis and periods of apnea; Arrhythmias; paralytic ileus.	Increased neuromuscular irritability; convulsions.

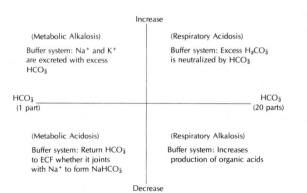

Increase

(Metabolic Alkalosis)

Buffer system: Na^+ and K^+ are excreted with excess HCO_3^-

(Respiratory Acidosis)

Buffer system: Excess H_2CO_3 is neutralized by HCO_3

HCO_3^-
(1 part)

HCO_3^-
(20 parts)

(Metabolic Acidosis)

Buffer system: Return HCO_3^- to ECF whether it joints with Na^+ to form $NaHCO_3^-$

(Respiratory Alkalosis)

Buffer system: Increases production of organic acids

Decrease

A Guide to Assessing a Rape Victim

CYNTHIA DEGAZON

LYNNE SORENSEN LOGATTO

The nurse must be objective, accurate, precise, and legible in recording her or his assessment on a rape victim. This information "is one of the strongest supportive documents of corroborating evidence to the victim's physical and emotional state."[1]

1. Determine the victim's priorities in the following areas:
    a. Physical—prevention of venereal disease and pregnancy
    b. Psychological—emotional support
    c. Legal—punish and protect
2. Determine nursing priorities
3. Begin data collection and adjust plan to meet the victim's primary need
    a. Nursing history
    b. Nursing assessment

NURSING PRIORITIES

1. Nursing History
    a. Circumstances of the assault
        • date, time, location of abuse
        • description of assailant

[1]Burgess, Ann W. and Laszlo, Anna T. "Courtroom Use of Hospital Records in Sexual Assault Cases." *American Journal of Nursing.* (January 1977), p. 68.

- acts committed
- presence of physical or verbal threats
- use of weapons
- injuries

b. Health history
  - chronic medical problems
  - medications used
  - allergies
  - LMP
  - contraceptive method, if any
  - last intercourse

c. Actions after the rape
  - clothes change
  - bath
  - douche

2. Nursing Assessment

a. General overview
  - description of the clothing (dirty, ripped)
  - broken or dirty fingernails
  - smeared make-up
  - disarrayed hair

b. Emotional status
  - expressions of fear, anger, withdrawal, and anxiety (fidgeting, crying, posture, being noncommunicative, avoidance of eye contact)
  - perception of the rape
  - availability of support systems

c. Physical assessment
  - signs and symptoms of trauma such as complaints of pain, lacerations, abrasions, contusions, teeth marks
  - carefully observe ears, face, mouth, neck, breasts, perineum, labia, and inner aspects of thighs

LABORATORY SPECIMENS ON RAPE VICTIMS

Specimen	Purpose
Vaginal smear and washing	To determine the presence of spermatozoa
Semen	To determine prostatic acid phosphatase levels that give support on the time the attack occurred
Client's clothes	To detect the presence of semen stains. A Woods lamp may be used. Clothing should be folded to prevent cracking or flaking of specimens
Fingernail scrapings	To identify the assailant or the location of the attack (dirt)
Head and pubic hair combings	To determine the presence of any foreign hair(s) and in an effort to collect a specimen from the alleged assailant
Saliva	May be obtained if oral sex abuse occurred to determine the presence of spermatozoa
Rectal washings, swabs, and slides	May be obtained if anal sexual abuse occured to determine the presence of spermatozoa
Sperm—ABO grouping	To identify the assailant

Suicidal Risk Index Assessment Sheet

NAME: _____ AGE/D.O.B.: _____

SEX: _____ ADDRESS: _____

DATE: _____

DIRECTIONS: Circle the one number that best matches the client's history for items A through D (See *Guide to Suicidal Risk Index*).

Historical Item	Total(s)			
A. Family suicidal history	1	2	3	4
B. Degree of family isolation	1	2	3	4
C. Presence of maturational crisis	1	2	3	4
D. Extent of suicidal plan and outcome fantasies	1	2	3	4
Total(s)				

SCORE INTERPRETATION: 0-7 = Low suicidal risk
8-10 = Possible suicidal risk
11-12 = Probable suicidal risk
13-16 = High suicidal risk

COMMENTS:

GUIDE TO SUICIDAL RISK INDEX

Historical Item	Number Value	Definition
A. Family suicidal history	1	Self destructive behavior of family member(s) (drug abuse, anorexia, etc.)
	2	Self destructive behavior of client (drug abuse, anorexia, etc.)
	3	Suicidal attempt of client, nuclear family, or extended family member.
	4	Suicide of nuclear family or extended family member
B. Degree of family isolation	1	Conflictual family relationships without issue resolution
	2	Conflictual family relationships without issue resolution and distance used in an attempt to end conflict
	3	No reported positive relationships within family
	4	No reported positive relationships within family or the community
C. Presence of maturational crisis	1	Life change (positive or negative) requiring new behaviors
	2	Life change requiring new coping mechanisms
	3	Geriatric or early adulthood adjustment
	4	Adolescent or middle years (particularly males age 35 to 50) adjustment
D. Extent of suicidal plan and outcome fantasies	1	Client verbalizes suicide as an option for coping
	2	Client has suicidal ideation
	3	Client reports suicidal plan without postsuicidal fantasy or suicidal note
	4	Client reports detailed suicidal plan with suicidal note and postsuicidal fantasies

Developed by Andrea Bretz Savitz, based on the lecture on "Suicide" delivered by Philip J. Guerin, Jr., M.D., at the Center for Family Learning, New Rochelle, New York, January 30, 1978.

The *Suicidal Risk Index* is presently being tested for validity and reliability.

Physical Assessment of the Elderly: Normal Findings

MARGARET MERVA

INTEGUMENTARY SYSTEM

Texture	Skin loses elasticity
	Wrinkles, folding, sagging, dryness
Color—pigmentation	Spotty pigmentation in areas exposed to sun
Temperature	Extremities cooler: perspiration decreases
Fat distribution	Less on extremities: greater on trunk
Hair color	Dull gray, white, or yellow
Hair distribution	Thinning on scalp, axilla, pubic area, upper and lower extremities, decreased facial hair in men
Nails	Normal decreased growth rate

GASTRO-INTESTINAL SYSTEM

Mastication	Impaired due to the decrease or absence of teeth and or malocclusive bite
Swallowing and carbohydrate digestion	Swallowing more difficult as salivary lubricating secretions decrease
	Reduced ptyalin production by the paratoid gland impairs starch digestion
Esophagus	Increased lower esophageal acidity and decreased esophageal peristalsis
	An increased incidence of hiatus hernia in the aged with accompanying gaseous distention
Digestive enzymes	Decreased production of HCL, pepsin and the pancreatic enzymes
	Achlorhydria prevents VIT B_{12}-absorption (Lamy, 1978)

Intestinal peristalsis	Reduced GI mobility accompanies aging; however, it has been shown that 90% of individuals over age 60 have at least one bowel movement per day (Malasanos et al., 1978)

MUSCLO-SKELETAL SYSTEM

Muscle strength and function	Decreases with loss of muscle mass as total body protein decreases with age
	Bony prominences are normal in the aged as muscle mass decreases
Bone structure	Normal demineralization of bones (calcium leeches out of bones) leaving them porous; hence, fractures occur more easily
	Shortening of body trunk occurs as intervertebral spaces narrow
Joints	Become less mobile as changes occur in joints with tightening and fixation
	Activity may maintain function longer
	Postural changes are normal
	Range of motion is impaired
Anatomical size and height	Total decrease in body size as loss of body protein and total body water decreases in proportion to decreases in basal metabolic rate
	Proportion of total fat to body weight increases with age, especially on trunk, while it diminishes on legs and arms
	Height may decrease 1–4 inches from early adult years (related to shortening of trunk)

GENITOURINARY AND REPRODUCTIVE SYSTEMS

Renal blood flow	Decreases due to diminished cardiac output, therefore reduction in filtration rate and renal efficiency occurs; subsequent increase in loss of proteins from the kidney can occur (Lamy, 1978)
Micturition	In males, frequency may increase due to prostatic enlargement
	In females, decrease in tone in perineal muscles leads to urgency and stress incontinence
	Nocturia increases with age
	Polyuria may be related to minimal diabetes
	Decreased volume may be related to decreased intake; evaluation is needed

Incontinence	Occurrence increases with age In 80% of the elderly, organic brain disease is the associated factor (Burnside, 1974)
Male reproduction	
Testestorone production	Decreased secretion with age with a decline in sexual energy Phases of intercourse are less intense with a slower excitement phase, longer duration of the plateau phase, and shorter orgasm Refractory phase lengthens
Frequency of intercourse	Change in libido and sexual satisfaction should not occur with aging, but frequency may decline to 1–2 times/week in men over 60 (Malasanos et al., 1978)
Testes	Decrease in size and are less firm Sperm count decreases and amount of viscosity of seminal fluid diminishes
Female Reproduction	
Estrogen	Production decreases beginning with menopause
Breasts	Diminished breast tissue as estrogen secretion decreases
Uterus	Decreases in size as well as the cervix; mucus secretions cease; uterine prolapse may be seen due to weakened musculature
Vagina	Epithelial lining of vaginal cavity atrophies; canal narrows and shortens with age
Vaginal secretions	Decreased estrogen production leads to increased alkalinity as glycogen content and acidity decline; pathogens can then grow more freely replacing protective Doderlien's bacilli (Malasanos et al., 1978)

RESPIRATORY CHANGES

Pulmonary blood flow and diffusion	Up to 33% decrease in blood flow to the pulmonary circulation; hence O_2 and CO_2 diffusion is decreased by 1/3 (Malasanos et al., 1978)
Anatomical structure	Increase in anterior–posterior diameter due to changes in calcium metabolism (barrel-chest appearance)
Respiratory accessory muscles	Degeneration and decrease in strength of these muscles and increased rigidity of chest wall

Internal pulmonic structure	Decrease in pulmonary elasticity leading to what has been called "senile emphysema"
	Shorter breaths are taken with decrease in maximum breathing capacity, vital capacity, residual volume, and functional capacity (Burnside, 1974)
	Airway resistance increases; there is less ventilation at the base of the lung than at the apex (Carotenuto and Bullock, 1978)
Respiratory character: shortness of breath on exertion	Decreased cardiac output leads to increased production of lactic acid and therefore decreased tolerance to oxygen debt (Carotenuto and Bullock, 1978)

CARDIOVASCULAR CHANGES

Cardiac output (product of heart rate and ventricular stroke volume)	Maximum decrease of 6.81 l/min to 3.81 l/min in populations over 65 (Carotenuto and Bullock, 1978)
Arterial circulation	Decrease in vessel compliance with increase in peripheral resistance to blood flow; occurs with generalized or localized arteriosclerosis
Venous circulation	Does not exhibit change with aging in the absence of disease (Carotenuto and Bullock, 1978)
Blood pressure	Significant increase in the systolic due to increase in peripheral resistance; diastolic should increase only slightly; pulse pressure will increase (Carotenuto and Bullock, 1978)
	Baroreceptor sensitivity decreases (Malasanos et al., 1978)
Physical exercise	Heart loses elasticity; therefore, heart contractility decreases in response to increased demands of exercise
	Conditioning will take longer in elderly, but will improve cardiovascular efficiency (Carotenuto and Bullock, 1978)
Heart	Dislocation of the apex occurs due to kyphoscolosis, hence location loses diagnostic significance (Malasanos, 1978)
Murmurs	60% of elderly have diastolic murmurs; the most common are heard at the base of the heart due to sclerotic changes on the aortic valves (Malasanos, 1978)
Peripheral pulses	Easily palpated due to increased narrowness of the arterial wall and loss of connective tissue; vessels may feel tortous and rigid (Malasanos et al., 1978)
	Pedal pulses may be weaker due to arteriosclerotic changes; clients may complain of cold lower ex-

	tremities, especially at night
	Feet and hands may be cold and have a mottled color
Heartrate	No changes with aging at normal rest

NERVOUS SYSTEM AND SPECIAL SENSES

Response to stimuli	All voluntary or automatic reflexes are slowed with decreased ability to respond to multiple stimuli (may be in relation to increased synaptic delay); decreased vascularity of the spinal cord (Carotenuto and Bullock, 1978)
Stimuli threshold	Threshold for light touch and pain is increased
	Ishemic parathesias in the extremities are common
Sleep patterns	Stage four sleep is reduced by 50% at age 50 in comparison to age 20
	Frequency of spontaneous awakening increases
	The elderly stay in bed longer but get less sleep
	Insomnia is common
Reflexes	Deep tendon reflexes remain responsive in the healthy elderly
Hearing	Higher frequency tones are less perceptable to the aged; hence, language understanding is greatly impaired, promoting confusion and seeming to affect increased rigidity in thought processes (Burnside, 1974)
Voice	Range, duration, and intensity of the voice diminish
	Voice may become high-pitched and monotonous (Carotenuto and Bullock, 1978)
Gustatory	Acuity decreases as taste buds atrophy
	May desire increased amount of seasoning such as salt and sugar on foods
Ambulation	Kinesthetic senses less efficient and the elderly frequently demonstrate an extrapyramidal Parkinson-like gait
	The basal ganglia of the nervous system are affected by the vascular changes and decreased O_2 supply

SENSE OF VISION

Peripheral vision	Decreases in the elderly
Lens accomodation	Decreases with age, requiring corrective lenses
Ciliary body	Atrophy in accomodation or lens focusing
Iris	Arcus senilus, an opaque white ring caused by fatty deposits

Choroid	Structure shows atrophy around the disc; a halo may be seen
Lens	Observe for opacitics—this may mean cataracts
	More light is necessary to see, especially at night
Color	Fades or disappears with age
Macula	Degeneration occurs with age, affecting visual activity
Conjunctiva	Thins and looks yellow with age
Tearing	Amount decreases with increased irritation and infection; this condition is treatable by an opthalmologist
Pupils	The two pupils may be different in size (aniscorea)
Cornea	Look for *arcus senilis,* deposition of fat in corneal layers but observed in iris
Retina	Vascular changes with aging can be seen here; however a skilled physician can best determine their diagnostic significance (e.g. look for thickened, constricted vessels, exudate, A–V nicking)

METABOLISM AND NUTRIENT BALANCE

Caloric requirements	Needs decreased due to lowered basal metabolism and decreased physical activity
	Thyroid gland reduces in size and in function (Malasanos, 1978)
	Suggested calories per kg. of body weight: 34 for men over 60, 29 for women (Lamy, 1978)
Protein requirements	Needs decrease as total body protein is decreased by 45% (Lamy, 1978)
Blood glucose levels (Minimal diabetes present in 50% of the elderly population)	Return to normal more slowly in the aged (Christakis, 1973) as insulin secretion time is lengthened (Malasanos, 1978)
Nutrient deficiencies	Complete vegetarians are subject to B_{12} and possibly iron deficiencies (Lamy, 1978)
Nutrient absorption	Medications can interfere with nutritional absorption or interfere with appetite, e.g., antacids lead to alkaline destruction of thiamine while barbiturates decrease vitamin B_{12}-absorption
	Calcium absorption is decreased due to achlorhydria (see *GI System*)
Primary malnutrition	Unbalanced nutrient intake leading to food excess or deficiency occurs with decreased income, isolation, and decreased mobility
Appetite	Medications can lead to anorexia
	Sense of taste decreases with a loss of 60% of taste buds (Lamy, 1978)

	Increased seasoning of food is common
	Olfactory acuity decreases with age
	Endentulous diet affects appetite as well as intake

BIBLIOGRAPHY FOR APPENDIX I

Bates, Barbara. *A Guide to Physical Examination.* Philadelphia: J. B. Lippincott Co., 1974.

Burnside, Irene Mortenson. "Developmental Reactions in Old Age." In *New Dimensions in Mental Health and Psychiatric Nursing.* New York: McGraw-Hill, 1974.

Carotenuto, Rosine, and Bullock, John. *Physiological Assessment of the Elderly.* Philadelphia: F. A. Davis Co. (for release 1979).

Christakis, George, ed. "Nutritional Assessment in Health Programs." *American Journal of Public Health* 63 (November 1973): supplement.

Jennings, Muriel; Nordstrom, Margene; and Shumake, Norine. "Physiologic Functioning in the Elderly." *Nursing Clinics of North America* 7 (June 1972): 237–252.

Lamy, Peter P. "Nutrition and Drug-Food Interactions in the Elderly." Paper presented at the annual spring meeting, Gerontological Society of New Jersey, Newark, N.J., April 15, 1978.

Lantz, John. "Assessment: A Beginning to Individualized Care." *Journal of Gerontological Nursing* 2 (November/December 1976): 34–40.

Malasanos, Lois et al. "Assessment of the Aging Client." In *Health Assessment,* St. Louis: C. V. Mosby Co., 1978.

Sana, Josephine. "The Elderly." In *Physical Appraisal Methods in Nursing Practice.* Edited by Josephine Sana and Richard D. Judge. Boston: Little, Brown and Company, 1975.

U.S. Department of Health, Education, and Welfare. *Working with Older People. Vol. 1: The Practitioner and the Elderly.* PHS Pubn. No. 1459 Washington, D.C.: Government Printing Office, 1971.

Index